FDA
REGULATORY
AFFAIRS

FDA
REGULATORY
AFFAIRS
A GUIDE FOR PRESCRIPTION DRUGS,
MEDICAL DEVICES, AND BIOLOGICS
SECOND EDITION

Edited by
Douglas J. Pisano
Massachusetts College of Pharmacy and Health Sciences
Boston, Massachusetts, USA
David S. Mantus
Cubist Pharmaceuticals, Inc.
Lexington, Massachusetts, USA

informa
healthcare

Informa Healthcare USA, Inc.
52 Vanderbilt Avenue
New York, NY 10017

© 2008 by Informa Healthcare USA, Inc.
Informa Healthcare is an Informa business

No claim to original U.S. Government works
Printed and bound in India by Replika Press Pvt. Ltd.
10 9 8 7 6 5 4 3 2

International Standard Book Number-10: 1-4200-7354-0 (Hardcover)
International Standard Book Number-13: 978-1-4200-7354-6 (Hardcover)

Library of Congress Cataloging-in-Publication Data

FDA regulatory affairs : a guide for prescription drugs, medical devices, and biologics / edited by Douglas J. Pisano, David S. Mantus. — 2nd ed.
   p. ; cm.
   Includes bibliographical references and index.
   ISBN-13: 978-1-4200-7354-6 (hb : alk. paper)
   ISBN-10: 1-4200-7354-0 (hb : alk. paper)   1. Drug development—United States. 2. United States Food and Drug Administration—Rules and practice. 3. Pharmaceutical industry—United States.   I. Pisano, Douglas J.   II. Mantus, David.
   [DNLM: 1. United States. Food and Drug Administration.   2. Drug Industry—standards—United States.   3. United States Government Agencies—United States. 4. Biological Products—standards—United States.   5. Equipment and Supplies—standards—United States.   6. Government Regulation—United States.   QV 1 F287 2008]
   RM301.25.F37 2008
   615′.19—dc22

                                                                        2008014296

For Corporate Sales and Reprint Permissions call 212-520-2700 or write to: Sales Department, 52 Vanderbilt Avenue, 7th floor, New York, NY 10017.

**Visit the Informa Web site at
www.informa.com**

**and the Informa Healthcare Web site at
www.informahealthcare.com**

Preface

This book is a roadmap to the U.S. Food and Drug Administration and drug, biologic, and medical device development. It is written in plain English, with an emphasis on easy access to understanding how this agency operates with respect to the practical aspects of U.S. product approval. It is meant to be a concise reference that offers current, real-time information. It has been written as a handy reference for use by students, staff, and professionals at corporations, organizations, and schools and colleges across the United States in need of a simple, concise text from which to learn and teach. The topics in *FDA Regulatory Affairs: A Guide for Prescription Drugs, Medical Devices, and Biologics, Second Edition* are covered in a straightforward format. It is a compilation and commentary of selected laws and regulations pertaining to the development and approval of drugs, biologics, and medical devices in the United States. It is *not* intended to take the place of an actual reading of the *Laws of the United States of America* or the regulations of the U.S. Food and Drug Administration, it's agencies or any body that regulates the development or approval of drugs, biologics, and medical devices in the United States.

Douglas J. Pisano
David S. Mantus

Contents

Contributors

Josephine C. Babiarz MS Program in Regulatory Affairs, Massachusetts College of Pharmacy and Health Sciences, Boston, Massachusetts, U.S.A.

Robert Blanks Idenix Pharmaceuticals, Inc., Cambridge, Massachusetts, U.S.A.

Bob Buckley Idenix Pharmaceuticals, Inc., Cambridge, Massachusetts, U.S.A.

Karen L. Drake Cubist Pharmaceuticals, Inc., Lexington, Massachusetts, U.S.A.

Vahé Ghahraman Regulatory Operations and Technology, Dyax Corporation, Cambridge, Massachusetts, U.S.A.

Alberto Grignolo PAREXEL Consulting, Lowell, Massachusetts, U.S.A.

Yolanda Hall Datafarm, Inc., Marlborough, Massachusetts, U.S.A.

Michael R. Hamrell MORIAH Consultants, Yorba Linda, California, U.S.A.

Timothy A. Keutzer Cubist Pharmaceuticals, Inc., Lexington, Massachusetts, U.S.A.

Steven R. Koepke SRK Consulting, LLC, Walkersville, Maryland, U.S.A.

Shylendra Kumar Datafarm, Inc., Marlborough, Massachusetts, U.S.A.

David S. Mantus Cubist Pharmaceuticals, Inc., Lexington, Massachusetts, U.S.A.

Christina A. McCarthy Cubist Pharmaceuticals, Inc., Lexington, Massachusetts, U.S.A.

Charles Monahan Regulatory Affairs, Molecular Insight Pharmaceuticals, Inc., Cambridge, Massachusetts, U.S.A.

Prabu Nambiar   Vertex Pharmaceuticals, Inc., Cambridge, Massachusetts, U.S.A.

Tan T. Nguyen   Food and Drug Administration, Center for Devices and Radiological Health, Rockville, Maryland, U.S.A.

Douglas J. Pisano   School of Pharmacy, Massachusetts College of Pharmacy and Health Sciences, Boston, Massachusetts, U.S.A.

Barry Sall   PAREXEL Consulting, Waltham, Massachusetts, U.S.A.

1

Overview of FDA and Drug Development

Josephine C. Babiarz

MS Program in Regulatory Affairs, Massachusetts College of Pharmacy and Health Sciences, Boston, Massachusetts, U.S.A.

Douglas J. Pisano

School of Pharmacy, Massachusetts College of Pharmacy and Health Sciences, Boston, Massachusetts, U.S.A.

INTRODUCTION

A single agency, the Food and Drug Administration (FDA), regulates a trillion dollars of products, ranging from 80% of the U.S. food supply to all human health care products, electronic products that emit radiation, animal products, and cosmetics. In 2006, that agency approved 101 new drugs, 10 biologic license applications, and 39 devices under the premarket approval process and cleared 3217 devices[1] and recalled 4266 products in all categories.[2] That single agency is responsible for shellfish, stents, over-the-counter (OTC) cough syrups, tetanus shots, artificial sweeteners, mammography standards, prescription drugs, vitamins, and lipsticks, not to mention the readability of calorie and trans-fat information on a bag of potato chips. The economic impact of the FDA is difficult to calculate, the scientific challenges and increasing medical needs overwhelming, and the expectations contradictory.

The FDA is expected to protect us and our pets from harm, but allow us access to unproven therapies that might cure or benefit us. The FDA is to act

---

[1] See www.fda.gov/oc/FDA's 2006 Accomplishments/healthcare.html.

[2] See www.fda.gov/ora/about/enf_story/ch10/FY96toFY06Recalls.pdf.

quickly to get products to market, but must be right the first time, and is criticized as being too permissive or lax if a drug or device must be recalled later for safety concerns or unpredicted adverse events. Given the pace of scientific advancement, this is no small demand.

The FDA's authority and influence are the product of compromise, evolving over time. It is an agency that is governed as much by law as by science. History shows us that the FDA's authority has grown commensurate with the magnitude of harm suffered by the public because of the food and drugs consumed, as well as the devices used. The agency and its statutory framework remain a work in progress. To better understand the FDA, its controlling laws, and its role in public health, a brief summary is in order.

Regulations and laws are central social constructs that provide guidance for all societies around the globe. Governments create laws in a number of ways with various intents for a myriad of purposes. In the United States, laws are created by the Congress, a body of officials elected by the citizenry, who are charged with the governance of the country by representing the common, public good. The Congress proposes and passes laws that are relatively general in nature and intended to address some particular issue in a fashion that can be consistently applied by all who are affected by them. Once passed, laws are remanded to the appropriate government or administrative agency, which then decides on how these laws are to be applied. These "applications of law" are called regulations. Regulations serve as the practical foundation from which citizens adhere to the law as it was originally intended.

In the United States, all food, drugs, cosmetics, and medical devices for both humans and animals are regulated under the authority of the Food, Drug, and Cosmetic Act (FDCA), which in turn establishes the FDA. The FDA and all of its regulations were created by the government in response to the pressing need to address the safety of public with respect to its foods and medicinals. The purpose of this chapter is to describe and explain the nature and extent of these regulations as they apply to medical products in the United States. A historical perspective is offered as a foundation for regulatory context. In addition, the chapter will discuss the FDA's regulatory oversight and that of other agencies, the drug approval and development process, the mechanisms used to regulate manufacturing and marketing, as well as various violation and enforcement schemas.

THE EVOLUTION OF THE FDA—HOW THE PURE FOOD AND DRUG ACT BECAME THE FOOD AND DRUG ADMINISTRATION AMENDMENTS OF 2007

The History—1902 to 1972

Prior to 1902, the U.S. government took a hands-off approach to the regulation of drugs. Many of the drugs available were so-called patent medicines, which were so named because each had a more or less descriptive or patent name. No laws, regulations, or standards existed to any noticeable extent, even though the

United States Pharmacopoeia (USP) became a reality in 1820 as the first official compendium of the United States. The USP set standards for strength and purity, which could be used by physicians and pharmacists who needed centralized guidelines to extract, compound, and otherwise utilize drug components that existed at the time.[3]

However, in 1848, the first American drug law, the Drug Importation Act, was enacted when American troops serving in Mexico became seriously affected when adulterated quinine, an antimalarial drug, was discovered. This law required laboratory inspection, detention, and even destruction of drugs that did not meet acceptable standards. Later, in 1902, the Virus, Serum, and Toxins Act (Biologics Control Act) was passed in response to tetanus-infected diphtheria antitoxin, which was manufactured by a small laboratory in St. Louis, Missouri. Ten school children died as a result of the tainted serum. No national standards were as yet in place for purity or potency. The act authorized the Public Health Service to license and regulate the interstate sale of serum, vaccines, and related biologic products used to prevent or treat disease.

This act also spurred Dr. Harvey W. Wiley, chief chemist for the Bureau of Chemistry, a branch of the United States Department of Agriculture (USDA) and the forerunner for today's FDA investigate the country's foods and drugs. He established the Hygienic Table, a group of young men who volunteered to serve as human guinea pigs and who would allow Dr. Wiley to feed them a controlled diet laced with a variety of preservatives and artificial colors. More popularly known as the "Poison Squad," they helped Dr. Wiley gather enough data to prove that many of America's foods and drugs were "adulterated," the products' strength or purity was suspect or "misbranded," or the products had inadequate or inaccurate labeling. Dr Wiley's efforts, along with publication of Upton Sinclair's *The Jungle* (a book revealing the putrid conditions in America's meat industry), were rewarded when Congress passed America's first food and drug law, in 1906, the United States Pure Food and Drug Act (PFDA) (also known as the Wiley Act). The Wiley Act prohibited interstate commerce of misbranded foods or drugs based on their labeling. It did not affect unsafe drugs in that its legal authority would only come to bear when a product's ingredients were falsely labeled. Even intentionally false therapeutic claims were not prohibited.

This began to change in 1911 with the enactment of the Sherley Amendment, which prohibited the labeling of medications with false therapeutic claims that were intended to defraud the purchaser. These amendments, however, required the government to find proof of intentional labeling fraud. Later, in 1937, a sentinel event occurred that changed the entire regulatory picture. Sulfa became the miracle drug of the time and was used to treat many life-threatening infections. It tasted bad and was hard to swallow, which led

---

[3] Valentino J. Practical uses for the USP: a legal perspective. In: Strauss's Federal Drug Laws and Examination Review. 5th ed. Lancaster, PA: Technomic Publishing Co., 1999:38.

entrepreneurs to seek a palatable solution. S.E. Massingill Co. of Bristol, Tennessee, developed what it thought was a palatable, raspberry-flavored liquid product. However, it used diethylene glycol to solublize the sulfa. Six gallons of this dangerous mixture, Elixir of Sulfanilamide, killed some 107 people, mostly children.

The result was the passage of one of the most comprehensive statutes in the history of American health law. The federal Food, Drug, and Cosmetic Act of 1938 (FDCA), repealed the Sherley Amendments and required that all new drugs be tested by their manufacturers for safety and that those tests be submitted to the government for marketing approval via a new drug application (NDA). The FDCA also mandated that drugs be labeled with adequate directions if they were shown to have had harmful effects. In addition, the FDCA authorized the FDA to conduct unannounced inspections of drug manufacturing facilities. Though amended many times since 1938, the FDCA is still the broad foundation for statutory authority for the FDA as it exists today.

However, a new crisis loomed. Throughout the late 1950s, European and Canadian physicians began to encounter a number of infants born with a curious birth defect called "phocomeglia," a defect that resulted in limbs that resembled "flippers," similar to those found on seals. These birth defects were traced back to mothers who had been prescribed the drug thalidomide in an effort to relieve morning sickness while pregnant. The manufacturer of this drug applied for the U.S. marketing approval as a sleep aid. However, because of the efforts of Dr. Frances O. Kelsey, the FDA's chief medical officer at the time, a case was made that the drug was not safe and therefore not effective for release in the U.S. marketplace.

Dr. Kelsey's efforts and decisive work by the U.S. Congress resulted in yet another necessary amendment to the FDCA, in 1962, the Kefauver-Harris Act. This act essentially closed many of the loopholes regarding drug safety in American law. These "Drug Efficacy Amendments" now required drug manufacturers to prove safety and efficacy of their drug products, register with the FDA and be inspected at least every two years, have their prescription drug advertising approved by the FDA (this authority being transferred from the Federal Trade Commission), provide and obtain documented "informed consent" from research subjects prior to human trials, and increase controls over manufacturing and testing to determine drug effectiveness.

In an effort to address these new provisions of the act, the FDA contracted with the National Academy of Sciences along with the National Research Council to examine some 3400 drug products approved between 1938 and 1962 on the basis of safety alone. Called the Drug Efficacy Study Implementation Review of 1966 (DESI), it charged these organizations to determine whether post-1938 drug products were "effective" for the indications claimed in their labeling, or "probably effective," "possibly effective," or "ineffective." Those products not deemed effective were removed from the marketplace, reformulated, or sold with a clear warning to prescribers that the product was not deemed effective.

Later, in 1972, the FDA began to examine OTC drug products. Phase II of the Drug Efficacy Amendments required the FDA to determine the efficacy of OTC drug products. This project was much larger in scope than the analysis of prescription drugs. In the America of the 1970s, consumers could choose from more than 300,000 OTC drug products. The FDA soon realized that it did not have the resources to evaluate each and every one. Hence, the FDA created advisory panels of scientists, medical professionals, and consumers who were charged with evaluating active ingredients used in OTC products within 80 defined therapeutic categories. After examining both the scientific and medical literature of the day, the advisory panels made decisions regarding active ingredients and their labeling. The result was a "monograph" that described in detail acceptable active ingredients and labeling for products within a therapeutic class. Products that complied with monograph guidelines were deemed category I: safe and effective, not misbranded. However, products not in compliance with monograph guidelines were deemed category II: not safe and effective or misbranded. Category II products were removed from the marketplace or reformulated. Products for which data were insufficient for classification were deemed category III and were allowed to continue in the market until substantive data could be established or until they were reformulated and were in compliance with the monograph. The OTC Drug Review took approximately 20 years to complete.

Although there were numerous other federal laws and regulations that were passed throughout the 1970s, many were based on regulating the professional practice of medical professionals or for the direct protection of consumers. For example, the federal Controlled Substances Act (CSA), part of the Comprehensive Drug Abuse and Prevention Act of 1970, placed drugs with a relatively high potential for abuse into five federal schedules along with a "closed record keeping system," designed to track federally controlled substances via a definite paper trail, as they were ordered, prescribed, dispensed, and utilized throughout the health care system.

1980—2004: AIDS, Orphans, Terrorism, and Economic Incentives

The 1980s also passed with significant regulatory changes. Biotechnology had begun on a grand scale and the pharmaceutical industry was on its cutting edge. Many of the medicinal compounds being discovered were shown to be very expensive and have limited use in the general U.S. population. However, these compounds could prove lifesaving to demographically small patient populations who suffered from diseases and conditions that were considered rare. In an effort to encourage these biotech pharmaceutical companies to continue to develop these and other products, Congress passed the Orphan Drug Act in 1983. The Act continues to allow manufacturers incentives for research, development, and marketing of drug products used to treat rare diseases or conditions that would otherwise be unprofitable via a system of market exclusivity, and substantial breaks and deductions in a manufacturer's corporate taxes. Though the success of the Orphan Drug Act proved of great medical benefit for a few, a scandal was looming in other parts of the pharmaceutical industry.

The generic pharmaceutical industry experienced steady growth as many of the exclusive patents enjoyed by major pharmaceutical companies for brand-named products were beginning to expire. Generic versions of these now freely copied products were appearing much more frequently in the marketplace. However, these generic copies were required to undergo the same rigorous testing that brand name, pioneer, or innovator products did, thereby increasing costs, duplicating test results, and substantially slowing the availability of less expensive but equivalent drugs. To speed access to cheaper therapies, Congress passed the Price Competition and Patent Restoration Act in 1984. This Act, also called the Waxman-Hatch Act after its sponsors, was designed to level the playing field in the prescription drug industry with regard to patent-protected prescription drug products and their generic copies.

The Waxman-Hatch Act was composed of two distinct parts or "titles." Title I was for the benefit of the generic pharmaceutical industry. It extended the scope of the Abbreviated NDA (ANDA) to cover generic versions of post-1962–approved drug products. It required that generic versions of pioneer or innovator drugs have the same relevant aspects as those with regard to bio-equivalence (rate and extent of absorption of the active drug in the human body) and pharmaceutical equivalence (same dosage form as the pioneer drug to which it is compared). Though somewhat simplified, the Waxman-Hatch Act permitted easier market access to generic copies of pioneer drugs, provided they were not significantly different from the pioneer drug in their absorption, action, and dosage form. In addition, Title II of the act was designed to aid and encourage research-based or innovator pharmaceutical companies in continuing their search for new and useful medicinal compounds by extending the patent life of pioneer drug products to compensate for marketing time lost during the FDA "review period."[4]

While the patent extension benefit has become somewhat moot because of an overall reduction in the FDA review time as a result of prescription drug user fees, the value of patent-protected drugs has skyrocketed, with so-called block-buster drugs garnering millions of dollars in sales in less than a year. Market exclusivity and patent extensions remain powerful motivators used to encourage orphan drug development and, as discussed below in the section "The Food and Drug Administration Amendments Act of 2007," pediatric testing.

Congress recognized that counterfeit drugs, as well as improper control over drug samples, and sales and marketing materials posed serious health

---

[4] No federal agency, including the FDA, can compel the manufacture of generic drugs once patent rights have expired. In recent times, the Waxman-Hatch Act has come under criticism for that reason. Under a free market system, companies that hold expired patents may, and some do, make "reverse payments" to potential competitors to keep generic drugs off the market. This practice clearly frustrates the spirit of the law; however, it is legal.

hazards. Accordingly, the Prescription Drug Marketing Act of 1988 requires that all drugs be distributed through legitimate commercial channels, that pharmaceutical sales representatives maintain detailed accounts of drug samples (giving birth to the term "detailer"), and that importation of drugs from foreign countries be restricted.[5]

Nineteen ninety was a year when Congress focused on devices and nutrition. The Safe Medical Devices Act of 1990 established a user reporting system to improve device safety. If a medical device probably caused or contributed to death, serious injury, or illness, representatives of the institution or facility where the incident occurred were required to file a report with the FDA. In turn, the device manufacturers were required to address or respond to the incident. The statute also gives FDA the power and authority to recall devices,[6] which it does not have in the case of drugs (drug recalls are voluntary actions by the manufacturers; FDA can and will seize drug lots, however). This Act also addressed combination products, establishing that the jurisdiction of the FDA centers would be based on the primary indication of the product. Nineteen ninety also brought regulation to food; the Nutrition Labeling and Education Act requires nutrition labeling and health claims to be consistent with the format and rules established by the FDA. This law brought new—and uniform—meaning to the words "low fat" and "light."[7]

Nineteen ninety-two saw three major laws enacted. An unintended side effect of the Waxman-Hatch Act was a very public scandal in which a few unscrupulous generic pharmaceutical companies took shortcuts in reporting data, submitted fraudulent samples, and offered bribes to the FDA officials to gain easy and rapid market approval of their products.[8] The Generic Drug Enforcement Act provided for debarment and other serious penalties for bribery, fraud, or misconduct, among other deterrents.[9] Congress also strengthened device oversight; the Medical Device Amendments of 1992 added penalties if a manufacturer did not comply with postmarketing surveillance testing and reporting.[10]

---

[5] Prescription Drug Marketing Act of 1988; Public Law 100–23. See www.fda.gov/opacom/backgrounders/miles.html.

[6] Ibid.

[7] Ibid.

[8] Sec. 306(k) of the FDCA [21 USC 335a(k)] requires that drug product applicants certify that they did not and will not use in any capacity the services of any debarred persons in connection with a drug product application. See www.fda.gov/cder/guidance/1700dft.pdf. Note that this certification applies to combination products that include any drug component; this certificate is commonly used by device manufacturers as well.

[9] Generic Drug Enforcement Act of 1992; Public Law 102–282; See www.fda.gov/ora/compliance_ref/debar/297_debar.htm.

[10]See http://thomas.loc.gov/cgi-bin/bdquery/z?d102:SN02783:@@@D&summ2=m&|TOM:/bss/d102query.html.|

The most significant change of that year came in the form of the first Prescription Drug User Fee Act (PDUFA).[11] The Act was intended to help the FDA generate additional funds to upgrade and modernize its operations and to accelerate drug approval. It authorized FDA to charge pharmaceutical manufacturers a "user fee" to accelerate drug review. These funds in turn are used by the FDA. Critics and supporters alike quickly point out that the user fee is fully paid when the FDA approves a product—not if the final clinical results do not prove the benefit outweighs the risk. This fee assessment has sparked a great deal of debate about the real conflict of interest present when the FDA reviewers are examining a product whose approval fees go directly to fund the reviewers' employment. As will be discussed later, there are checks and balances in this system, as Congress appropriates funds to cover FDA administration, including reviewers' salaries.[4]

As a result of PDUFA, FDA has hired more personnel and reduced approval time of new pharmaceutical products from greater than 30 months to approximately 13 to 15 months today. However, the first act had a "sunset" provision, which limited FDA's authority to charge user fees to the year 1997. The Act was so successful that PDUFA has been reauthorized and extended three additional times, and the fee concept has been expanded to include medical devices and biologics (Medical Device User Fee and Modernization Act of 2002, MDUFMA),[12] as well as voluntary review fees for television advertisements. The most recent reauthorization, PDUFA IV, is part of the Food and Drug Administration Amendments Act of 2007, discussed at length below.

Congress relaxed the regulation of certain industries. The Dietary Supplement Health and Education Act (DSHEA) of 1994 shifted the burden of proof from industry to the FDA. For drugs, devices, and biologics, a sponsor or manufacturer must prove that the product is safe and effective for the indication claimed. The opposite is true of dietary supplements; thanks to this law, FDA "bears the burden of proof...to show that a dietary supplement is adulterated."[13]

Congress continued to expand and enhance the scope and powers of the FDA. One example is the FDA Modernization Act (FDAMA) of 1997.[14] FDMA not only extended user fee provisions but also waived some fees for small companies and for developers of orphan products, manufacturers of pediatric applications, and certain biologics. FDAMA also gave FDA authority to conduct "fast track" product reviews to speed lifesaving drug therapies to market, permitted an additional six-month patent exclusivity for pediatric prescription drug products and required the National Institutes of Health (NIH) to build a

---

[11] Public Law 102–571; 21 USC 379g and ff.

[12] Public Law 107–250; 21 USC 379F et seq.

[13] See www.fda.gov/opacom/laws/dshea.htmo#sec4.

[14] Public Law 105–115; 21 USC 301 et seq.

publicly accessible database on clinical studies of investigational drugs or life-threatening diseases.

FDAMA addressed the real dilemma of terminally ill patients, who were routinely denied access to experimental drugs because of the lack of safety and efficacy data on the drugs; FDA had no authority to allow the use of such drugs outside enrollment in a controlled clinical investigation. However, pressures from acquired immunodeficiency syndrome (AIDS) activists in particular moved Congress to change the rules. Under FDAMA, there was expanded access to unapproved drug and devices, specifically therapies and diagnostics for serious diseases or life-threatening conditions.[15] Individuals not enrolled in a formal clinical trial could obtain unapproved products—i.e., products covered by an investigational new drug (IND) or investigational device exemption (IDE)— during emergencies or for personal use. Unapproved drugs are available under "expanded access" or "compassionate use,"[16] experimental devices are available under the humanitarian device exemptions.[17]

FDAMA addressed, albeit briefly, issues of "off-label" promotion. Generally, a manufacturer may only advertise those claims and indications that are stated in the label; any deviation can be prosecuted as misbranding.[18] FDA took the position that certain publications directed at prescribers were in fact off-label promotion. Various critics, including the Washington Legal Foundation, felt that this position violated the right of freedom of speech, guaranteed by the First Amendment to the United States Constitution. A federal court agreed with the foundation,[19] and Congress was forced to address the issue. The fundamental question was and remains how can the public be adequately protected if a manufacturer is allowed to promote all the uses of a product and not only those that FDA has determined to be supported by scientific evidence?

The compromise Congress crafted was to allow dissemination of information on unapproved uses of products to a limited group of professionals— i.e., physicians, insurance companies, and other health care practitioners. This provision has expired,[20] and the battlefront has shifted to the arena of post-marketing surveillance and drug database registries, discussed below in the section "The Food and Drug Administration Amendments Act of 2007."

Imitation is the sincerest compliment—the success of PDUFA gave birth to the Medical Device User Fee and Modernization Act (MDUFMA) in 2002. MDUFMA was enacted "in order to provide the FDA with the resources necessary to better review medical devices, to enact needed regulatory reforms so that medical

---

[15] See 21 USC section 360bbb and following.

[16] See www.fda.gov/cder/guidance/3647fnl.pdf.

[17] See www.fda.gov/cdrh/ode/guidance/1381.html.

[18] See 21 USC section 331 and following.

[19] See Washington Legal Foundation v. Henney; Federal Appellate District DC US Court of Appeals, Decided Feb 11, 2000; No. 99-5304.

[20] See 21 USC section 360aaa and following.

device manufacturers can bring their safe and effective devices to the American people at an earlier time, and to ensure that reprocessed medical devices are as safe and effective as original devices."[21] MDUFMA continues to be strengthened and is now reauthorized through 2012. This same fee scheme has been adapted by veterinary medicines with ADUFA, the Animal Drug User Fee Act of 2003.[22]

In 2002 and again in 2003, Congress addressed the untested use of adult drugs for pediatric indications, by passing the Best Pharmaceuticals for Children Act in 2002.[23] This law extended the six-month patent exclusivity, as a reward for manufacturers who tested the formulation in pediatric indications, and strengthened Health and Human Services (HHS) executive powers with respect to pediatrics. This law was followed in 2003 by the Pediatric Research Equity Act,[24] which mandates that new drugs and biologics be tested in children if they can be used by children; FDA can grant a waiver for this mandatory testing. FDA takes the position that prescribing adult formulations for children without adequate studies is off-label and in effect, constitutes unapproved and unmonitored ongoing drug trials.

The events of 9/11 also impacted the FDA. The Public Health Security and Bioterrorism Preparedness and Response Act of 2002[25] requires the stockpiling of certain drugs and enhances protection of the food supply, among the measures that address national emergency situations. The Project Bioshield Act of 2004[26] will "... provide protections and countermeasures against chemical, radiological, or nuclear agents that may be used in a terrorist attack against the United States ... [by] streamlining the Food and Drug Administration approval process of countermeasures."

The Food and Drug Administration Amendments Act of 2007

The Food and Drug Administration Amendments Act of 2007[27] is broad detailed legislation that impacts each pressure point, not only in drug and device development but also throughout the FDA's purview. The law extends PDUFA and MDUFMA, addresses pediatrics in drugs and devices, and establishes new and robust requirements for postmarketing surveillance. It creates the Regan-Udall Foundation, whose mission is to spur public-private partnerships, modernize the development of products regulated by the FDA, and accelerate medical

---

[21] See www.fda.gov/cdrh/mdufma/whitepaper.html, citing *Medical Device User Fee and Modernization Act* of 2002, Report 107–728 (October 7, 2002), p. 21.

[22] Public Law 108–130 (Feb 20, 2003).

[23] Public Law 107–109 (Jan 4 2002).

[24] Public Law 108–155 (Dec 3, 2003).

[25] Public Law 107–188 (June 12, 2002); See http://thomas.loc.gov/home/gpoxmlc110/h3580_rds.xml#toc-H5597472044A142FBB29600862048CB39 for an electronic, linked version.

[26] Public Law 108–276 (July 21, 2004).

[27] Public Law 110–85 (Sept 27, 2007), H.R. 3580.

innovation. It improves food safety. Six months after its passage, the FDA and industry are still learning its language and sections. A brief summary is in order. Recapping the sections of this Act:[28]

1. The act reauthorized and expanded PDUFA. Under PDUFA of 2007, the government estimates user fees for prescription drugs and biologics at $392 million annually, an increase of $87 million over current fees, and a tripling of fees for postmarketing surveillance. The total PDUFA increase over five years is estimated to be $225 million.

2. Additionally, the Act authorizes the collection of user fees to review direct to consumer (DTC) television advertisements, which are voluntarily submitted to the FDA for review. As of this print date, this provision is moot because drug manufacturers did not file sufficient requests for review to meet the minimum threshold.

3. The Act expands FDA's implementation of guidance for product review, and FDA is to develop in particular, guidelines for industry on clinical trial design.

4. The fees will help move FDA and industry to all electronic environments.

5. Regarding devices, MDUFMA of 2007 also extended fees and appropriations, estimated to generate $287 million by 2012. For the Center for Devices and Radiological Health (CDRH), this Act allows accredited outside firms to conduct manufacturing inspections, shifting FDA resources to high-risk products. There will also be new guidance on in-vitro diagnostic device development.

6. Two major pediatric initiatives, the Pediatric Research Equity Act and the Best Pharmaceuticals Act are extended and a new one, the Pediatric Medical Device Safety Act, is added. Under this new initiative, medical devices must include a description of pediatric populations; FDA is to track the number and type of devices specifically approved for children and/or pediatric conditions. Additionally, FDA will report on approval times for pediatric devices and humanitarian device exemptions. Manufacturers will still have the additional six-month exclusivity as incentive for the FDA-requested studies.

7. The FDA is to set up an electronic surveillance system for using e-health records and electronic health data sources for surveillance of adverse events. This system will be implemented over time.

8. It improves clinical trial databases, a responsibility shared between the FDA and NIH. The databases will be expanded in three phases. New medications and devices must provide clinical trial registry information, going beyond the currently published categories of serious, life-threatening illness and will cover all trials beyond phase 1. Sponsors will be required to post basic trial results on the databases for approved drugs and devices; the

---

[28] Summary taken from www.fda.gov/bbs/transcripts/transcript092707.pdf.

purpose of the law is to make trial results transparent to the public. An area to be determined is the inclusion of all adverse event information and potentially information of adverse events from on-going trials of unapproved products.

9. The act emphasizes postmarketing surveillance across all fields. There is no new requirement for health care professionals but rather a mandate that the FDA work with the health care system to get data that are in electronic form and much more complete. Currently, the FDA estimates that 1 of 10 serious adverse events are reported now by health care professionals. Having access to the health care databases improves reporting significantly because there are more patients and better epidemiologic information.

Specific sections of the Amendments Act merit review; this law is in effect now. Section 303 expands the humanitarian device exemption to pediatric applications, including persons aged 21 years or younger at the time of diagnosis or treatment. Under the Pediatric Research Equity Act, all marketed drugs must have a pediatric label unless a waiver is granted. However, there are "workarounds" in the law. Section 505B allows a sponsor to extrapolate pediatric effectiveness from adequate and well-controlled studies in adults, supplemented with other information obtained in pediatric patients, e.g., pharmacokinetic studies, and also allows the extrapolation of data from one pediatric age group to another age group. Pediatric studies themselves can be deferred if the adult form is ready before pediatric studies are complete or until additional safety and effectiveness data have been collected. The law provides for full and partial waivers from pediatric studies if they are impossible or impractical, if there is strong evidence that the product is ineffective or unsafe in all pediatric age groups, or if the new product does not have a meaningful benefit over existing pediatric treatments and is not likely to be used in a substantial number of pediatric patients, provided, however, that the product label reflects that the product would be ineffective or unsafe in pediatric populations.

There are changes to the Best Pharmaceuticals Act, starting at Section 505A. The market exclusivity for new drugs has been extended, and market exclusivity for already-marketed drugs has been added. The FDA may request a sponsor to conduct ethnically and racially diverse pediatric studies, of both approved and unapproved uses. If a sponsor disagrees with this request on the basis that it is not possible to develop a pediatric formulation, but gives no other reason, then the drug labeling must clearly state it is unsafe/untested for pediatric use. If the sponsor agrees to test, the sponsor must provide not only all postmarket adverse event reports regarding the drug but also those generated during the pediatric trial. Additionally, the law requires the publication of pediatric labeling changes, including both on and off-label indications and study results of both. If the FDA and sponsor cannot agree on the labeling change, the matter will be referred to the Pediatric Advisory Committee, which can make recommendations but not bind the agency. Changes required by the FDA but not made by the manufacturer means the product is misbranded. If the FDA does not determine that a drug is safe and effective, or the data are inconclusive, the labeling must reflect that information.

Regarding dissemination of pediatric information at subsection (k), the law requires FDA to publish the medical, statistical, and clinical pharmacology reviews of pediatric studies. It also provides that subject to funding, NIH may conduct pediatric studies; if the drug has no listed patents, the Public Health Services shall conduct the studies. The law requires that NIH and FDA award funds to conduct pediatric trials of prioritized drugs.

Section 701 revisits conflicts of interest and advisory committee panels. A member cannot participate in a matter if that member or an immediate family member has a financial interest that could be affected by the advice given, subject to standard financial exceptions. There are waivers granted, with the conflicted member participating but not voting.

Clinical trial databases are the subject of Section 80. The statute generally exempts inclusion of information for drugs in phase 1 and devices in feasibility or prototype trials. However, the NIH clinical trial registry has been expanded to include most types of clinical trial results, where a clinical trial is the primary basis of an efficacy claim or if the trial is conducted after the drug is approved or the device is cleared. This means that devices studied under a 501(k), premarket approval application, or humanitarian device exemption are now reportable, as are pediatric postmarketing studies. The reportable elements are extensive and will include the product, the indications being studied, eligibility criteria, and links to existing results. Over the next three years, FDA is to issue regulations over a broad number of topics, expanding the information available to the public. The agency must determine whether or not information on unapproved or uncleared products will be included and the format of all submissions and guidelines for writing entries in language understandable to patients. The results of these clinical trials must be disclosed when a drug or device is initially approved, when there is a new previously off-label use, and where the product is not approved or cleared. Serious adverse events and frequent adverse events are also reportable. The law is clear that this information is to be available via the Internet.

The greatest changes were demanded by the public. Section 901 greatly strengthens the FDA's authority over and resources in conducting postmarket surveillance. This law applies to drugs and biologics but not to veterinary drugs. Under the law now, a responsible person may not introduce or deliver a new drug if that person has not (*i*) conducted postapproval studies or postapproval clinical trials on the basis of scientific data selected by the FDA or (*ii*) not made safety labeling changes requested by the FDA.

The purposes of the study or clinical trial are to (*i*) assess a known, serious risk related to the use of the drug involved; (*ii*) to assess signals of serious risk related to the use of the drug; and (*iii*) to identify an unexpected serious risk when available data indicate the potential for serious risks. Regarding the safety labeling changes, there is a discussion and dispute resolution procedure, but the Secretary of HHS wields considerable power in the outcome.[29]

The Act also requires a risk evaluation and mitigation strategy before certain new drugs are marketed; failure to conduct the aforementioned post-market studies when required, constitutes a violation of this law.

A "risk determination" is necessary to "ensure that the benefits of the drug outweigh the risks of the drug." Criteria to be used to determine when the evaluation is necessary are:

- the estimated size of the population likely to use the drug involved,
- the seriousness of the disease or condition to be treated with the drug,
- the expected benefit of the drug,
- the expected or actual duration of treatment,
- the seriousness of any known or potential adverse events that may be related to the drug and the background incidence of such events in the population likely to use the drug, and
- whether the drug is a new molecular entity.

The law specifically extends the postapproval requirements to drugs approved before the effective date of the Act of 2007 if the FDA "becomes aware of new safety information and makes a determination that such a strategy is necessary to ensure that the benefits of the drug outweigh the risks of the drug." The law brings its own definitions of "adverse events" and "new safety information," among others.

An adverse drug experience occurs when an adverse event (AE) is associated with drug use, whether or not drug related, including instances of overdose, abuse, withdrawal, or failure of pharmacological action. The term "new safety information" is broadly defined to include information obtained from a clinical trial, adverse event reports, postapproval studies, or notably, peer-reviewed biomedical literature and data derived from the postmarket risk identification and analysis system or other scientific data that reveal a serious risk or an unexpected serious risk associated with use of the drug that has been unearthed since the drug was approved, the risk evaluation was filed, or the last assessment. Other terms are redefined for these purposes to capture negative experiences or harmful side effects, whether due directly to the drug or attributable to the treatment experience.

The risk assessment strategies are keyed to timetables—the first assessment is due 18 months after initial approval of the strategy, the second at three years, and the third at seven years. It can be basically eliminated if the agency is satisfied that all risks have been identified and managed. The strategy also contemplates new Medication Guides for patients, package inserts, and enhanced health care professional communications.

---

[29] The law actually vests the Secretary of HHS with these powers, not the FDA; for the sake of expediency, the text refers to the FDA.

The Act ratify earlier risk management programs of FDA, allowing enhanced patient monitoring, patient registries, and increased training and licensing for prescribing or dispensing professionals. These risk evaluation and mitigation rules are truncated for generic drugs undergoing the ANDA process, in that a generic must only comply with the revised Medication Guide requirements, and may use a single, shared system, such as a registry.

The Act establishes a Drug Safety Management Board, whose job is to advise the Secretary on the decisions required under this Act. The FDA employees who have participated in the drug review may not sit on the Board.

The Act significantly changes television drug advertisements. A company may be required to submit its advertisements 45 days before airing, to make changes in the advertisement to protect consumers, or to be consistent with prescribing information. The Secretary may only require changes in advertising material that is false or misleading without a specific disclosure about a serious risk listed in the labeling of the drug involved and may require inclusion of such disclosure in the advertisement. In all DTC advertisements, the major statement relating to side effects and contraindications shall be presented in a clear, conspicuous, and neutral manner. The law requires that all DTC advertisements contain this statement: "You are encouraged to report negative side effects of prescription drugs to the FDA. Visit www.fda.gov/medwatch, or call 1–800-FDA-1088." The penalties for violation of these provisions have been revised and increased.

The Act has added a section on Active PostMarket Risk Identification, which contemplates that a database will be established, including 25 million patients, by 2010 and 100 million patients by 2012. This system will actively survey existing databases, such as Medicare, Veterans Administration, and private insurance carriers, for adverse event monitoring and other information.

Finally, the law prohibits food to which drugs or biological products have been added, assures pharmaceutical safety by strengthening controls against counterfeit, diverted, misbranded, or adulterated drugs, and establishes a specific Internet Web site for dissemination of drug and safety-related information. A separate section dealing with food safety has been enacted, and there are new protections for safe pet food, undoubtedly a response to the various poisons found in dog food made with imported ingredients earlier in 2007. There are numerous other sections with relatively minimal impact on drugs, devices, and biologics.

SUMMARY

Federal oversight of prescription drugs, devices, and biologics has come quite far since the early 1900s. Today, scientific breakthroughs, new diseases, and the general expectation that every disease can be "cured" all guarantee that the expectations of the FDA ratchet ever higher. There is obvious need for continued congressional oversight, to maintain the precious balance between the commercial motivation of pharmaceutical industry and the deployment of safe medical products. The overriding regulatory challenge that the FDA will face will be to keep current, through regulation and policy, with future technological advances by the science and the industry.

AGENCY ROLE AND ORGANIZATION

The primary responsibility for the regulation and oversight of pharmaceuticals and the pharmaceutical industry lies with the US FDA. The FDA was created in 1931 and is one of several branches within the U.S. Department of HHS. The FDA's counterparts within HHS include agencies such as the Centers for Disease Control and Prevention (CDC), the NIH, and the Centers for Medicare and Medicaid Services (CMS), formerly the Healthcare Financing Administration (HCFA).

The FDA is organized into a number of offices and centers headed by a commissioner who is appointed by the President with consent of the Senate. It is a scientifically based law enforcement agency whose mission is to safeguard the public health and to ensure honesty and fairness between health-regulated industries, i.e., pharmaceutical, device, and biologic, and the consumer.[30] It licenses and inspects manufacturing facilities, tests products, evaluates product submissions, assesses postmarket safety and effectiveness, evaluates claims and prescription drug advertising, monitors research, and creates regulations, guidelines, standards, and policies.

The following chart underscores the complexity of the administrative operations:[31]

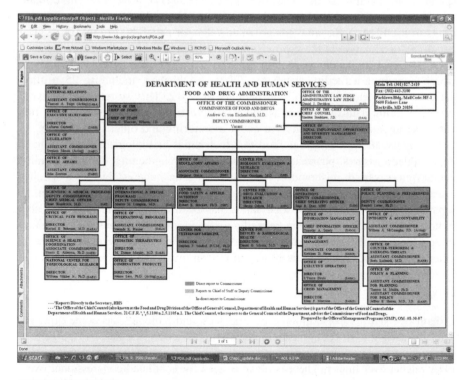

---

[30] Strauss S. Food and Drug Administration: an overview. In: Strauss's Federal Drug Laws and Examination Review, 5th ed. Lancaster, PA: Technomic Publishing Co., 1999:323.

[31] Chart found at www.fda.gov/oc/orgcharts/FDA.pdf.

The most familiar entities are located at the FDA headquarters in Rockville, Maryland. These are the five centers: the Center for Drug Evaluation and Research (CDER), Center for Biologics Evaluation and Research (CBER), Center for Devices and Radiological Health (CDRH), Center for Food Safety and Applied Nutrition (CFSAN), and the Center for Veterinary Medicine (CVM). Along with the Office of Regulatory Affairs, these report directly to the commissioner.

Other frequently noted resources include the Office of Combination Products and the Office of Pediatric Therapeutics, both located under the Office of International and Special Programs; the Office of the Ombudsman, which "reports directly to the associate commissioner for External Relations in the FDA's Office of the Commissioner. The office works to resolve problems with the FDA or to provide information to individuals or companies to enable them to proceed independently if they choose. The office can assist in determining an appropriate path to problem resolution by presenting the available options,"[32] and the Office of Orphan Products Development, which is not a mail stop but a clearinghouse for orphan product information.[33]

The Office of Generic Drugs, not surprisingly, is located within CDER. The Offices of Special Health Issues, Women's Health, and Women's Health Updates are consumer oriented, with a strong Web presence.

The Office of Regulatory Affairs is the lead office for all field activities; on its Web site (www.fda.gov/ora/default.htm), one can find the Regulatory Procedures Manual, which contains instructions that the FDA staff is to use when inspecting a facility, various enforcement reports, and other very useful information.

In addition to these centers and offices, the FDA has from time to time various programs. Of note is the Good Clinical Practice Program (www.fda.gov/oc/gcp/default), which is a centralized resource for all things under clinical investigation, including information for industry, consumers, subjects, and practitioners.

Each of these entities has a defined role, though sometimes their authorities overlap. For example, if a pharmaceutical company submits a drug that is contained and delivered to a patient during therapy by a device not comparable to any other, CDER and CDRH may need to coordinate that product's approval. Though most prescription drugs are evaluated by CDER, any other center or office may become involved with its review. One of the most significant resources to industry and consumers is the FDA's Web site, www.fda.gov. Easily accessible and navigable, each center and office has its own link within the site.

The FDA isn't the only agency within the U.S. government with a stake in pharmaceutical issues. The Federal Trade Commission (FTC) has authority over business practices in general, such as deceptive and anticompetitive practices, i.e., false advertising. In addition, FTC regulates the advertising of OTC drugs,

---

[32] See www.fda.gov/oc/ombudsman/whencon.htm.

[33] See www.fda.gov/orphan/index.htm.

medical devices, and cosmetics. To a lesser degree, the Consumer Product Safety Commission (CPSC) regulates hazardous substances and containers of poisons and other harmful agents; the Environmental Protection Agency (EPA) regulates pesticides used in agriculture and FDA-regulated food products; the Occupational Safety and Health Administration (OSHA) regulates the working environment of employees who may use FDA-regulated commodities, i.e., syringes, chemotherapy, and chemical reagents; the CMS (formerly the HCFA) regulates the federal Medicaid and Medicare programs as well as the State Children's Health Insurance Program (SCHIP), and the Drug Enforcement Administration (DEA) enforces the federal Controlled Substances Act (CSA) and is charged with controlling and monitoring the flow of licit and illicit controlled substances. Additionally, there are various state and local drug control agencies, which establish their own regulations and procedures for manufacturing, research, and development of pharmaceuticals.

NEW DRUG DEVELOPMENT AND APPROVAL SUMMARY

Prior to any discussion of how pharmaceuticals make their way through the FDA for market approval, one must understand what a "drug" is. A drug is a substance which exerts an action on the structure or function of the body by chemical action or metabolism and is intended for use in the diagnosis, cure, mitigation, treatment, or prevention of disease.[34] Many different elements are metabolized, but it is that intended use—diagnosis, treatment, mitigation—which is the core of the drug "indication" and the basis of the claims and labeling, once proved. The concept of "new drug" stems from the Kefauver-Harris Amendments to the FDCA. A new drug is defined as one that is not generally recognized as safe and effective for the indications proposed.[35] However, this definition has much greater reach than simply a "new" chemical entity. The term "new drug" also refers to a drug product already in existence, though never approved by the FDA for marketing in the United States; new therapeutic indications for an approved drug; a new dosage form; a new route of administration; a new dosing schedule; or, any other significant clinical differences than those approved.[36] Therefore, any chemical substance intended for use in humans or animals for medicinal purposes, or any existing chemical substance that has some significant change associated with it, is considered a new drug and not safe or effective until proper testing and FDA approval is met.

FDA approval is generally a lengthy and, almost always, an expensive process. While PDUFA has authorized fast track and "accelerated approvals," these procedures do not eliminate any phases of testing. As discussed in later

---

[34] 21 USC Sec. 321(g)(1).

[35] 21 USC Sec 321(p).

[36] Strauss S. Food and Drug Administration: an overview. In: Strauss' Federal Drug Laws and Examination Review, 5th ed. Lancaster, PA: Technomic Publishing Co., 1999:176,186.

chapters, these procedures essentially allow for multitasking in clinical trials, allowing for some overlap of clinical investigation planning.

For a pharmaceutical manufacturer to place a product on the market for human use, a multiphase procedure must be followed. It must be remembered that the mission of the FDA is to protect the public and the agency takes that charge very seriously. Hence, all drug products must at least follow the sequence of steps in the review process.

These steps begin with a number of preclinical or "before human" studies, followed usually by three phases of human testing. Drugs are also subject to a fourth phase, known as postmarket surveillance, which may include additional formal trials. The nature and scope of postmarket surveillance has been dramatically increased by provisions in the Food and Drug Administration Amendments Act of 2007, as discussed below.

FDA has published extensive information on the Drug Development Process; the following chart clearly demonstrates not only the significant interaction between the agency and the sponsor, but also the interrelation between the various stages of investigation and the continuing nature of FDA review throughout the drug development and deployment process.[37]

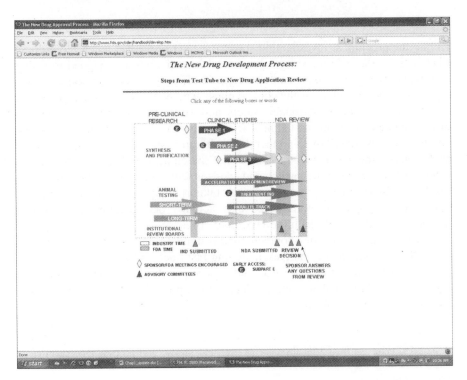

---

[37] See www.fda.gov/cder/handbook/develop.htm.

PRECLINICAL INVESTIGATION

Human testing of new drugs cannot begin until there is solid evidence that the drug product can be used with reasonable safety in humans. This phase is called "preclinical investigation." The basic goal of preclinical investigation is to assess potential therapeutic effects of the substance on living organisms and to gather sufficient data to determine reasonable safety of the substance in humans through laboratory experimentation and animal investigation.[38] The FDA requires no prior approval for investigators or pharmaceutical industry sponsors to begin a preclinical investigation on a potential drug substance. Investigators and sponsors are, however, required to follow Good Laboratory Practices (GLP) regulations.[39] GLPs govern laboratory facilities, personnel, equipment, and operations. Compliance with GLPs requires procedures and documentation of training, study schedules, processes, and status reports, which are submitted to facility management and included in the final study report to the FDA. Preclinical investigation usually takes one to three years to complete. If at that time enough data are gathered to reach the goal of potential therapeutic effect and reasonable safety, the product sponsor must formally notify the FDA of its wishes to test the potential new drug on humans.

INVESTIGATIONAL NEW DRUG APPLICATION

Unlike the preclinical investigation stage, the IND phase has much more direct FDA activity throughout. Since a preclinical investigation is designed to gather significant evidence of reasonable safety and efficacy of the compound in live organisms, the IND phase is the clinical phase where all activity is used to gather significant evidence of reasonable safety and efficacy data about the potential drug compound in humans. Clinical trials in humans are carefully scrutinized and regulated by the FDA to protect the health and safety of human test subjects and to ensure the integrity and usefulness of the clinical study data.[40] Numerous meetings between both the agency and sponsor will occur during this time. As a result, the clinical investigation phase may take as many as 12 years to complete. Only one in five compounds tested may actually demonstrate clinical effectiveness and safety and reach the U.S. marketplace.

(Note that the total development time is not the same as actual FDA review time. PDUFA and other initiatives, including fast track and accelerated approval, have shortened the drug approval and, consequently, the drug development cycle, with the result that some products are approved within a year of commencement of human testing.)

---

[38] Strauss S. Food and Drug Administration: an overview. Strauss' Federal Drug Laws and Examination Review. 5th ed. Lancaster, PA: Technomic Publishing Co., 1999:176,186.

[39] See 21 CFR Part 58.

[40] Pinna K, Pines W. The DRUGS/BIOLOGICS APPROVAL PROCESS. A Practical Guide to Food and Drug Law and Regulation. Washington, DC: FDLI, 1998:98.

The sponsor will submit the IND to the FDA. The IND must contain information and information of the study on the compound itself. All INDs must have the same basic components: a detailed cover sheet, a table of contents, an introductory statement and basic investigative plan, an investigator's brochure, comprehensive investigation protocols, the compound's actual or proposed chemistry, manufacturing and controls, any pharmacology and toxicology information, any previous human experience with the compound, and any other pertinent information the FDA deems necessary. After submission, the sponsor company must wait 30 days to commence clinical trials. FDA does not "approve" an IND; rather, if the FDA does not object within that period, the trials may begin.

Prior to the actual commencement of the clinical investigations, however, a few ground rules must be established. For example, a clinical study protocol must be developed, proposed by the sponsor, and reviewed by an Institutional Review Board (IRB). An IRB is required by regulation[41] and is a committee of medical and ethical experts designated by an institution such as a university medical center, in which the clinical trial will take place. The charge of the IRB is to oversee the research to ensure that the rights of human test subjects are protected and that rigorous medical and scientific standards are maintained.[42] IRBs must approve the proposed clinical study and monitor the research as it progresses. Each IRB must develop written procedures of its own regarding its study review process and its reporting of any changes to the ongoing study as they occur. In addition, an IRB must also review and approve documents for informed consent prior to commencement of the proposed clinical study. Regulations require that potential participants be informed adequately about the risks, benefits, and treatment alternatives before participating in experimental research.[43] An IRB's membership must be sufficiently diverse to review the study in terms of the specific research issue, community and legal standards, and professional and conduct and practice norms. All of its activities must be well documented and open to FDA inspection at any time.

Once the IRB is satisfied that the proposed trial is ethical and proper, the testing may begin. The clinical trial phase has three steps or phases. Each has a purpose, requires numerous patients, and can take more than one year to complete.

Phase I

A Phase I study is relatively small, less than 100 subjects, and brief (1 year or less). Its purpose is to determine toxicology, metabolism, pharmacologic actions, and, if possible, any early evidence of effectiveness. The results of the Phase I study are used to develop the next step, Phase II.

---

[41] 21 CFR Part 56; 21 CFR Part 312.66.

[42] See generally www.fda.gov/cder/about/smallbiz/humans.htm.

[43] 21 CFR Part 50, Human Subject Protection.

Phase II

Phase II studies are the first controlled clinical studies using several hundred subjects who are afflicted with the disease or condition being studied. The purpose of Phase II is to determine the compound's possible effectiveness against the targeted disease or condition and its safety in humans at that dosing. Phase II may be divided into two subparts: Phase IIa is a pilot study, which is used to determine initial efficacy, and Phase IIb, which uses controlled studies on several hundred patients. At the end of the Phase II studies, the sponsor and the FDA will usually confer to discuss the data and plans for Phase III.

Phase III

Phase III studies are considered "pivotal" trials, which are designed to collect all of the necessary data to meet the safety and efficacy standards that FDA requires to approve the compound for the U.S. marketplace. Phase III studies are usually very large, consisting of several thousand patients in numerous study centers with a large number of investigators who conduct long-term trials over several months or years. Also, Phase III studies establish final formulation, marketing claims and product stability, and packaging and storage conditions. On completion of Phase III, all clinical studies are complete, all safety and efficacy data has been analyzed, and the sponsor is ready to submit the compound to the FDA for market approval. This process begins with submission of an NDA.

NEW DRUG APPLICATION

An NDA is a regulatory mechanism that is designed to give the FDA sufficient information to make a meaningful evaluation of a new drug.[44] Although the quantity of information and data contained in an NDA is dependent on the drug testing, all NDAs contain essentially the same information, organized and delivered in a very precise way. The goals of the NDA are to provide enough information to permit the FDA reviewer to reach the following key decisions:

- Whether the drug is safe and effective in its proposed use(s), and whether the benefits of the drug outweigh the risks.
- Whether the drug's proposed labeling (package insert) is appropriate, and what it should contain.
- Whether the methods used in manufacturing the drug and the controls used to maintain the drug's quality are adequate to preserve the drug's identity, strength, quality, and purity.[45]

---

[44] 21 CFR Part 314.

[45] See www.fda.gov/cder/regulatory/applications/nda/htm.

The NDA is supposed to tell the drug's whole story, including what happened during the clinical tests, what the ingredients of the drug are, the results of the animal studies, how the drug behaves in the body, and how it is manufactured, processed, and packaged.[46] The NDA starts with an index and summary, moves on to chemistry, manufacturing, and controls, and then to preclinical laboratory and animal data, human pharmacokinetic and bioavailability data, clinical data, including tabulations of individual subject case report forms, safety data, packaging, a description of the drug product and substance, a list of relevant patents for the drug, its manufacture or claims, any proposed labeling, and any additional information the FDA considers relevant.

Traditionally, NDAs consisted of hundreds of volumes of information, in triplicate, all cross-referenced. Since 1999, the FDA has continued to move toward electronic filings; today, electronic submissions are encouraged but not required. These electronic submissions facilitate ease of review and possible approval.[47]

The NDA must be submitted complete, in the proper form, and with all critical data. On receipt, the FDA first determines whether an application is "filable." FDA screens the document to determine if the application is complete, justifying the time it will take to review the application. FDA must notify the sponsor within 60 days of its "refuse-to-file" decision. Otherwise, the review process begins.

The next steps require in-depth review, and the sponsor may be required to submit additional information. The purpose of an NDA from the FDA's perspective is to ensure that the new drug meets the criteria to be "safe and effective." FDA makes the safety and effectiveness and risk versus benefit determinations on the basis of the data; the data from the Phase III pivotal studies are given most weight.

Also, the NDA must be very clear about the manufacture and marketing of the proposed drug product. The application must define and describe manufacturing processes, validate Current Good Manufacturing Practices (cGMPs), provide evidence of quality, purity, strength, identity, and bioavailability (a preinspection of the manufacturing facility will be conducted by FDA). Finally, FDA will review all product packaging and labeling for content and clarity. Statements on a product's package label, package insert, media advertising, or professional literature must be reviewed. Of note, "labeling" refers to all of the above and not just the label on the product container.

FDA is required to review the application within 180 days of filing, but in practice, this time frame is frequently extended. The FDA's actual goals are to review priority applications within six months and standard applications within 10 months.[48] There are three possible results of a review, each reported through an "action letter." An "approval letter" signifies that all substantive requirements

---

[46] Ibid.

[47] See www.fda.gov/cder/guidance/index.htm#electronic_submissions.

[48] See www.fda.gov/ope/pdufa/report2005/PDUFA05perfrpt.pdf.

for approval are met and that the sponsor company can begin marketing the drug as of the date on the letter.

An "approvable letter" signifies that the application substantially complies with the requirements but has some minor deficiencies, which must be addressed before an approval letter is sent. Generally, these deficiencies are minor in nature and the product sponsor must respond within 10 days of receipt. At this point, the sponsor may amend the application and address the agency's concerns, or request a hearing with the agency, or withdraw the application entirely.

A "nonapprovable letter" signifies that FDA has major concern with the application and will not approve the proposed drug product for marketing as submitted. The remedies available to a sponsor for this type of action letter are similar to those in the approvable letter.

PHASE IV AND POSTMARKETING SURVEILLANCE

Pharmaceutical companies who successfully gain marketing approval for their products are not exempted from further regulatory requirements. In addition to the extensive postmarketing changes made by the Acts of 2007, compliance efforts take center stage. All producers must be registered and inspected, file various safety reports, meet import and export requirements, and maintain cGMPs. Many products are approved for market on the basis of a continued submission of clinical research data to the FDA. These data may be required to further validate efficacy or safety, detect new uses or abuses for the product, or to determine the effectiveness of labeled indications under conditions of widespread usage.[49] The FDA may also require a Phase IV study for drugs approved under FDAMA's fast track provisions.

Any changes to the approved product's indications, active ingredients, manufacture, or labeling require the manufacturer to submit a supplemental NDA (SNDA) for agency approval. Also, as emphasized in the section "The Food and Drug Administration Amendments Act of 2007," "adverse drug reports" must be reported to the agency. All reports must be reviewed by the manufacturer promptly, and if found to be serious, life threatening, or unexpected (not listed in the product's labeling), the manufacturer is required to submit an "alert report" within 15 working days of receipt of the information.

ORPHAN DRUGS

Orphan drugs are approved using many of the same processes as any other application. However, there are several significant differences. An orphan drug as defined under the Orphan Drug Act of 1993 is a drug used to treat a "rare disease," which would not normally be of interest to commercial manufacturers in the ordinary course of business. A rare disease is defined in the law as any

---

[49] Pinna K, et al. p. 111.

disease that affects fewer than 200,000 persons in the United States or one in which a manufacturer has no reasonable expectation of recovering the cost of its development and availability (e.g. manufacturing and marketing) in the United States. The Act creates a series of financial incentives for manufacturers. For example, the Act permits grant assistance for clinical research, tax credits for research and development, and a seven-year market exclusivity to the first applicant who, to obtain market approval for a drug, is designated as an orphan. This means that if the sponsor gains approval for an orphan drug, FDA will not approve any application by any other sponsor for the same drug for the same disease or condition for seven years from the date from the first applicant's approval, provided certain conditions are met, such as an assurance of sufficient availability of drug to those in need or a revocation of the drugs' orphan status.[50,51]

ABBREVIATED NEW DRUG APPLICATIONS

ANDAs are used when a patent has expired on a product that has been in the U.S. market and a company wishes to market a copy. In the United States, a drug patent is for 20 years. Subsequently, a manufacturer is able to submit an abbreviated application for that product, provided that it certifies that the product patent in question has already expired, is invalid, or will not be infringed.

The generic copy must meet certain other criteria as well. The drug's active ingredient must have already been approved for the conditions of use proposed in the ANDA, and nothing should have changed to call into question the basis for approval of the original drug's NDA.[52] Sponsors of ANDAs are required to prove that their version meets with standards of bio- and pharmaceutical equivalence. FDA publishes a list of all approved drugs called, "Approved Drug Products with Therapeutic Equivalence Evaluations," also called the "Orange Book" because of its orange-colored cover. It lists marketed drug products that are considered by FDA to be safe and effective and provides information on therapeutic equivalence evaluations for approved multisource prescription drug products[53] monthly. The Orange Book rates drugs on the basis of their therapeutic equivalence. For a product to be considered therapeutically equivalent, it must be both pharmaceutically equivalent (i.e., the same dose, dosage form, strength, etc.), and bioequivalent (i.e., rate and extent of its absorption is not significantly different than the rate and extent of absorption of the drug with which it is to be interchanged).

Realizing that there may be some degree of variability in patients, FDA allows pharmaceuticals to be considered bioequivalent in either of two methods. The first method studies the rate and extent of absorption of a test drug, which

---

[50] The Orphan Drug Act of 1982, Public Law 97–414.

[51] The Orphan Drug Amendments of 1985, Public Law 99–91.

[52] Pinna K, et al. p. 119.

[53] USP/DI, Volume III, 13th Edition, Preface, v.

may or may not be a generic variation, and a reference or brand name drug under similar experimental conditions and in similar dosing schedules where the test results do not show significant differences. The second approach uses the same method and from the results determine that there is a difference in the test drug's rate and extent of absorption, except, the difference is considered to be medically insignificant for the proper clinical outcome of that drug.

> "Bioequivalence of different formulations of the same drug substance involves equivalence with respect to the rate and extent of drug absorption. Two formulations whose rate and extent of absorption differ by 20% or less are generally considered bioequivalent. The use of the 20% rule is based on a medical decision that, for most drugs, a 20% difference in the concentration of the active ingredient in blood will not be clinically significant."[54]

The FDA's Orange Book uses a two letter coding system, which is helpful in determining which drug products are considered therapeutically equivalent. The first letter, either an "A" or a "B", indicates a drug product's therapeutic equivalence rating. The second letter describes dose forms and can be any one of a number of different letters.

The A codes are described in the Orange Book as follows:

> "Drug products that the FDA considers to be therapeutically equivalent to other pharmaceutically equivalent products, i.e., drug products for which
>
> 1. there are no known or suspected bioequivalence problems. These are designated **AA, AN, AO, AP,** or **AT,** depending on the dose form; or
> 2. actual or potential bioequivalence problems have been resolved with adequate in vivo and/or in vitro evidence supporting bioequivalence. These are designated **AB**."[55]

The B codes are a much less desirable rating when compared with a rating of A. Products, which are rated B, may still be commercially marketed, however, they may not be considered therapeutically equivalent. The Orange Book describes B codes as follows:

> "Drug products that the FDA at this time does not consider to be therapeutically equivalent to other pharmaceutically equivalent products, i.e., drug products for which actual or potential bioequivalence problems have not been resolved by adequate evidence of bioequivalence. Often the problem is with specific dosage forms rather than with the active ingredients. These are designated **BC, BD, BE, BN, BP, BR, BS, BT,** or **BX.**"[56]

---

[54] USP/DI, p. I/7.

[55] USP/DI, p. I/9.

[56] USP/DI, p. I/10.

The FDA has adopted an additional subcategory of B codes. The designation "B*" is assigned to former A minus-rated drugs "if the FDA receives new information that raises a significant question regarding therapeutic equivalence."[57] Not all drugs are listed in the Orange Book. Drugs obtainable only from a single manufacturing source, DESI –drugs or drugs manufactured prior to 1938 are not included. Those that do appear are listed by generic name.

OVER-THE-COUNTER REGULATIONS

The 1951 Durham-Humphrey Amendments of the FDCA specified three criteria to justify prescription-only status. If the compound is shown to be habit forming, requires a prescriber's supervision, or has an NDA prescription-only limitation, it will require a prescription. The principles used to establish OTC status (nonprescription required) are a wide margin of safety, method of use, benefit to risk ratio, and adequacy of labeling for self-medication. For example, injectable drugs may not be used OTC, with certain exceptions such as insulin. OTC market entry is less restrictive than that for Rx drugs and does not require premarket clearance; these pose fewer safety hazards than Rx drugs because they are designed to alleviate symptoms rather than disease. Easier access far outweighs the risks of side effects, which can be adequately addressed through proper labeling.

As previously discussed, OTC products underwent a review in 1972. Because agency review of the 300,000 plus OTC drug products in existence at the time would be virtually impossible, the FDA created OTC advisory panels to review data based on some 26 therapeutic categories. OTC drugs would only be examined by active ingredient within a therapeutic category. Inactive ingredients would only be examined, provided they were shown to be safe and suitable for the product and not interfering with effectiveness and quality.

This review of active ingredients would result in the promulgation of a regulation or a monograph, which is a "recipe" or set of guidelines applicable to all OTC products within a therapeutic category. OTC monographs are general and require that OTC products show "general recognition of the safety and effectiveness of the active ingredient." OTC products do not fall under prescription status if their active ingredients (or combinations) are deemed by FDA to be "generally recognized as safe and effective" (GRASE). The monograph system is a public system with a public comment component included after each phase of the process. Any products for which a final monograph has not been established may remain on the market until one is determined.

There are four phases in the OTC monograph system. In Phase I, an expert panel was selected to review data for each active ingredient in each therapeutic category for safety, efficacy, and labeling. Its recommendations were made in the Federal Register. A public comment period of 30 to 60 days was permitted and supporting or contesting data accepted for review. Then the panel reevaluated the

---

[57] USP/DI, p. I/12.

data and published a "proposed monograph" in the Federal Register, which publicly announced the conditions for which the panel believes that OTC products in a particular therapeutic class are GRASE and not misbranded. A tentative "final monograph" was then developed and published stating the FDA's position on safety and efficacy of a particular ingredient within a therapeutic category and acceptable labeling for indications, warnings, and directions for use. Active ingredients were deemed: category I—GRASE for claimed therapeutic indications and not misbranded; category II—not GRASE and/or misbranded; or category III—insufficient data for determination.

After public comment, the final monograph was established and published with the FDA's final criteria for which all drug products in a therapeutic class become GRASE and not misbranded. Following the effective date of the final monograph, all covered drug products that fail to conform to its requirements are considered misbranded and/or an unapproved new drug.[58]

However, since monograph panels are no longer convened, many current products are switched from prescription status. A company who wishes to make this switch and offer a product to the U.S. marketplace can submit an amendment to a monograph to the FDA who will act as the sole reviewer. The company may also file an SNDA, provided that it has three years of marketing experience as a prescription product, can demonstrate a relatively high use during that period, and can validate that the product has a mild profile of adverse reactions. The last method involves a "citizens petition," which is rarely used.[59]

BIOLOGICS

Biologics are defined as substances derived from or made with the aid of living organisms, which include vaccines, antitoxins, serums, blood, blood products, therapeutic protein drugs derived from natural sources (i.e., antithrombin III) or biotechnology (i.e., recombinantly derived proteins), and gene or somatic cell therapies.[60] As with the more traditionally derived drug products, biologics follow virtually the same regulatory and clinical testing schema with regard to safety and efficacy. Manufacturers of biologics for introduction into interstate commerce must hold a license for the products, which are issued by CBER. A Biologics License Application (BLA) is used rather than an NDA, though the official BLA form is designated 356h and is identical to the NDA form. The sponsor merely indicates in check box if the application is for a drug or a biologic. Compounds characterized as biologics are reviewed by CBER.[61]

CDER has certain responsibilities for certain therapeutic biologic products that were transferred from CBER. CDER's duties include premarket review and

---

[58] Strauss S. p. 285.

[59] Ibid.

[60] 42 USC Sec 262.

[61] See Form FDA 356h.

oversight; however, despite this transfer, the products continue to be regulated as licensed biologics. Some of the transferred products include growth factors and enzymes. CBER regulates xenotransplantation and has a large regulatory role in vaccine development, tissue safety, and blood.

DEVICES

Devices range from the simplest of products that fall under FDA jurisdiction because they are sold with a therapeutic claim, such as a toothbrush and sterile gauze, to the most complex of surgical instruments, such as a drug-eluting stent, to diagnostic machines like MRIs. The statutory definition of device is the same as that of a drug, except that the device "... does not achieve its primary intended purposes through chemical action within or on the body of man or other animals and which is not dependent upon being metabolized for the achievement of its primary intended purposes."[62]

Devices are classified by the risk they pose to users. Class I is the simplest and subject to the least oversight and regulation. Class III includes all devices of the highest risk, which support or sustain human life, and are subjected to the strictest of testing standards, the premarket approval, which usually involves testing in Phases I, II, and III. Class II devices are everything that are not Class I or III and are reviewed using the so-called 510(k) premarket notification, where the sponsor proves that the device is substantially equivalent to a predicate (existing, cleared device); within 90 days of submission, CDRH will notify the sponsor whether the device is cleared or not.

Devices are subject to quality system requirements rather than current good manufacturing practices. Devices are also subject to stringent adverse event reporting and postmarket surveillance. All device manufacturing facilities should expect to be inspected every two years.

REGULATING DRUG AND DEVICE MARKETING

FDA has jurisdiction over prescription drug advertising and promotion. The basis for these regulations lies within the 1962 Kefauver-Harris Amendments. Essentially, any promotional information, in any form, must be truthful, fairly balanced, and fully disclosed. FDA views this information as either "advertising" or "labeling." Advertising includes all traditional outlets in which a company places an advertisement. Labeling includes everything else such as brochures, booklets, lectures, slide kits, letters to physicians, and company-sponsored magazine articles, etc. All information must be truthful and not misleading. All material facts must be disclosed in a manner that is fairly balanced and accurate. If any of these requirements are violated, the product is considered misbranded for the indications for which it was approved under its NDA. FDA

---

[62] 21 USC Sec 321(h).

is also sensitive to the promotion of a product for "off-label use." Off-label use occurs when a product is in some way presented in a manner that does not agree with or is not addressed in its approved labeling. Also, provisions of the Prescription Drug Marketing Act (PDMA) of 1987 apply. The Act prohibits company representatives from directly distributing or reselling prescription drug samples. Companies are required to establish a closed system of record keeping, which will be able to track a sample from their control to that of a prescriber in order to prevent diversion. Prescribers are required to receive these samples and record and store them appropriately.[63]

Additionally, television, Internet, and print advertisements must comply with standards set by law and regulation. The Division of Drug Marketing, Advertising, and Communications (DDMAC), within CDER, reviews such advertisements; the advertisements may not be false or misleading, present a "fair balance" between side effects, contraindications, and effectiveness information, and presumably, neutrality under the Acts of 2007, reveal material facts, and include established, scientific, and brand names in specified font ratios.[64]

Although there are fewer regulations and guidances regarding device and biologic marketing and advertisement, these are still regulated activities and the same concepts apply.

VIOLATIONS AND ENFORCEMENT

FDA has the power to enforce the regulations for any product as defined under the FDCA. It has the jurisdiction to inspect a manufacturer's premises and its records. After a facilities inspection, an agency inspector will issue an FDA form 483, which describes observable violations. Response to the finding as described in this form must be made promptly. A "warning letter" may be used when the agency determines that one or more of a company's practices, products, and procedures are in violation of the FDCA. The FDA district has 15 days to issue a warning letter after an inspection. The company has 15 days in which to respond. If the company response is satisfactory to the agency, no other action is warranted. If the response is not, the agency may request a "recall" of the violated products. However, the FDA has no authority to force a company to recall a drug product. But, it may force removal of a product through the initiation of a seizure.

Recalls can fall into one of three classes. A Class I recall exists when there is a reasonable possibility that the use of a product will cause either serious adverse effects on health or death. A Class II recall exists when the use of a product may cause temporary or medically reversible adverse effects on health, or where the probability of serious adverse effects on health is remote. A Class III recall exists when the use of a product is not likely to cause adverse health

---

[63] 21 USC Sec 301 and ff.

[64] See 21 CFR 202.

consequences. Recalls are also categorized as consumer level, where the products are requested to be recalled from the consumers' homes or control, a retail level, where the products are to be removed from retail shelves or control, and wholesale level, where the products are to be removed from wholesale distribution. Companies who conduct a recall of their products are required to conduct "effectiveness checks" to determine the effectiveness of recalling the product from the marketplace.

If a company refuses to recall the product, the FDA will seek an injunction against the company.[65] An injunction is recommended to the Department of Justice (DOJ) by the FDA. The DOJ takes the request to federal court who issues the order that forbids a company from carrying out a particular illegal act, such as marketing a product that the FDA considers a violation of the FDCA. Companies can either comply with the order or sign a "consent agreement" that will specify changes required by the FDA for the company to continue operations or to litigate.

The FDA may also initiate a seizure of violative products.[66] A seizure is ordered by the federal court in the district that the products are located. The seizure order specifies products, their batch numbers, and any records as determined by the FDA as violative. The U.S. Marshals carry out this action. The FDA institutes a seizure to prevent a company from selling, distributing, moving, or otherwise tampering with the product.

The FDA may also debar individuals or firms from assisting or submitting an ANDA or directly providing services to any firm with an existing or pending drug product application. Debarment may last for up to 10 years.[67]

However, one of the more powerful deterrents that the FDA uses is adverse publicity. The agency has no authority to require a company to advertise adverse publicity. It does publish administrative actions against a company in any number of federal publications such as the *Federal Register*, the *FDA Enforcement Report*, the *FDA Medical Bulletin*, and *the FDA Consumer*. Additionally, letters detailing a company's or a person's violation of regulation can be found at the warning letters link from the FDA home page, www.fda.gov.

SUMMARY

The laws and regulations that govern the U.S. pharmaceutical industry are both vast and complicated. Interpretation of the FDCA is in a constant state of flux. FDA is charged with this interpretation on the basis of the rapid technology changes that are everyday occurrences within the industry. Many may suggest that more rapid drug approval places the citizenry in greater danger of adverse

---

[65] 21USC302, et seq.

[66] 21USC304, et seq.

[67] Fundamentals of Regulatory Affairs, Regulatory Affairs Professionals Society, 1999, p. 199.

events. Others may reply that technology offers newer and more effective therapies for deadly disease.

Historically, the U.S. Congress has passed laws governing our medication on the basis of a reaction to a crisis. The Pure Food and Drug Act, the FDCA, and the Price Competition and Patent Restoration Act are to name a few. One hopes that this method of regulation will not continue as the norm. We can be proud of proactive legislation such as the Kefauver-Harris Amendments, the Orphan Drug Act, PDUFA, FDAMA, and now, the Administration Amendments Act of 2007. These Acts have paved the way for meaningful change within the drug investigation process as we continue in our battle against disease. The U.S. system of investigating new drugs, devices, and biologics is one that continues to have merit by allowing enough time to investigate benefit versus risk and remains the gold standard throughout the world. The American public can look forward to great advances from the industry and should be comfortable that the FDA is watching.

2

What Is an IND?

Michael R. Hamrell
MORIAH Consultants, Yorba Linda, California, U.S.A.

WHAT IS AN IND?

The Federal Food, Drug, and Cosmetic Act (FD&C Act) requires that all drugs have an approved marketing application [new drug application (NDA) or abbreviated new drug application (ANDA)] before they can be shipped in interstate commerce. An IND, or investigational new drug application, is a submission to the U.S. Food and Drug Administration (FDA) requesting permission to initiate a clinical study of a new drug product in the United States. From a legal perspective, the IND is a request for exemption from the act's prohibition from introducing any new drug into interstate commerce without an approved application. The IND allows you to legally ship an unapproved drug, or import the new drug from a foreign country.

In reality, the IND is much more than a legal tool allowing a company to ship an investigational new drug. The IND application allows a company to initiate and conduct clinical studies of their investigational drug product. The IND application provides the FDA with the data necessary to decide whether the new drug and the proposed clinical trial pose a reasonable risk to the human subjects participating in the study. The act directs the FDA to place investigations on *clinical hold* if the drug involved presents unreasonable risk to the safety of the subjects. The safety of the clinical trial subjects is always the primary concern of the FDA when reviewing an IND, regardless of the phase of

Based on the original chapter by Robert G. Pietrusko and Thomas Class Millennium Pharmaceuticals, Inc., Cambridge, Massachusetts, U.S.A.

the clinical investigation. In later phases (phases 2 and 3), the FDA also evaluates the study design in terms of demonstrating efficacy; but safety of the subjects is critical throughout the drug development process. When preparing an IND, and throughout the drug development process, the primary goal of the sponsor should be to demonstrate to the FDA that the new drug, the proposed trial, and the entire clinical development plan described in the IND is designed to minimize risk to the trial subjects.

IND Term

Clinical hold—an order issued by the FDA to the sponsor to delay a proposed clinical investigation or to suspend an ongoing investigation. Subjects may not be given the investigational drug or the hold may require that no new subjects be enrolled into an ongoing study. The clinical hold can be issued before the end of the 30-day IND review period to prevent a sponsor from initiating a proposed protocol or at any time during the life of an IND.

When Do I Need an IND?

Simply put, an IND is required anytime you want to conduct a clinical trial of an unapproved drug in the United States. However, what is actually considered a new or unapproved drug and how the act defines a drug often makes the decision about filing an IND more complicated. The act defines a drug, in part, as "articles intended for use in the diagnosis, cure, mitigation, treatment, or prevention of disease in man or other animals; and articles (other than food) intended to affect the structure or any function of the body of man or other animals."[1] The act further defines a new drug, in part, as "any drug the composition of which is such that such drug is not generally recognized as safe and effective for use under the conditions prescribed, recommended, or suggested in the labeling."[2] Because of these legal definitions, an approved drug can be considered a new drug and would require an IND to conduct a study. An IND would be required to conduct a clinical trial if the drug is

- a new chemical entity,
- not approved for the indication under investigation,
- in a new dosage form,
- being administered at a new dosage level, and
- in combination with another drug and the combination is not approved.

---

[1] Federal Food, Drug & Cosmetic Act Chapter II Section 201(g)(1).

[2] Federal Food, Drug & Cosmetic Act Chapter II Section 201(g)(1).

A less obvious situation in which a clinical study must be conducted under the authority of an IND is when the chemical compound is being used as a "clinical research tool" but will not be developed for therapeutic use. Sometimes these "tools" are administered to human subjects to elicit specific physiologic responses that are being studied. In this context, these compounds are considered drugs because the act states that compounds intended to affect the structure or any function of the body of man or other animals are drugs. There is no exemption from the IND requirements in the act or regulations for studies conducted with compounds considered drugs that are not being developed for a therapeutic use. All clinical studies where an unapproved drug is administered to human subjects, regardless of whether the drug will be commercially developed, require an IND.

When Don't I Need an IND?

An IND is not required to conduct a study if the drug

- is not intended for human subjects, but is intended for in vitro testing or laboratory research animals (nonclinical studies) and
- is an approved drug and the study is within its approved indication for use.

The regulations also exempt studies of *approved* drugs if *all* of the following criteria are satisfied.[3]

- The study will not be reported to the FDA in support of a new indication or other change in labeling or advertising for the product.
- The study will not involve a route of administration, dose level, or patient population that increases the risks associated with the use of the drug.
- The studies will be conducted in compliance with IRB and informed consent regulations.
- The studies will not be used to promote unapproved indications.

The FDA will generally not accept an IND application for investigations that meet these exemption criteria. The IND regulations also provide an exemption for studies that use placebos,[4] as long as the study would not otherwise require submission of an IND. The use of a placebo in a clinical study does not automatically necessitate an IND.

In January of 2004, the FDA published a final guidance document clarifying under what circumstances an IND would not be required for the study of marketed cancer drugs.[5] The guidance specifically discusses how investigators

---

[3] Code of Federal Regulations Title 21 Section 312.2.

[4] Code of Federal Regulations Title 21 Section 312.2 (b)(5).

[5] FDA Draft Guidance for Industry: IND Exemptions for Studies of Lawfully Marketed Cancer Drug or Biologic Products. FDA, Rockville, MD, January 2004.

assess increased risk to cancer patients when there is scientific literature or other clinical experience available to support the proposed uses. The guidance states that studies may be considered exempt from the IND requirements if the studies involve a new use, dosage, schedule, route of administration, or new combination of marketed cancer drugs in a patient population with cancer if the four exemption criteria for approved products listed above are met. They also clarified that as a basis for assessing whether there is an increased risk associated with the proposed use, the investigators and the Institutional Review Boards (IRBs) must determine that on the basis of scientific literature and generally known clinical experience, there is no significant increase in the risk associated with the use of the drug product. The guidance also provides a clarification for drug manufacturers who provide approved cancer drugs to sponsor investigators for clinical study. Providing an approved cancer drug for an investigator-sponsored trial would not, in and by itself, be considered promotional activity on the part of the manufacturer if it were for a bona fide clinical investigation.

Whenever a sponsor or investigator considers conducting a clinical study, careful consideration should be given to the need for an IND. Companies should consult with their regulatory affairs staff to determine if an IND is required, and investigators can consult with the IRB at their institution. If after consultation it is still unclear whether an IND is required, potential sponsors should contact the FDA for advice. Conducting a study without an IND when one is required can lead to regulatory action by the FDA.

IND Term

Institutional Review Board—a board or committee formally designated by an institution to review and approve the initiation of biomedical research involving human subjects. The primary purpose of the IND is to protect the rights and welfare of human subjects.

IND Facts

In 2006, the Center for Drug Evaluation & Research at the FDA received 1863 original INDs (including therapeutic biologics in CDER). Of these, 713 were commercial INDs and 1150 were noncommercial INDs. At the close of the 2006 calendar year, there were 14,117 active INDs (5445 commercial and 8672 noncommercial).

PRE-IND MEETING

Frequent meetings between the sponsor and the FDA are useful in resolving questions and issues raised during the preparation for an IND. The FDA encourages such meetings to the extent that they aid in the solution of scientific problems and to the extent that the FDA has available resources. To promote efficiency, all issues related to the submission of the IND should be included to the extent practical, since the FDA generally expects to grant only one pre-IND meeting. On occasion, when there are complex manufacturing issues, a separate chemistry, manufacturing, and controls (CMC) meeting can be granted. Meetings at this stage regarding CMC information are often unnecessary when the project is straightforward. A pre-IND meeting is considered a type B meeting. It is a "formal" meeting requiring a written request that includes, among other things, a list of specific objectives and outcomes and a list of specific questions, grouped by discipline. Most issues and questions usually are related to the design of animal studies needed to initiate clinical trials as well as the scope and design of the initial study in humans. Type B meetings should be scheduled to occur within 60 days of the FDA's receipt of the written request for the meeting. A briefing document is required at least four weeks before the meeting. The briefing document should provide summary information relevant to the product and supplementary information that the FDA can use to provide responses to the questions that have been identified by the sponsor for the IND submission. There should be full and open communication about the scientific or medical issue to be discussed during the meeting. The meeting may be a face-to-face one or the FDA may prefer to have a telephonic conference call to serve as the meeting. Typically, the FDA will have a pre-meeting to address the issues that have been raised and may provide initial feedback before the meeting. The attendance at the pre-IND meeting is multidisciplinary, involving FDA personnel in clinical, pharmacology/toxicology, biopharmaceutics, chemistry, statistics, microbiology, and other disciplines. At the conclusion of the meeting, there should be a review of all the issues, responses, and agreements. An assigned individual from the FDA, usually the project manager, will prepare the minutes of the meeting, and the FDA's version of the minutes are considered the official version, so they should be reviewed carefully to assure that all discussion points and agreements were captured properly. In general, they should be available to the sponsor within 30 days after the meeting but are often made available just before the meeting to form the basis for any discussion. It is most important that all issues and agreements be addressed in the IND submission. There are other meetings that can be held during the IND phases of development and include an end-of-phase 1 meeting (generally for fast track products), an end-of-phase 2 meeting, and a pre-NDA or pre-BLA (biologic license application) meeting.

THE CONTENT AND FORMAT OF AN IND APPLICATION

The content and format of an initial IND is laid out in 21 Code of Federal Regulations (CFR) Part 312 and in numerous guidance documents published by FDA. This section outlines the required content and format of an initial IND based on CFR requirements and the published guidance. In addition, since the FDA has adopted the common technical document (CTD) format for NDAs, it is also possible and encouraged that sponsors consider submitting the IND in the CTD format. This provides better consistency for reviewers and facilitates the later preparation of the NDA application, since everything is already in the proper format. The initial IND application to the FDA can be for a phase 1 first in human study, or it can be for a later-phase study where clinical studies of the compound have already been conducted in another country. Although the basic content is the same, the expected level of detail is different. The information expected in later-phase studies is based on the phase of investigation, the amount of human experience with the drug, the drug substance, and the dosage form of the drug. In the outline, requirements will be addressed both for INDs for phase 1 studies as well as initial INDs for later-stage studies. This section is not intended to be a recitation of CFR 312.23 or the guidance documents, but an overview of the key elements of the initial IND, regardless of the phase of the proposed study. The specific references to section 312.23 for each of the sections of an IND are included for reference.

Cover Sheet—312.23(a)(1) FDA Form 1571—IND

The Form 1571 (Fig. 1) is a required part of the initial IND and every subsequent submission related to the IND application. Each *IND Amendment, IND Safety Report, IND Annual Report,* or general correspondence with the FDA regarding the IND must include a 1571. The Form 1571 serves as a cover sheet for IND submissions and provides the FDA with basic information about the submission—name of the sponsor, IND number, name of the drug, type of submission, serial number, and the contents of the application. Each submission to the IND must be consecutively numbered, starting with the initial IND application, which is numbered 0000. The next submission (response to clinical hold, correspondence, amendment, etc.) should be numbered 0001, with subsequent submissions numbered consecutively in the order of submission. It is important to note that the FDA expects that every submission, even the most routine correspondence, be made with a completed Form 1571 and have a serial number. The FDA tracks all IND submissions on the basis of serial numbers and files them according to the serial number on receipt. If more than one group within a company submits IND amendments (e.g., a pharmacovigilance group may submit safety reports directly to the FDA), it is essential that the serial numbers be consecutive.

The 1571 Form provides a section for the sponsor to state whether a contract research organization (CRO) will conduct any parts of the clinical study and if any sponsor obligations will be transferred to the CRO. If sponsor responsibilities are to be transferred, a list of the obligations transferred and the name and address of the CRO must be attached to the 1571 form. Although the sponsor may transfer some or all of its obligations to a CRO, the sponsor of

DEPARTMENT OF HEALTH AND HUMAN SERVICES FOOD AND DRUG ADMINISTRATION	Form Approved: OMB No. 0910-0014. Expiration Date: May 31, 2009 See OMB Statement on Reverse.
INVESTIGATIONAL NEW DRUG APPLICATION (IND) *(TITLE 21, CODE OF FEDERAL REGULATIONS (CFR) PART 312)*	**NOTE:** No drug may be shipped or clinical investigation begun until an IND for that investigation is in effect (21 CFR 312.40).

1. NAME OF SPONSOR	2. DATE OF SUBMISSION
3. ADDRESS *(Number, Street, City, State and Zip Code)*	4. TELEPHONE NUMBER *(Include Area Code)*
5. NAME(S) OF DRUG *(Include all available names: Trade, Generic, Chemical, Code)*	6. IND NUMBER *(If previously assigned)*

7. INDICATION(S) *(Covered by this submission)*

8. PHASE(S) OF CLINICAL INVESTIGATION TO BE CONDUCTED:
☐ PHASE 1 ☐ PHASE 2 ☐ PHASE 3 ☐ OTHER_____
(Specify)

9. LIST NUMBERS OF ALL INVESTIGATIONAL NEW DRUG APPLICATIONS (21 CFR Part 312), NEW DRUG OR ANTIBIOTIC APPLICATIONS (21 CFR Part 314), DRUG MASTER FILES (21 CFR Part 314.420), AND PRODUCT LICENSE APPLICATIONS (21 CFR Part 601) REFERRED TO IN THIS APPLICATION.

10. *IND submission should be consecutively numbered. The initial IND should be numbered "Serial number: 0000." The next submission (e.g., amendment, report, or correspondence) should be numbered "Serial Number: 0001." Subsequent submissions should be numbered consecutively in the order in which they are submitted.*   SERIAL NUMBER ____ ____ ____

11. THIS SUBMISSION CONTAINS THE FOLLOWING: *(Check all that apply)*
☐ INITIAL INVESTIGATIONAL NEW DRUG APPLICATION (IND)   ☐ RESPONSE TO CLINICAL HOLD

PROTOCOL AMENDMENT(S):	INFORMATION AMENDMENT(S):	IND SAFETY REPORT(S):
☐ NEW PROTOCOL	☐ CHEMISTRY/MICROBIOLOGY	☐ INITIAL WRITTEN REPORT
☐ CHANGE IN PROTOCOL	☐ PHARMACOLOGY/TOXICOLOGY	☐ FOLLOW-UP TO A WRITTEN REPORT
☐ NEW INVESTIGATOR	☐ CLINICAL	

☐ RESPONSE TO FDA REQUEST FOR INFORMATION   ☐ ANNUAL REPORT   ☐ GENERAL CORRESPONDENCE

☐ REQUEST FOR REINSTATEMENT OF IND THAT IS WITHDRAWN, INACTIVATED, TERMINATED OR DISCONTINUED   ☐ OTHER _____ *(Specify)*

CHECK ONLY IF APPLICABLE

JUSTIFICATION STATEMENT MUST BE SUBMITTED WITH APPLICATION FOR ANY CHECKED BELOW. REFER TO THE CITED CFR SECTION FOR FURTHER INFORMATION.

☐ TREATMENT IND 21 CFR 312.35(b)   ☐ TREATMENT PROTOCOL 21 CFR 312.35(a)   ☐ CHARGE REQUEST/NOTIFICATION 21 CFR 312.7(d)

FOR FDA USE ONLY

CDR/DBIND/DGD RECEIPT STAMP	DDR RECEIPT STAMP	DIVISION ASSIGNMENT:
		IND NUMBER ASSIGNED:

FORM FDA 1571 (4/06)   PREVIOUS EDITION IS OBSOLETE.   **PAGE 1 OF 2**
PSC Graphics: (301) 443-1090   EF

Figure 1   *(Continued on next page)* Form 1571—IND Application Form.

the IND is ultimately responsible for the conduct of the clinical investigation and all the regulatory and legal requirements pertaining to a clinical trial.

When signing the 1571 Form, the sponsor is also making three important commitments to the FDA, which are outlined on page 2 of the form.

```
12.                        CONTENTS OF APPLICATION
                This application contains the following items: (Check all that apply)

☐  1. Form FDA 1571 [21 CFR 312.23(a)(1)]
☐  2. Table of Contents [21 CFR 312.23(a)(2)]
☐  3. Introductory statement [21 CFR 312.23(a)(3)]
☐  4. General Investigational plan [21 CFR 312.23(a)(3)]
☐  5. Investigator's brochure [21 CFR 312.23(a)(5)]
☐  6. Protocol(s) [21 CFR 312.23(a)(6)]
        ☐  a. Study protocol(s) [21 CFR 312.23(a)(6)]
          ☐  b. Investigator data [21 CFR 312.23(a)(6)(iii)(b)] or completed Form(s) FDA 1572
          ☐  c. Facilities data [21 CFR 312.23(a)(6)(iii)(b)] or completed Form(s) FDA 1572
            ☐  d. Institutional Review Board data [21 CFR 312.23(a)(6)(iii)(b)] or completed Form(s) FDA 1572
☐  7. Chemistry, manufacturing, and control data [21 CFR 312.23(a)(7)]
        ☐  Environmental assessment or claim for exclusion [21 CFR 312.23(a)(7)(iv)(e)]
☐  8. Pharmacology and toxicology data [21 CFR 312.23(a)(8)]
☐  9. Previous human experience [21 CFR 312.23(a)(9)]
☐ 10. Additional information [21 CFR 312.23(a)(10)]
```

13. IS ANY PART OF THE CLINICAL STUDY TO BE CONDUCTED BY A CONTRACT RESEARCH ORGANIZATION? ☐ YES ☐ NO

IF YES, WILL ANY SPONSOR OBLIGATIONS BE TRANSFERRED TO THE CONTRACT RESEARCH ORGANIZATION? ☐ YES ☐ NO

IF YES, ATTACH A STATEMENT CONTAINING THE NAME AND ADDRESS OF THE CONTRACT RESEARCH ORGANIZATION, IDENTIFICATION OF THE CLINICAL STUDY, AND A LISTING OF THE OBLIGATIONS TRANSFERRED.

14. NAME AND TITLE OF THE PERSON RESPONSIBLE FOR MONITORING THE CONDUCT AND PROGRESS OF THE CLINICAL INVESTIGATIONS

15. NAME(S) AND TITLE(S) OF THE PERSON(S) RESPONSIBLE FOR REVIEW AND EVALUATION OF INFORMATION RELEVANT TO THE SAFETY OF THE DRUG

I agree not to begin clinical investigations until 30 days after FDA's receipt of the IND unless I receive earlier notification by FDA that the studies may begin. I also agree not to begin or continue clinical investigations covered by the IND if those studies are placed on clinical hold. I agree that an Institutional Review Board (IRB) that complies with the requirements set fourth in 21 CFR Part 56 will be responsible for initial and continuing review and approval of each of the studies in the proposed clinical investigation. I agree to conduct the investigation in accordance with all other applicable regulatory requirements.

16. NAME OF SPONSOR OR SPONSOR'S AUTHORIZED REPRESENTATIVE

17. SIGNATURE OF SPONSOR OR SPONSOR'S AUTHORIZED REPRESENTATIVE   **Sign**

18. ADDRESS (Number, Street, City, State and Zip Code)

19. TELEPHONE NUMBER (Include Area Code)

20. DATE

(WARNING: A willfully false statement is a criminal offense. U.S.C. Title 18, Sec. 1001.)

Public reporting burden for this collection of information is estimated to average 100 hours per response, including the time for reviewing instructions, searching existing data sources, gathering and maintaining the data needed, and completing reviewing the collection of information. Send comments regarding this burden estimate or any other aspect of this collection of information, including suggestions for reducing this burden to:

Department of Health and Human Services
Food and Drug Administration
Center for Drug Evaluation and Research (HFD-143)
Central Document Room
5901-B Ammendale Road
Beltsville, MD 207052-1266

Department of Health and Human Services
Food and Drug Administration
Center for Biologics Evaluation and Research (HFM-99)
1401 Rockville Pike
Rockville, MD 20852-1448
Please DO NOT RETURN this application to this address.

"An agency may not conduct or sponsor, and a person is not required to respond to, a collection of information unless it displays a currently valid OMB control number."

FORM FDA 1571 (4/06)   PAGE 2 OF 2

Figure 1 *(Continued)*

1. The sponsor is committing not to initiate the clinical study until 30 days after the FDA receives the IND, unless otherwise notified by the FDA, and not to begin or continue clinical studies covered by the IND if they are placed on clinical hold.

2. The sponsor is committing to ensure that an IRB will be responsible for initial and continuing review and approval of each study in the proposed clinical investigation.
3. The sponsor is committing to conduct the investigation in accordance with all other applicable regulatory requirements.

These are significant commitments and the sponsor should be aware that signing the 1571 Form is more than a formality. Making a willfully false statement on the 1571 Form or accompanying documentation is a criminal offense. Detailed information on completing the 1571 form can be found on the FDA Web site,[6] in section 312.23(a)(1) and from the FDA review division responsible for reviewing the IND.

IND Term

IND amendment—*A submission to the IND file that adds new or revised information. Every submission adds to, revises, or affects the body of information within the IND and is, therefore, considered an IND amendment. Protocol amendments and information amendments are two examples of information that is filed to an IND in the course of clinical development. A protocol amendment is submitted when a sponsor intends to conduct a new study, wishes to modify the design or conduct of a previously submitted study protocol, or adds a new investigator to a protocol. An information amendment is used to submit new CMC, toxicology, pharmacology, clinical, or other information that does not fall within the scope of a protocol amendment, annual report, or IND safety report.*

IND Term

IND safety report—*An expedited report sent to the FDA and all participating investigators of a serious and unexpected adverse experience associated with use of the drug or findings from nonclinical studies that suggest a risk to human subjects.*

---

[6] FDA Center for Drug Evaluation and Research Information for Sponsor-Investigators Submitting Investigational New Drug Applications. Available at: http://www.fda.gov/cder/forms/1571-1572-help. html.

IND Term

IND annual report—A brief report to the FDA on the progress of the clinical investigations. It is submitted each year within 60 days of the anniversary date that the IND went into effect.

Table of Contents—Section 312.23(a)(2)

This should be a comprehensive listing of the contents of the IND broken down by section, volume, and page number. The table of contents should include all required sections, appendices, attachments, reports, and other reference material. The table of contents must be accurate and building the table should not be a last minute task. An accurate, well laid out table of contents will allow the FDA reviewers to quickly find the information they need and ultimately speed up review of the IND application. Many sponsors begin planning the IND submission by laying out the table of contents first. This allows the team to clearly see what information is required for the submission and how the document will be structured, and it allows the table of contents to be updated as the application is being built.

Introductory Statement and General Investigational Plan— Section 312.23(a)(3)

This section should provide a brief, three- to four-page overview of the investigational drug and the sponsor's investigational plan for the coming year. The goal of this section is simply to provide a brief description of the drug and lay out the development plan for the drug. For a phase 1 first-in-person (FIP) submission, two to three pages may be sufficient if the sponsor is attempting to determine early pharmacokinetic and pharmacodynamic properties of the drug. The sponsor should not attempt to develop and present a detailed development plan that will, in all likelihood, change considerably should the product proceed to further development.[7]

    The introductory statement should begin with a description of the drug and the indication(s) to be studied and include the pharmacologic class of the compound, the name of the drug and all active ingredients, the structural formula of the drug, the dosage form, and the route of administration. This section must

---

[7] FDA Guidance for Industry: Content and Format of Investigation New Drug Applications (INDs) for Phase I Studies of Drugs, Including Well-Characterized, Therapeutic, Biotechnology drugs. FDA, Rockville, MD, November 1995.

also describe the sponsor's plan for investigating the drug during the following year and should include a rationale for the drug and the research study proposed, the general approach to be followed in studying the drug, the indication(s) to be studied, the type of clinical studies to be conducted, the estimated number of patients receiving the drug, and the risks anticipated on the basis of nonclinical studies or prior studies in humans.

If the drug has been previously administered to humans, the introductory statement should include a brief summary of human clinical experience to date, focusing mainly on safety of the drug in previous studies and how that supports studies proposed in the IND. If the drug was withdrawn from investigation or marketing in any country for safety reasons, the name of the country and the reasons for withdrawal should also be briefly discussed in the introductory statement.

Investigator's Brochure—Section 312.23(a)(5)

The content and format of the investigator's brochure (IB) is described in 21 CFR section 312.23(a)(5) and in greater detail in the International Conference on Harmonization (ICH) E6 Good Clinical Practice Guidance document.[8] An exhaustive discussion of the IB is not presented here, preferring to focus more broadly on the purpose of the document and the general content required by the regulations.

The investigator's brochure is a key document provided to each clinical investigator and the institutional review board at each of the clinical sites. The IB presents, in summary form, the key nonclinical (safety), clinical, and CMC (quality) data that support the proposed clinical trial. The IB provides the clinical investigators with the information necessary to understand the rationale for the proposed trial and to make an unbiased risk-benefit assessment of the appropriateness of the proposed trial.[8]

IND Term

CMC (chemistry, manufacturing and controls)—describes the chemical structure and chemical properties of the compound, the composition, manufacturing process and control of the raw materials, drug substance, and drug product that ensure the identity, quality, purity and potency of the drug product. The ICH guidance refers to this as the Quality section of the file.

---

[8] Guidance for Industry: ICH E6 Good Clinical Practice: Consolidated Guidance. May 1997.

The type and extent of information provided in the IB will be dependent on the stage of development of the drug product, but the IB must contain the following information.

1. A brief summary of CMC information, including the physical, chemical, and pharmaceutical properties of the drug and the chemical name and chemical structure, if known. It should also include a description of the formulation and how the drug is supplied and the storage and handling requirements.
2. A summary of all relevant nonclinical pharmacology, toxicology, pharmacokinetic, and drug metabolism information generated to support human clinical studies. It should include a tabular summary of each nonclinical study conducted, outlining the methodology used and the results of each study.
3. If human clinical studies have been conducted with the drug, a summary of information relating to safety and efficacy should be presented, including any information from those studies on the metabolism, pharmacokinetics, pharmacodynamics, dose response, or other pharmacologic activities.
4. A summary of data and guidance for the investigator in the management of subjects participating in the trial. An overall discussion of the nonclinical and clinical data presented in the IB and a discussion of the possible risks and adverse reactions associated with the investigational drug product and the specific tests, observations and precautions that may be needed for the clinical trial.

It is important to remember that the IB is a living document and must be updated by the sponsor as new information becomes available from ongoing clinical and nonclinical studies. Keep in mind though, that the document must be a readable and useful document, so it is recommended that the IB should ideally not exceed 75 to 80 pages. At a minimum, the IB should be reviewed and updated annually. However, important safety information should be communicated to the investigator, the IRB and the FDA, if required, before it is included in the IB.

Clinical Protocol—Section 312.23(a)(6)

As with the IB, the content and format of the protocol is described in 21 CFR section 312.23 and in greater detail in the ICH E6 *Good Clinical Practice Guidance Document*[8] and will not be presented here.

A clinical protocol describes how a particular clinical trial is to be conducted. It describes the objectives of the study, the trial design, the selection of subjects, and the manner in which the trial is to be carried out. The initial IND is required to have a clinical protocol for the initial planned study. However, the IND regulations specifically allow phase 1 protocols to be less detailed and more flexible than protocols for phase 2 or 3 studies.[7] The regulations state that phase 1 protocols should be directed primarily at providing an outline of the investigation: an estimate of the number of subjects to be included; a description of safety exclusions; and a description of the dosing plan, including duration, dose, or method to be used in determining dose. Phase 1 protocols should specify in detail only those elements for the study that are critical to subject safety, such as necessary monitoring of vital signs and blood chemistries, and toxicity-based stopping, or dose adjustment rules.[7]

Although the regulations allow Phase 1 protocols to be less detailed, the sponsor cannot submit a protocol summary in lieu of a complete protocol as part of the initial IND. A protocol summary may be acceptable in some instances, but submission of a summary should be discussed and agreed to by the reviewing division at the FDA during the pre-IND meeting. Later-phase protocols should be more detailed than a Phase 1 protocol and reflect that stage of development of the drug. It should contain efficacy parameters, the methods, and timing for assessing and analyzing the efficacy parameters and detailed statistical sections, describing the statistical methods to be employed and the timing of any planned interim analysis.

The regulations require any protocol submitted as part of an IND to contain the following elements.

1. A statement of the objectives and the purpose of the study.
2. The name, address, and qualifications (curriculum vitae) of each investi-gator and each sub-investigator participating in the study; the name and address of each clinical site; and the name and address of each institutional review board responsible for reviewing the proposed study. The required information regarding all investigators is collected on the FDA Form 1572—statement of investigator (Fig. 2). The 1572 Form collects basic information about the investigator, such as the name and address of the investigator, a description of the education and training of the investigator (a copy of the investigator's CV is usually attached), the name and address of the IRB at the site and the names of any sub-investigators at the site. The 1572 Form includes a series of commitments (see box 9 in Fig. 2) that the investigator agrees to by signing the form. These commitments include, among others, agreeing to conduct the study according to the protocol, agreeing to personally conduct or supervise the investigation, agreeing to report adverse events (AEs) to the sponsor, agreeing to maintain accurate records, and agreeing to comply with all other obligations and require-ments outlined in the regulations. Investigators and sponsors should be aware that making willfully false statements on the 1572 Form is a criminal offense.
3. The criteria for study subject inclusion and exclusion and an estimate of the number of subjects to be enrolled in the study.

DEPARTMENT OF HEALTH AND HUMAN SERVICES FOOD AND DRUG ADMINISTRATION	Form Approved: OMB No. 0910-0014. Expiration Date: May 31, 2009. *See OMB Statement on Reverse.*
STATEMENT OF INVESTIGATOR *(TITLE 21, CODE OF FEDERAL REGULATIONS (CFR) PART 312)* (See instructions on reverse side.)	**NOTE:** No investigator may participate in an investigation until he/she provides the sponsor with a completed, signed Statement of Investigator, Form FDA 1572 (21 CFR 312.53(c)).

1. NAME AND ADDRESS OF INVESTIGATOR

2. EDUCATION, TRAINING, AND EXPERIENCE THAT QUALIFIES THE INVESTIGATOR AS AN EXPERT IN THE CLINICAL INVESTIGATION OF THE DRUG FOR THE USE UNDER INVESTIGATION. ONE OF THE FOLLOWING IS ATTACHED.

☐ CURRICULUM VITAE   ☐ OTHER STATEMENT OF QUALIFICATIONS

3. NAME AND ADDRESS OF ANY MEDICAL SCHOOL, HOSPITAL OR OTHER RESEARCH FACILITY WHERE THE CLINICAL INVESTIGATION(S) WILL BE CONDUCTED.

4. NAME AND ADDRESS OF ANY CLINICAL LABORATORY FACILITIES TO BE USED IN THE STUDY.

5. NAME AND ADDRESS OF THE INSTITUTIONAL REVIEW BOARD (IRB) THAT IS RESPONSIBLE FOR REVIEW AND APPROVAL OF THE STUDY(IES).

6. NAMES OF THE SUBINVESTIGATORS *(e.g., research fellows, residents, associates)* WHO WILL BE ASSISTING THE INVESTIGATOR IN THE CONDUCT OF THE INVESTIGATION(S).

7. NAME AND CODE NUMBER, IF ANY, OF THE PROTOCOL(S) IN THE IND FOR THE STUDY(IES) TO BE CONDUCTED BY THE INVESTIGATOR.

FORM FDA 1572 (5/06)   PREVIOUS EDITION IS OBSOLETE.   **PAGE 1 OF 2**

PSC Graphics (301) 443-1090   EF

Figure 2   *(Continued on next page)* Form 1572—statement of investigator.

4. A description of the study design, control groups to be used, and methods employed to minimize bias on the part of the subjects, investigators, and analysts.
5. The planned maximum dose, the duration of patient exposure to the drug, and the methods used to determine the doses to be administered.

8. ATTACH THE FOLLOWING CLINICAL PROTOCOL INFORMATION:
☐ FOR PHASE 1 INVESTIGATIONS, A GENERAL OUTLINE OF THE PLANNED INVESTIGATION INCLUDING THE ESTIMATED DURATION OF THE STUDY AND THE MAXIMUM NUMBER OF SUBJECTS THAT WILL BE INVOLVED.
☐ FOR PHASE 2 OR 3 INVESTIGATIONS, AN OUTLINE OF THE STUDY PROTOCOL INCLUDING AN APPROXIMATION OF THE NUMBER OF SUBJECTS TO BE TREATED WITH THE DRUG AND THE NUMBER TO BE EMPLOYED AS CONTROLS, IF ANY; THE CLINICAL USES TO BE INVESTIGATED; CHARACTERISTICS OF SUBJECTS BY AGE, SEX, AND CONDITION; THE KIND OF CLINICAL OBSERVATIONS AND LABORATORY TESTS TO BE CONDUCTED; THE ESTIMATED DURATION OF THE STUDY; AND COPIES OR A DESCRIPTION OF CASE REPORT FORMS TO BE USED.

9. COMMITMENTS:

I agree to conduct the study(ies) in accordance with the relevant, current protocol(s) and will only make changes in a protocol after notifying the sponsor, except when necessary to protect the safety, rights, or welfare of subjects.

I agree to personally conduct or supervise the described investigation(s).

I agree to inform any patients, or any persons used as controls, that the drugs are being used for investigational purposes and I will ensure that the requirements relating to obtaining informed consent in 21 CFR Part 50 and institutional review board (IRB) review and approval in 21 CFR Part 56 are met.

I agree to report to the sponsor adverse experiences that occur in the course of the investigation(s) in accordance with 21 CFR 312.64.

I have read and understand the information in the investigator's brochure, including the potential risks and side effects of the drug.

I agree to ensure that all associates, colleagues, and employees assisting in the conduct of the study(ies) are informed about their obligations in meeting the above commitments.

I agree to maintain adequate and accurate records in accordance with 21 CFR 312.62 and to make those records available for inspection in accordance with 21 CFR 312.68.

I will ensure that an IRB that complies with the requirements of 21 CFR Part 56 will be responsible for the initial and continuing review and approval of the clinical investigation. I also agree to promptly report to the IRB all changes in the research activity and all unanticipated problems involving risks to human subjects or others. Additionally, I will not make any changes in the research without IRB approval, except where necessary to eliminate apparent immediate hazards to human subjects.

I agree to comply with all other requirements regarding the obligations of clinical investigators and all other pertinent requirements in 21 CFR Part 312.

INSTRUCTIONS FOR COMPLETING FORM FDA 1572
STATEMENT OF INVESTIGATOR:

1. Complete all sections. Attach a separate page if additional space is needed.
2. Attach curriculum vitae or other statement of qualifications as described in Section 2.
3. Attach protocol outline as described in Section 8.
4. Sign and date below.
5. FORWARD THE COMPLETED FORM AND ATTACHMENTS TO THE SPONSOR. The sponsor will incorporate this information along with other technical data into an Investigational New Drug Application (IND).

10. SIGNATURE OF INVESTIGATOR	11. DATE

(WARNING: A willfully false statement is a criminal offense. U.S.C. Title 18, Sec. 1001.)

Public reporting burden for this collection of information is estimated to average 100 hours per response, including the time for reviewing instructions, searching existing data sources, gathering and maintaining the data needed, and completing reviewing the collection of information. Send comments regarding this burden estimate or any other aspect of this collection of information, including suggestions for reducing this burden to:

Department of Health and Human Services
Food and Drug Administration
Center for Drug Evaluation and Research (HFD-143)
Central Document Room
5901-B Ammendale Road
Beltsville, MD 20705-1266

Department of Health and Human Services
Food and Drug Administration
Center for Biologics Evaluation and Research (HFM-99)
1401 Rockville Pike
Rockville, MD 20852-1448

"An agency may not conduct or sponsor, and a person is not required to respond to, a collection of information unless it displays a currently valid OMB control number."

Please DO NOT RETURN this application to this address.

FORM FDA 1572 (5/06)   PAGE 2 OF 2

Figure 2 *(Continued)*

6. A description of the measurements and observations to be made to achieve the study objectives.
7. A description of the clinical procedures and laboratory tests planned to monitor the effects of the drug in the subjects.

Chemistry Manufacturing and Controls Information—Section 312.23(a)(7)

This key section of an IND describes the quality information, comprising the composition, manufacturing process and control of the drug substance and drug product. The CMC section must provide sufficient detail and information to demonstrate the identity, quality, purity, and potency of the drug product. The amount of information needed to accomplish this is based on the phase of the proposed study, the duration of the study, the dosage form of the investigational drug, and the amount of additional information available.[7] For a phase 1 IND the CMC information provided for the raw materials, drug substance, and drug product should be sufficiently detailed to allow the FDA to evaluate the safety of the subjects participating in the trial. A safety concern or lack of data, which make it impossible for the FDA to conduct a safety evaluation, are the only reasons for a clinical hold based on the CMC section. Safety concerns may include the following:

1. Product is made with unknown or impure components.
2. Product has a chemical structure(s) of known or highly likely toxicity.
3. Product does not remain chemically stable throughout the testing program.
4. Product has an impurity profile indicative of a potential health hazard or an impurity profile insufficiently defined to assess potential health hazard.
5. Master or working cell bank is poorly characterized.[7]

A key aspect to assuring the safety of the subjects participating in clinical trials is adherence to current good manufacturing practices (cGMP). The FDA requires that any drug product intended for administration to humans be manufactured in conformance with cGMP. Adherence to GMP provides a minimum level of control over the manufacturing process and final drug product and helps ensure the identity, quality, purity, and potency of the clinical trial material. The GMP controls used to manufacture drug products for clinical trials should be consistent with the stage of development, and they should be manufactured in suitable facilities, using appropriate production and control procedures to ensure the quality of the drug product.[9]

INDs for later-phase studies must contain the CMC information outlined in section 312.23, but the focus should be on safety issues relating to the proposed phase and expanded scope of the investigation. The FDA expects that the CMC section for a later-phase IND will be more detailed than a phase 1 study and demonstrate a higher level of characterization of the drug substance and drug product and greater control over the raw materials and manufacturing process. For phase 2 studies, the sponsor should be able to document that the manufacturing

---

[9] FDA Guidance for Industry: ICH Q7A Good Manufacturing Practice Guidance for Active Pharmaceutical Ingredients. FDA, Rockville, MD, August 2001.

process is controlled at predetermined points and yields products that meet the tentative acceptance criteria.[10]

The regulations require the CMC section of an IND to contain the following sections:

1. CMC introduction

    This section should provide a brief overview of the investigational drug product. In this section, the sponsor should state whether there are any signals of potential risk to human subjects because of the chemistry of the drug substance or drug product or the manufacturing process for the drug substance or drug product. If potential risks are identified, the risks should be discussed and steps to monitor for the risks should be described or the reasons the potential risks are acceptable should be presented. In the introduction, the sponsor should also describe any differences between the drug product to be used in the proposed study and the drug product used in the nonclinical toxicology studies that support the clinical investigations. How these differences affect the safety profile should be discussed, and if there are no differences, those should be stated.

2. Information on the drug substance in the form of a summary report containing the following information.

    *   A brief description of the drug substance and evidence to support its chemical structure. INDs for later-phase trials should include a more complete description of the physical, chemical, and biological characteristics of the drug substance and provide additional supporting evidence characterizing the chemical structure.
    *   The name and address of the manufacturer.
    *   A brief description of the manufacturing process. The description should include a detailed flow diagram of the process and a list of all the reagents, solvents, and catalysts used in the process. INDs for later-phase trials will include a more detailed description of the manufacturing process and the controls. A process flow diagram that includes chemical structures and configurations and significant side products should be included, and the acceptance criteria for the product described.
    *   A brief description of the acceptable limits (specifications) and analytical methods used to assure the identity, strength, quality, potency, and purity of the drug substance. This section should include a description of the test methods used and outline the proposed acceptance criteria. The proposed acceptance criteria should be based on analytical data (e.g., IR spectrum to prove identity, and HPLC

---

[10] FDA Guidance for Industry: INDs for Phase 2 and Phase 3 Studies. Chemistry, Manufacturing, and Controls Information. FDA, Rockville, MD, May 2003.

chromatograms to support purity level, and impurities profile).[7] Validation data and established specifications are not required for phase 1 studies; however, a certificate of analysis for the lot(s) of clinical trial material should be included with the initial IND. Initial INDs for later-phase studies should provide the same type of information as for earlier-phase studies, but analytical procedures and acceptance criteria should be better defined and validation data should be available if requested by the FDA.

- Data to support the stability of the drug substance. For a phase 1 IND, a brief description of the stability studies conducted and the methods used to monitor stability should be provided, including a table outlining stability data from representative lots of material. For later-phase studies, a stability protocol should be submitted, including a list of all tests, analytical procedures, sampling time points for each test and the duration of the stability studies. Preliminary stability data should be submitted along with stability data from clinical material used in earlier-phase studies.

3. Information on the drug product in the form of a summary report containing the following information.

- A list of all components used in the manufacture of the drug product, including components intended to be in the drug product and those that may not appear, but are used in the manufacturing process. The components should be identified by their established name (chemical name) and their compendial status [National Formulary (NF), United States Pharmacopoeia (USP)] should be listed, if it exists. Analytical procedures and acceptance criteria should be presented for noncompendial components. If applicable, the quantitative composition of the drug product should be summarized and any expected variations should be discussed. The same type of information should be presented in an IND for a later-phase study.
- The name and address of the manufacturer of the drug product.
- A brief, step-by-step description of the manufacturing and packaging procedures including a process flow diagram. For sterile products, a description of the sterilization process should be included. The same type of information should be included in an IND for a later-phase study.
- A description of the proposed acceptable limits (specifications) for the drug product and the test methods used. Validation data and established specifications are not required in the phase 1 IND; however, a complete description of the analytical procedures and validation data should be available on request for later-phase studies. For sterile products, sterility and endotoxin tests should be submitted in the initial

IND. A certificate of analysis for the drug product lot(s) to be used in the proposed investigation should also be provided.

- A description of the proposed container closure system and a brief description of the stability study and test methods. Stability data on representative material should be presented in a tabular format. A copy of the stability protocol is not required for a phase 1 study. An initial IND for a later-phase study should include a copy of the stability protocol that includes a list of tests, analytical procedures, sampling time points, and the expected duration of the stability program. When applicable, stability data on the reconstituted drug product should be included in the initial IND.

4. Information on any placebo or comparator product that will be utilized in the proposed clinical study. This should include a brief written description of the composition, manufacture and control of the placebo. Process flow diagrams and tabular summaries can be used in the description.

5. Copies of all proposed product labels and any other proposed labeling that will be provided to the investigators. Mock-ups of the proposed labeling are acceptable or actual printed labeling can be submitted. The investigational drug must be labeled with the caution statement: "Caution: New Drug—Limited by Federal (or United States) law to investigational use."[11]

6. A claim for categorical exclusion from an environmental assessment. The National Environmental Policy Act of 1969 (NEPA) requires all Federal agencies to assess the environmental impacts of their actions and to ensure that the interested and affected public is informed of environmental analyses.[12] The FDA is required to consider the environmental impacts of approving drug and biologic applications and requires all such applications to include an environmental assessment or a claim for categorical exclusion. IND applications are generally categorically excluded from the requirement to prepare and submit an environmental assessment.[13] In this section of the IND, the sponsor should state that the action requested (approval of an IND application) qualifies for categorical exclusion in accordance with 21 CFR section 25.31(e) and that, to the sponsor's knowledge, no extraordinary circumstances exist (21 CFR section 25.15(d)).

Pharmacology and Toxicology Information—Section 312.23(a)(8)

The decision to proceed to the initial administration of the investigational drug to humans must include the careful conduct and review of the data from nonclinical in vivo and in vitro studies. These data must provide a good level of confidence

---

[11] Code of Federal Regulations Title 21 Section 312.6(a).

[12] FDA Guidance for Industry: Environmental Assessment of Human Drug and Biologics Applications. FDA, Rockville, MD, July 1998.

[13] Code of Federal Regulations Title 21 Section 25.31(e).

that the new drug product is reasonably safe for administration to human subjects at the planned dosage levels. The goals of the nonclinical safety testing include characterization of toxic effects with respect to target organs, dose dependence, relationship to exposure, and potential reversibility. Nonclinical safety information is important for the estimation of an initial safe starting dose for human trials and the identification of parameters for clinical monitoring for potential AEs.[14]

The pharmacology and toxicology section of the IND includes the nonclinical safety data that the sponsor generated to conclude that the new drug is reasonably safe for clinical study. The amount and type of nonclinical data needed to support a new drug product depends on the class of the new drug, the duration of the proposed clinical trials, and the patient population that will be exposed to the drug. Generally, the following nonclinical safety studies are required before initiating phase 1 studies and the results of these studies must be included in the IND:

- Safety pharmacology studies (often conducted as part of the toxicity studies).
- Single dose and repeat dose toxicity studies (duration of the repeat dose studies should equal or exceed the duration human clinical trials).
- Genotoxicity studies (in vitro studies evaluating mutations and chromosomal damage).
- Reproduction toxicity studies (Nonclinical animal studies conducted to reveal any effects the investigational drug may have on mammalian reproduction). These studies are needed before including women of childbearing potential in any clinical study and are usually not needed for an initial phase 1 study in normal male volunteers.
- Other supplementary studies may be needed if safety concerns are identified. The FDA and ICH are proposing that nonclinical studies evaluating the potential of the new drug to delay ventricular repolarization (QT interval prolongation) be conducted prior to initiation of phase 1 studies.[15,16]

The CDER guidance documents Web page[17] provides access to all of the key guidance documents discussing required nonclinical testing for new drugs. The pharmacology and toxicology information or safety section of the initial IND should contain the following sections.

1. A summary report describing the pharmacologic effects and mechanism of action of the drug and information on the absorption, distribution,

---

[14] FDA Guidance for Industry: ICH M3 Nonclinical Safety Studies for the Conduct of Human Clinical Trials for Pharmaceuticals. FDA, Rockville, MD, July 1997.

[15] FDA Guidance for Industry: ICH E14 Clinical Evaluation of QT/QTc Interval Prolongation and Proarrhythmic Potential for Non-Antiarrhythmic Drugs. FDA, Rockville, MD, October 2005.

[16] FDA Guidance for Industry: ICH S7B Safety Pharmacology Studies for Assessing the Potential for Delayed Ventricular Repolarization by Human Pharmaceuticals. FDA, Rockville, MD, October 2005.

[17] FDA Center for Drug Evaluation and Research Guidance Documents. Available at: http://www.fda.gov/cder/guidance/index.htm

metabolism, and excretion (ADME) of the drug. If this information is not known at the time the initial IND is submitted, it should be stated. Lack of this information should not generally be a reason for a phase 1 IND to be placed on clinical hold.[7] However, most sponsors will have at least early pharmacologic data, including exposure, half-life of the drug, and an understanding of the major factors that influence the pharmacokinetics of the drug, e.g., the enzymes responsible for metabolism of the drug. Initial INDs for later-phase studies should be able to provide this pharmacology information and it may be derived from earlier-phase clinical investigations.

2. An integrated summary of the toxicologic effects of the drug in animals and in vitro. The summary presents the toxicologic findings from completed animal studies that support the safety of the proposed human investigation. The integrated summary is usually 10 to 20 pages long, includes text and tables, and should contain the following information:

- A brief description of the design of the trials and any deviations from the design in the conduct of the studies, including the dates the studies were conducted.
- A "systematic" presentation of the findings from the animal toxicology and toxicokinetic studies. This data should be presented by organ system (cardiovascular, renal, hepatic, etc.) and if a particular body system was not assessed, it should be noted.
- The names and qualifications of the individuals who evaluated the animal safety data and concluded it to be reasonably safe to begin the proposed human studies.
- A statement of where the studies were conducted and where the study records are stored and available for inspection.
- A declaration that each nonclinical safety study reported in the IND was performed in full compliance with good laboratory practices (GLP) or if a study was not conducted in compliance with GLP, a brief statement of why it was not, and a discussion on how this might affect the interpretations of the findings.

The integrated summary can be developed on the basis of unaudited draft toxicology reports of the completed animal studies. Final, fully quality assured individual study reports are recommended, but not required for submission of an initial IND. If the integrated summary is based on unaudited draft reports, the toxicology reports should be finalized, and an update to the summary submitted to the FDA within 120 days after submission of the original integrated summary.[18] The updated summary, as well as the final study reports, should identify any differences found in the preparation of the final, fully quality assured study reports and the

[18] FDA Guidance for Industry Q&A: Content and Format of INDs for Phase 1 Studies of Drugs, Including Well-Characterized, Therapeutic, Biotechnology-Derived Products. FDA, Rockville, MD, October 2000.

information submitted in the initial integrated summary. If there were no differences found, that should be stated in the update. The final reports must be available to the FDA upon request or by the 120-day timeframe. In any case, the final reports are submitted with the NDA.

3. Full data tabulations for each animal toxicology study supporting the safety of the proposed trial. This should be a full tabulation of the data suitable for detailed review and consists of line listings of individual data points, including laboratory data for each animal in the trials and summary tabulations of the data points. This section will also include either a brief technical report or abstract for each study or a copy of the study protocol and amendments. These are provided to help the FDA reviewer interpret the data included in the line listings. Many sponsors will include copies of the final toxicology study reports in this section in lieu of the technical report or protocol. However, this is not required, and submission of the initial IND does not need to be delayed until final fully quality-assured study reports are available.

Good Laboratory Practice (GLP)

A quality system, that applies to the conduct of nonclinical safety studies used to support an IND, NDA, BLA, or other regulatory submission. GLP regulations set standards for the organization of the laboratory, facilities, personnel, and operating procedures. Clinical studies with human subjects, basic exploratory studies to determine potential utility of a compound, or tests to determine the chemical or physical characteristics of a compound are not subject to GLP regulations.

Previous Human Experience—Section 312.23 (a)(9)

This section should contain an integrated summary report of all previous human studies and experiences with the drug. When the planned study will be the first administration to humans, this section should be indicated as not applicable. However, if initial clinical investigations have been conducted in other countries before the U.S. IND is filed, this section could be extensive. The summary should focus on presenting data from previous trials that are relevant to the safety of the proposed investigation (e.g., PK and PD data, the observed AE profile in previous studies or other experiences, and ADME data) and any information from previous trials on the drug's effectiveness for the proposed investigational use. Any published material relevant to the safety of the proposed investigation or assessment of the drug's effectiveness in the proposed indication should be provided in the IND. Other published material may be listed in a bibliography.

If the drug is marketed outside of the United States, or was previously, a list of those countries should be provided as well as a list of any countries where the drug was withdrawn from marketing because of safety or efficacy issues.

Additional Information—Section 312.23(a)(10)

This section is used to present information on special topics. The following topics should be discussed, if relevant, in this section.

1. Drug dependence and abuse potential. If the drug is a psychotropic or otherwise shows potential for abuse, data from clinical studies or animal studies that may be relevant to assessment of the investigational drug.
2. Radioactive drugs. Data from animal or human studies that allow calculation of radiation-absorbed dose to the whole body and critical organs upon administration to human subjects.
3. Pediatric studies. Any plans the sponsor has for assessing the safety and efficacy of the drug in the pediatric population.
4. Other information. Any other relevant information that might aid in the evaluation of the proposed clinical investigations.

Relevant Information—Section 312.23(a)(11)

Any information specifically requested by the FDA that is needed to review the IND application. It is common to place the meeting minutes from any pre-IND meeting or discussion in this section. This is especially useful if the information is referenced elsewhere in the IND.

Other Important Information about the Submission of an IND

- For clinical studies that will be submitted as part of an NDA or BLA, an IND sponsor must collect *financial disclosure* information from each investigator or subinvestigator who is directly involved in the treatment or evaluation of clinical trial subjects. Each investigator or subinvestigator must supply sufficient and accurate financial information that will allow the sponsor to eventually submit certification or disclosure statements in an NDA or BLA. Each investigator or subinvestigator must commit to update this information if any changes occur during the course of the investigation and for one year following completion of the study. Most Phase 1 studies, large open safety studies conducted at multiple sites, treatment protocols and parallel track protocols are exempted from financial disclosure requirements.[19,20,21]

---

[19] Code of Federal Regulations Title 21 Section 312.53 (c)(4).

[20] Code of Federal Regulations Title 21 Part 54—Financial Disclosure by Clinical Investigators.

[21] FDA Guidance for Industry: Financial Disclosure by Clinical Investigators. FDA, Rockville, MD, March 2001.

IND Term

Financial Disclosure—When submitting a marketing application for a drug, device, or biologic product, the applicant is required to include a list of all clinical investigators who conducted clinical studies and certify and/or disclose certain financial arrangements that include certification that no financial arrangements with an investigator have been made where study outcome could affect compensation; that the investigator has no proprietary interest in the product; that the investigator does not have significant equity interest in the sponsor; and that the investigator has not received significant payments of other sorts; and/or disclose specified financial arrangements and any steps taken to minimize the potential for bias. By collecting the financial disclosure information at the start of a study, the sponsor will be aware of potential conflicts and will be able to consult with the FDA early on and take steps to minimize the potential for bias. The thresholds for disclosure are defined in the regulation in 21 CFR part 54.

- Although not a required component of an IND, some FDA review divisions may ask the sponsor to submit a copy of the informed consent form for the study. This is often requested by CBER for INDs for biologic products, especially for new technology such as gene or cellular therapy studies.
- Within the IND application a sponsor may include references to other information pertinent to the IND that may have been previously submitted to the FDA, for instance in another IND or in a marketing application. Another IND might be referenced if the sponsor is submitting a treatment use protocol that references the technical sections of an open IND for the same drug, or a sponsor might be conducting a clinical study of an approved drug but for a new indication. In this instance, the sponsor may reference the nonclinical and CMC sections of the NDA instead of submitting the same information in a new IND.
- The sponsor may also reference a drug master file (DMF) in the IND application that contains important information necessary to complete review of the IND. A DMF might contain proprietary information about a unique excipient, component, technology, or specialized drug delivery device that the owner of the information does not want to share with the sponsor of the IND. In this case, the company will submit a DMF to the FDA and allow the sponsor to reference it in the IND. Reference to any DMF or other information submitted by an entity other than the sponsor must include a letter authorizing the sponsor to make

the reference and giving the FDA permission to review the DMF in support of the IND.

> ### *Drug Master File*
>
> *A Drug Master File (DMF) is a submission to the FDA that is used to provide confidential detailed information about processes, or articles used in the manufacturing, processing, packaging, and storing of one or more human drugs. The information contained in the DMF may be used to support an IND, an NDA, an ANDA, another DMF, an export. Application, or amendments and supplements to any of these.*

- Reports or journal articles in a foreign language must be accompanied by a complete and accurate English translation.
- Each IND submission must include a four-digit serial number. The initial IND must be numbered 0000 and each subsequent submission (correspondence, amendment, safety report) must be numbered consecutively. This serial number is included on the 1571 Form, any cover letter included with the submission and on any labels affixed to the binders containing submission.
- The FDA requires sponsors to submit the original and two copies of all IND submissions, including the initial IND application and any amendments, correspondence or reports if submitted by paper. For electronic submissions, only a single electronic version is required. The FDA can request that a sponsor submit additional copies of a particular submission at any time.
- The initial IND and all subsequent submissions more than one page in length should be fully paginated, including all appendices and attachments.
- All paper IND submissions should be printed on good quality 8.5 × 11 inch paper with a 1.25 inch left margin to allow for binding. Individual volumes should be no more than approximately 2 inches thick and bound in pressboard type binders. Three ring binders are not used. The FDA requires the following types of binders for specific sections of IND submissions:
  - One copy of the submission will serve as an archive copy and should be bound in a red polyethylene binder.
  - The CMC section should be bound in a green pressboard binder.
  - Microbiology information should be bound in an orange pressboard binder.
  - The pharmacology/toxicology information should be bound in an orange pressboard binder.

Each volume should be labeled with permanent adhesive labels printed in permanent black ink. The labels should contain the volume number of the submission (vol. X of XX vols.), name of drug, the IND number, and the sponsor's name.[22] Specifications for the binders for a variety of FDA submissions, including INDs, can be found on the FDA Web page (http://www.fda.gov/cder/ddms/binders.htm).

- For complete traceability and adequate documentation, the initial IND application, and subsequent submissions to the IND should be sent to the FDA, using a delivery service that documents delivery (i.e., FedEx, UPS, or DHL). Many of these services also offer e-mail notification to the sender upon delivery and other customer service tools that make routine shipments easier. Sponsors should keep records of receipt for all IND submissions as documented proof of submission should questions arise.

FDA Review of the IND

When the initial IND submission is made to the FDA, it is logged in the Document Management Room and assigned an IND number. A sponsor can call in advance of the submission and receive the number and this number can then be used within the submission document. Many companies commonly call ahead to receive this information. Once the IND is stamped as received, it is sent to the appropriate review division within CDER or CBER. If there is any question about which division the IND will reside, the ombudsman office is contacted. Once the IND arrives at the review division, it is critically evaluated by several reviewers of chemistry, biopharmaceutics, medical, statistics, microbiology, and pharmacology/toxicology sections, as appropriate. All these areas review the data submitted with the primary purpose of ensuring appropriate safety of the individuals who will be enrolled in the study.

Once an IND is submitted, the study cannot be initiated until a period of 30 calendar days has passed, or if the FDA has given agreement to start the study before the 30-day period expires. The usual practice is to contact the FDA shortly before the 30-day period has expired to see if there are any issues rather than going ahead at day 30 if nothing is heard from the FDA. If there are any major issues relating to the safety of the volunteers or patients in the proposed study, the FDA can institute a clinical hold [*Manual of Policies and Procedures* (MaPP) 6030.1]. A clinical hold is an order issued by the FDA to the sponsor of an IND to delay or to suspend a clinical investigation. A clinical hold may be either a "complete clinical hold"—a delay or suspension of *all* clinical work requested under an IND or a "partial clinical hold"—a delay or suspension of only part of the clinical work (e.g., a specific protocol or part of a protocol. If a clinical hold is imposed, the specific reasons for the clinical hold will be

---

[22] FDA Center for Drug Evaluation and Research IND, NDA, ANDA or Drug Master File Binders. Available at: (http://www.fda.gov/cder/ddms/binders.htm.

specified in the clinical hold letter to the sponsor of the IND. If the FDA concludes that there may be grounds for imposing a clinical hold, the agency will attempt to discuss and satisfactorily resolve the matter before issuing a clinical hold letter. A sponsor must respond to all clinical hold issues before the FDA will review the responses. When the FDA receives all responses from the sponsor, it has another 30 calendar days to review and respond in writing. Under no circumstances can the study be initiated unless the FDA lifts the clinical hold. Review divisions differ in the frequency of clinical holds that are imposed.

MAINTAINING AN IND—IND AMENDMENTS AND OTHER REQUIRED REPORTS

Clinical development of a new drug will take a number of years and can take as many as 10 or 12 years, all the time requiring an active IND to conduct the necessary clinical studies. Because of the long development times, the IND is continuously updated with new information and new protocols as the drug moves from one phase of investigation to the next. The IND regulations discuss two types of amendments, protocol amendments and information amendments and two types of required reports, safety reports and annual reports. Most other routine communication with the FDA regarding an IND is referred to as general correspondence. It is important to remember, however, that the FDA considers any submission to the IND an amendment and every submission must be labeled with the next sequential four-digit serial number. Even if the sponsor does not assign a submission the next serial number, the FDA will and this very often leads to confusion in future submissions. The Form 1571 cover sheet has an area for the sponsor to include the serial number and an area to designate specifically what type of submission it is they are submitting. Sponsors who maintain multiple INDs and other regulatory filings use electronic archiving systems that have powerful searching and cross-referencing capabilities. This allows for searching a database on the basis of key words or serial numbers.

In this section, we will discuss the most common types of amendments and reports to the IND, and review the required content and timing for the submissions.

The IND Safety Report

The sponsor of an IND is responsible for continuously reviewing the safety of the investigational drug(s) under investigation. IND regulations require each sponsor to review and investigate all safety information obtained about the drug regardless of the source of the information. Safety information can come from a wide variety of sources, including the clinical studies being conducted under the IND, animal studies, other clinical studies, marketing experience, and reports in scientific journals and unpublished reports. These can be foreign or domestic sources and may be information that is not generated by the sponsor. The ongoing safety review is also a critical component of the sponsor's responsibility to keep all participating investigators updated on new observations regarding the investigational drug, especially any information regarding potential AEs.

The FDA regulations (21 CFR §312.32) and the ICH E6 guidance[8] define an AE as any unfavorable and unintended sign (including an abnormal laboratory finding), symptom, or disease temporally associated with the use of the investigational product, whether or not related to the investigational product. The regulations further defines a serious adverse drug reaction as any AE at any dose that

- results in death,
- is life threatening,
- requires inpatient hospitalization or prolongation of an existing hospitalization,
- results in persistent or significant disability/incapacity, or
- is a congenital anomaly/birth defect.

An AE that does not result in death, is not life threatening, or does not require hospitalization may still be considered serious, if in the opinion of the investigator, the event may have jeopardized the subject and medical intervention may be necessary to prevent one of the outcomes that defines a serious AE. The final key definition related to IND safety reports is what constitutes an unexpected AE. The IND regulations define an unexpected AE as any adverse drug experience, the specificity or severity of which is not consistent with the current investigator's brochure.[23] Essentially, what this means is an adverse experience is unexpected if that event was not listed in the investigator's brochure as a possible side effect of the drug (not observed previously), or the event that occurred was listed in the brochure but it occurred in a more severe way than was expected.

Much of the safety information obtained by the sponsor will relate to safety data that the sponsor was already aware of and included in the investigator's brochure or is nonserious in nature and does not require immediate notification of the investigators or the FDA; however, all new safety information should be included in the sponsor's safety database regardless of the reporting requirements.

The IND regulations also require sponsors to notify all investigators and the FDA of certain types of safety events in an IND safety report. The IND regulations discuss two types of safety reports, a 15-day report, and a more urgent 7-day report. When a reported adverse experience is considered related to the use of investigational drug and is a serious and unexpected event, the sponsor is required to notify all of the investigators in the study and the FDA within 15 calendar days of learning of the event. A 15-day safety report is submitted to the FDA on the FDA form 3500A or in a narrative format and foreign events may

---

[23] Code of Federal Regulations Title 21 Section 312.32(a).

be submitted on a Council for International Organizations of Medical Sciences (*CIOMS*) *I form*. IND safety reports are sent to the reviewing division at the FDA with jurisdiction over the IND. The reports should be submitted in triplicate (one original and two copies) with a 1571 form cover sheet and serial number. The more urgent safety report, the 7-day report is required when any unexpected fatal or life threatening event associated with the use of the drug occurs. The FDA must be notified by telephone or facsimile within 7 calendar days of learning of a fatal or life threatening event and followed up with a written report on form 3500A (or CIOMS I) within 15 days of learning of the event. The telephone/facsimile report should be made to the FDA review division with jurisdiction over the IND. Other safety information that does not meet the requirements for expedited reporting should be submitted to the IND in the annual report.

IND Term

CIOMS 1 Form—A standardized international reporting form used to report individual cases of serious, unexpected adverse drug reactions.

CIOMS, the Council for International Organizations of Medical Sciences is an international, nongovernmental, nonprofit organization established jointly by WHO and UNESCO in 1949. CIOMS has established a series of working groups that develop safety requirements for drugs and standardized guidelines for assessment and monitoring of adverse drug reactions.

The FDA interprets when the sponsor learns of the event to mean anyone in the employ of the sponsor or engaged by the sponsor's initial receipt of the information. If the sponsor's clinical research associate learns of a serious AE while visiting a site, the 15-day clock begins as soon as the associate learns of the event and not when the associate reports the event to the clinical affairs or pharmacovigilance groups. The sponsor must have strict procedures and timelines in place for employees to report potential AE.

It is important to remember that these events may not come strictly from the sponsor's ongoing clinical trials. The IND regulations require 15-day IND safety reports for adverse findings from nonclinical studies that may indicate a risk to human subjects in the ongoing clinical trials. These could be adverse findings from carcinogenicity studies, reproductive toxicology studies, or any other nonclinical studies being conducted to support clinical trials.

The sponsor must continue to investigate the adverse experience after the IND safety report is submitted. Any additional or follow up information obtained as part of the investigation must be submitted to the FDA as soon as the new information becomes available. In practice, most sponsors will submit follow up information to the FDA within a 15-day timeframe, as with the original safety report.

Submission of an IND safety report does not mean that the sponsor or the FDA has concluded that the information being reported constitutes an admission that the drug caused or contributed to the event. In fact, the IND regulations state that a sponsor need not admit, and may deny, that the report or information submitted constitutes an admission that the drug caused or contributed to an AE.[24]

In the Federal Register of March 14, 2003, the FDA published a proposed rule[25] to amend the pre- and postmarketing safety reporting regulations for human drug and biological products. The proposed rule will harmonize the U.S. safety reporting requirements with international standards developed by CIOMS and ICH and provides new standards, definitions, and reporting formats. A final rule on these safety reporting requirements is still pending.

The Protocol Amendment

A protocol amendment is submitted to the FDA when a sponsor wants to initiate a new clinical study that is not described in the existing IND or when the sponsor makes changes to an existing protocol, including adding a new investigator to a trial. New protocols are submitted when clinical development of the drug advances to the next phase, e.g., from Phase 1 to Phase 2, or when an additional study is needed during the same phase of development, e.g., an additional Phase 2 study to evaluate dosing or a clinical study to evaluate potential differences in pharmacokinetics or pharmacodynamics in response to changes in the formulation or route of administration of the investigational drug.

A protocol amendment for a new protocol must include a copy of the new protocol and a brief description of the most clinically significant differences between the new and previous protocols. Although not specified in the regulations, the FDA also expects Phase 2 and Phase 3 protocol submissions to include information on how the data will be collected (case report forms) to ensure that the study will achieve its intended scientific purposes. When submitting a new protocol to an active IND, the sponsor may initiate the study once the IRB has approved the protocol and it has been submitted to the FDA. There is no 30-day review period for the FDA, and a sponsor can initiate a study once the protocol is submitted, if IRB approval is in place. However, the FDA can still place the study on clinical hold if it believes there is a safety issue or the protocol design is insufficient to meet the stated objective. Sponsors may want to request feedback from the FDA or specifically request in the amendment that the FDA notify the sponsor if there are no objections to the proposed trial.

---

[24] Code of Federal Regulations Title 21 Section 312.32(e).

[25] Safety reporting requirements for human drug and biological products: proposed rule. Federal Register 2003; 68(50): 12406–12497.

A protocol amendment is also required if a sponsor makes significant changes to an existing protocol. For Phase 1 protocols, an amendment is required if the changes may affect the safety of the subjects participating in the study. Other modifications that do not affect the safety of the subjects can be submitted in the IND annual report and not in a protocol amendment. In the case of a Phase 2 or Phase 3 protocol, a protocol amendment should be submitted for any change that may affect the safety of the subjects, changes the scope of the trial, or affects the scientific validity of the study.

When submitting a protocol amendment for a change to a protocol, the submission should include a description of the change, a brief discussion of the reason, and justification for the change and reference (date and serial number) to the submission that contained the protocol and other references to specific technical information in the IND or other amendments that supports the proposed change.

The IND regulations allow a sponsor to immediately implement a change to a protocol if the change is intended to eliminate an immediate hazard to the clinical trial subjects. In this case, the FDA must be notified of the change by a protocol amendment as soon as possible and the IRB at each site must also be notified of the change.

A protocol amendment is required when a new investigator or sub-investigator is added to conduct the clinical trial at a new or an existing site. The investigator is the person with overall responsibility for the conduct of the clinical trial at a trial site and a subinvestigator is any individual member of the clinical trial team designated and supervised by the investigator to perform trial-related procedures or make trial-related decisions (e.g., associates, residents, research fellows).[26] The required information regarding the new investigators is collected on the FDA Form 1572, statement of investigator (Fig. 2), and the sponsor must notify the FDA of new investigators and subinvestigators or changes to the submitted information by submitting Form 1572 as a protocol amendment within 30 days of the investigator being added to the study. An investigator may not participate in a study until he or she provides the sponsor with a completed and signed statement of investigator Form 1572.[27] Protocol amendments to add new investigators or to add additional information about an investigator or subinvestigator can be grouped and submitted at 30-day intervals.

All protocol amendments must be clearly labeled and identify specifically which type of protocol amendment is included, e.g., "Protocol Amendment: New Protocol or Protocol Amendment: New Investigator", and as with all IND submissions, a Form 1571 cover sheet should be included with the submission. The appropriate box on the Form 1571 should be marked, indicating that the submission is a protocol amendment.

---

[26] FDA Draft Guidance for Industry: Protecting the Rights, Safety, and Welfare of Study Subjects—Supervisory Responsibilities of Investigators. FDA, Rockville, MD, May 2007.

[27] Code of Federal Regulations Title 21 Section 312.53.

Information Amendments

Information amendments are used to submit important information to the IND that is not within the scope of a protocol amendment, annual report, or IND safety report. An information amendment may include new toxicology or pharmacology information, final study reports for completed nonclinical or other technical studies, new chemistry manufacturing and controls information, notice of discontinuation of a clinical study, or any other information important to the IND. An information amendment can also include information that is specifically requested by the FDA. As with the protocol amendment, the FDA requests that information amendments be identified on the cover as an information amendment with the type of information being provided, e.g. "Information Amendment: Toxicology" and as with all IND submissions, a Form 1571 cover sheet should be included. Information amendments should be submitted as needed but not more than once every 30 days, if possible.

Information typically submitted in an information amendment may also be required to support another type of amendment; for instance, a new protocol may require additional CMC information because of a change in formulation or change in manufacturing of the investigational drug. In these cases, it is not necessary to submit a separate protocol amendment and a separate information amendment with two different serial numbers. All of the protocol and CMC information can be submitted in the same amendment, but it should be clearly separated within the submission (by tabs or title pages), the submission should be labeled as containing a protocol amendment and an information amendment (Protocol Amendment: New Protocol and Information Amendment: CMC).

IND Annual Reports

The IND regulations[28] require IND sponsors to submit an annual report that provides the FDA with a brief update on the progress of all investigations included in the IND. The regulations provide clear instruction as to the specific content and format of the annual report so we will only briefly summarize the content here. The annual report must contain the following information:

- Individual study information—a brief summary of the status of each study in progress including the title of the study, total number of subjects enrolled to date, total number of subjects who completed the study, the number of subjects who dropped out for any reason, and a brief description of any study results if known.
- Summary Information—nonclinical and clinical information obtained during the previous year. This section will include a table summarizing the

---

[28] Code of Federal Regulations Title 21 Section 312.33.

most frequent and most serious AEs, a listing of all IND safety reports submitted during the past year, a list of subjects who died during the investigation, including cause of death, a list of patients who dropped out of the study because of AEs, any new information about the mechanism of action, dose response or bioavailability of the drug, a list of ongoing and completed nonclinical studies, and a list of any manufacturing changes made during the previous year.

- The general investigational plan for the coming year.
- A list of the changes along with a copy of the new brochure, if the investigator brochure was modified during the year.
- Any changes made to the protocol not reported in a protocol amendment, if there is a phase 1 protocol.
- A listing of any significant foreign marketing developments with the drug, e.g., approval in another country or withdrawal or suspension of marketing approval.
- A log of any outstanding business for which the sponsor requests or expects a reply, comment, or meeting with the FDA.

As mentioned, the content of an annual report is well defined in the regulations and sponsors should not use the annual report as a substitute for an information amendment. Final nonclinical or clinical study reports, major CMC changes or other important PK or PD data should be submitted in an information amendment and not held until the annual report. Information of this nature must be submitted to the IND when it becomes available, which allows the FDA to review it in a timely fashion, not several months after the information first became available. The annual report should not be used to report new information, e.g., new serious and unexpected AEs, that could change the risk/benefit profile of the investigation, perhaps necessitating a clinical hold. The annual report is a summary of the progress of the study over the past year and provides the general investigational plan for the coming year. The annual report must be submitted to the FDA review division with jurisdiction over the IND within 60 days of the anniversary date that the IND went into effect.

OTHER TYPES OF INDs

In addition to the IND submitted by the commercial sponsor, there are investigator-sponsored INDs. They usually involve a single investigator who is performing a clinical trial. The investigator usually seeks permission from a commercial sponsor to "cross-reference" manufacturing data and nonclinical pharmacology and toxicology data. Letters from the commercial supplier of the product are required to allow the FDA to review the data contained in the supplier's IND or DMF.

Additionally, there are Treatment INDs. These are reserved for investigational products for serious or immediately life-threatening diseases where no satisfactory alternative therapy is available. This IND would allow use in patients not in the formal clinical trials in accordance with a treatment protocol or Treatment IND.[29] Special procedures apply for these INDs.

Another type of IND is the screening IND (MaPP 6030.4) or exploratory IND.[30] Generally, the FDA encourages separate INDs for different molecules and dosage forms. However, in the early phases of development, exploratory studies may be conducted on a number of closely related compounds to choose the preferred compound or formulation. These studies may be most efficiently conducted under a single IND. Its main benefit is the use of a single IND to avoid duplicative paperwork and to alert the FDA that the IND will be used to screen multiple compounds. The CMC and nonclinical pharmacology and toxicology data for each active moiety in the screening IND should be in accord with appropriate FDA guidances. These INDs only allow limited dosing with microdoses of drug to determine essential properties in humans before proceeding with the lead candidate for development. Once the lead compound is identified, the exploratory IND is closed and a full IND submitted for the drug candidate.

PROMOTION AND CHARGING FOR INVESTIGATIONAL DRUGS

Promotion of Investigational Drug Products

The determination of safety and efficacy is made by the FDA on the basis all of the information submitted in a marketing application, and a drug cannot be represented as safe or effective until the FDA has approved the product for sale. Therefore, IND regulations specifically prohibit a sponsor or investigator from promoting or commercializing an investigational drug or stating that an investigational drug is safe or effective for the indication(s) under investigation. This includes commercial distribution of the investigational drug or test marketing the drug.[31] Sponsors must be particularly aware of this prohibition when issuing press releases about ongoing or completed clinical trials. The sponsor is often eager to publicly release positive information from trials, particularly pivotal trials, but a press release cannot state that the drug is safe or effective for its intended use, no matter how positive the results of the trial may be. The FDA will consider statements like this in a press release or other public statements, promotion of an unapproved drug. Sponsors can also run into trouble at professional meetings and trade shows. Company representatives cannot make claims about the safety or efficacy of an investigational drug either verbally or in writing or appear to be promoting an investigational drug in any way.

---

[29] Code of Federal Regulations Title 21 Section 312.34.

[30] FDA Guidance for Industry, Investigators, and Reviewers—Exploratory IND Studies. FDA, Rockville, MD, January 2006.

[31] Code of Federal Regulations Title 21 Section 312.7(a).

These prohibitions are not intended to restrict the dissemination of scientific information about the drug in scientific meetings, journals, or other lay media. The results of clinical studies can be published in peer reviewed scientific journals, presented at medical or scientific meetings, and announced publicly in press releases. The information presented in these forums should be limited to scientific information and the actual results of a clinical study. Presenting the number of patients that met the primary efficacy measurements or other study outcomes is permissible, as long as there is no conclusion of safety and efficacy based on the reported results.

Charging for Investigational Drugs

Charging for an investigational drug product in a clinical trial conducted under an IND is prohibited unless the sponsor has submitted a written request to the FDA, seeking permission to charge for the drug and the FDA has issued a written approval.[32] In the request the sponsor must justify why charging for the drug is necessary to initiate or continue the trial and why the cost of providing the investigational product to trial subjects should not be considered a normal part of the cost of developing the drug. Although the regulations provide this mechanism, it is rare that a sponsor will charge for an investigational drug.

The regulations do permit a sponsor to charge for an investigational drug being administered under a Treatment protocol or Treatment IND if certain conditions are met.[33] If the FDA allows the sponsor to charge for the drug, the price must not be greater than the costs of handling, distribution, manufacture, and research and development of the drug. The FDA can withdraw authorization to charge for an investigational drug if it finds that any of the conditions of the authorization are no longer valid, e.g., the price being charged is greater than costs associated with the drug.

MORE INFORMATION ABOUT INDs

There is a great deal of additional information available about the IND application and much of it is now easily available via the Internet. The most complete source of information about the IND application is the FDA Web site itself (www.fda.gov). The CDER and CBER Web sites contain a wealth of important information about preparing, submitting, and maintaining INDs. The most important documents to be familiar with are the guidance documents (guidance for industry) but there is significantly more IND information available on the FDA site than just the guidance documents. The FDA Web site section below outlines a number of Web pages that provide significant information about INDs,

---

[32] Code of Federal Regulations 312.7(d)(1).

[33] Code of Federal Regulations Title 21 Section 312.7(d)(2).

how the FDA processes them, meeting with the FDA, and the drug development process in general.

The following list provides a selection of other IND resources found on the Web, in journal articles, and in books.

The FDA Web sites

1. Compilation of laws enforced by the U.S. FDA (www.fda.gov/opacom/laws/lawtoc.htm).
2. Title 21 Code of Federal Regulations (www.accessdata.fda.gov/scripts/cdrh/cfdocs/cfcfr/cfrsearch.cfm).
3. CDER guidance documents (www.fda.gov/cder/guidance/index.htm).
4. CBER guidance documents (www.fda.gov/cber/guidelines.htm).
5. The CDER handbook (www.fda.gov/cder/handbook/).
6. IND form help—information for sponsor-investigators submitting INDs (www.fda.gov/cder/forms/1571-1572-help.html).
7. Office of drug evaluation IV (ODE IV)—pre-IND consultation program. A program offered by the ODE IV designed to facilitate early informal communications between ODE IV and sponsors of new therapeutics for the treatment of bacterial infections, HIV, opportunistic infections, transplant rejection, and other diseases (www.fda.gov/cder/Regulatory/default.htm#Regulatory).
8. *CDER* MaPPs (www.fda.gov/cder/mapp.htm).
    a. MaPP 6030.1 IND—process and review procedures.
    b. MaPP 6030.2 INDs—review of informed consent documents.
    c. MaPP 6030.4 INDs—screening INDs.
    d. MaPP 6030.8 INDs—exception from informed consent requirements for emergency research.
9. CBER *Manual of Regulatory Standard Operating Procedures and Policies* (SOPPs) (www.fda.gov/cber/regsopp/regsopp.htm).
    a. SOPP 8201 issuance of and response to clinical hold letters for INDs.
10. Good clinical practice in FDA-regulated clinical trials (www.fda.gov/oc/gcp/default.htm).

Other Web sites

1. RegSource.com (www.regsource.com/default.html). A comprehensive site that contains a wealth of information on many topics within regulatory affairs including INDs.

Further Reading

1. Mathieu M. New Drug Development: A Regulatory Overview. 7th ed. Waltham, MA: Parexel International, 2005.

3

The New Drug Application

Charles Monahan

Regulatory Affairs, Molecular Insight Pharmaceuticals, Inc.,
Cambridge, Massachusetts, U.S.A.

Josephine C. Babiarz[1]

MS Program in Regulatory Affairs, Massachusetts College of Pharmacy and
Health Sciences, Boston, Massachusetts, U.S.A.

OVERVIEW

The New Drug Application (NDA) is the single most important filing necessary to obtain marketing approval for a drug in the United States. When complete, the NDA contains thousands of pages of nonclinical, clinical, and drug chemistry information. It is the basis for the decision by the Food and Drug Administration (FDA) to approve or refuse permission to market the drug. The information contained in the NDA supports the proposed labeling of the drug under which the applicant intends to market the product.

The NDA is organized into specific, technical sections, which are evaluated by specialized review teams of highly qualified experts. Together, the review teams will make a decision to approve or disapprove the NDA.

This assessment by the review team is guided by the axiom that no drug is truly safe but that the benefits to the patients outweigh the risks of using it. While

---

[1] The authors gratefully thank and acknowledge the substantial and invaluable contributions of David Pizzi and Janet Rae, authors of the predecessor chapter.

the statute governing the NDA process requires that the article be "safe for use" and "effective for use,"[2] it does not define these terms.[3] The U.S. Supreme Court interpreted these requirements as follows:[4]

> A drug is effective if there is general recognition among experts, founded on substantial evidence, that the drug in fact produces the results claimed for it under prescribed conditions. Effectiveness does not necessarily denote capacity to cure. In the treatment of any illness, terminal or otherwise, a drug is effective if it fulfills, by objective indices, its sponsor's claims of prolonged life, improved physical condition, or reduced pain . . . Few if any drugs are completely safe in the sense that they may be taken by all persons in all circumstances without risk. Thus, [the FDA] generally considers a drug safe when the expected therapeutic gain justifies the risk entailed by its use.

The FDA has not only adopted this interpretation but has also developed content requirements for an NDA that implement these principles. The required content of an NDA is outlined in the Food, Drug, and Cosmetic Act and Title 21 of the U.S. Code of Federal Regulations (CFR). Applicants should follow these requirements to assure that their NDA provides enough information to enable the FDA reviewers to reach the following key decisions:[5]

* Whether the drug is safe and effective in its proposed use(s) and whether the benefits of the drug outweigh the risks.
* Whether the drug's proposed labeling (package insert) is appropriate and what it should contain.
* Whether the methods used in manufacturing the drug and the controls used to maintain the drug's quality are adequate to preserve the drug's identity, strength, quality, and purity.

To facilitate the review process, the information in the NDA should be presented clearly and consistently throughout the application. Applicants should prepare the NDA according to the regulations and guidances established by the FDA, preferably in an electronic format.

---

[2] 21 USC Section 355. New Drugs.

[3] FDA guidance, found at www.fda.gov/cder/guidance/old039fn.pdf, notes that "safe" is proven through adequate scientific evidence, while "effective" is determined by substantial objective evidence. CDER's main guidance page is at www.fda.gov/cder/guidance/index.htm#drug%20safety.

[4] United States v. Rutherford, 442 US 544 (1979).

[5] See www.fda.gov/cder/regulatory/applications/nda.htm.

The Center for Drug Evaluation and Research (CDER) is the group at the FDA charged with reviewing NDAs for drugs and some biologic products. Although this chapter concentrates on drugs, some of the information discussed here is applicable to biologics.

Other chapters in this book deal in detail with the preclinical and clinical testing requirements. For the purposes of this chapter, we assume that the precursor steps in the drug development process have been completed and the applicant believes that the pivotal trials have successfully shown the drug to be both safe and effective. The remaining tasks will be to compile the information into an NDA to enable FDA to arrive at the same conclusions.

LAWS, REGULATIONS, AND GUIDANCES

The FDA's authority to require and review an NDA (prior to an applicant marketing the product in the United States) is clearly stated in section 505 of the Food, Drug, and Cosmetic Act [21 USC 355].

The Act requires that the application contain:

(A) full reports of investigations which have been made to show whether or not such drug is safe for use and whether such drug is effective in use; (B) a full list of the articles used as components of such drug; (C) a full statement of the composition of such drug; (D) a full description of the methods used in, and the facilities and controls used for, the manufacture, processing, and packing of such drug; (E) such samples of such drug and of the articles used as components thereof as the Secretary may require; (F) specimens of the labeling proposed to be used for such drug and (G) any assessments required under section 505B. The applicant shall file with the application the patent number and the expiration date of any patent which claims the drug for which the applicant submitted the application or which claims a method of using such drug and with respect to which a claim of patent infringement could reasonably be asserted if a person not licensed by the owner engaged in the manufacture, use, or sale of the drug.

This requirement has broad application; the regulations at 21 CFR Part 310 include under the scope of "new drug" any changes to a molecular entity, no matter how small, which have not been the subject of an approved NDA or "grandfathered" (those drugs sold prior to 1938). Consequently, articles that are "new" and not marketable without further testing include a new substance, even a coating, excipient or carrier of the drug; a new combination, even of individually approved drugs or if the proportion of ingredients in the combination has changed; a new use; or a new dosage, duration, or method of administration.

The regulations at 21 CFR Part 314 titled "Applications for FDA Approval to Market a New Drug" can most easily be found using the e-CFR page of the

Government Printing Office.[6] The purpose of this regulation, as outlined in Part 314.20, is to establish an efficient and thorough drug review process to (*i*) facilitate the approval of drugs shown to be safe and effective and (*ii*) ensure the disapproval of drugs not shown to be safe and effective. These regulations are also intended to establish an effective system for FDA's surveillance of marketed drugs. These regulations shall be construed in light of these objectives.[7]

Of particular relevance to this chapter is 21 CFR Part 314.50, which outlines the primary content and format of the NDA, discussed in greater detail later in the chapter.

In addition to the regulations, numerous guidance documents have been established by the FDA that represent its current thinking on the content and format of an NDA. The guidance documents can be best accessed through the FDA Web site, http://www.fda.gov/opacom/morechoices/industry/guidedc.htm.

These guidances reflect major legislative changes that have been made over the past decade, especially the Prescription Drug User Fee Act (PDUFA) (see chap. 1, Overview of FDA and Drug Development supra). PDUFA requires the FDA to conduct speedier, more efficient reviews and establishes time frames for FDA's response to the applicant. This timetable starts when an NDA comes into the Controlled Document Room. On receipt, the FDA has 60 days to decide whether to review the NDA. The FDA can refuse to review an application that is incomplete. For example, some required studies may be missing.[8] Any deficiencies can stop the FDA review clock; delays can be very costly.

Once the application has been accepted for review, or "filed," there are three possible outcomes. An application can be "approvable," meaning that the sponsor must resolve additional issues, and then can market it, or the application can be "approved," meaning that the drug is marketable subject to the other provisions of the Food, Drug, and Cosmetic Act, as amended. FDA does post certain portions of the approved NDAs online at "Drugs@FDA." Lastly, the application can be "non-approvable."

In order to file an NDA and begin the review process, the sponsor must pay the Prescription Drug User Fee, currently at $1,178,000, for an application requiring clinical data, $589,000 for applications not requiring clinical data, and the same for a supplemental application requiring clinical data; these amounts are effective from October 1, 2007, through September 30, 2008, and shall increase thereafter.[9] There are no fees payable if the FDA refuses to file the NDA.[10] All fees are assessed under the Prescription Drug User Fee Act, which

---

[6] The main e-CFR page for FDA regulations is found at http://ecfr.gpoaccess.gov/cgi/t/text/text-idx?sid=714370aae2160c833d37224fbba5001e&c=ecfr&tpl=/ecfrbrowse/Title21/21tab_02.tpl.

[7] See http://ecfr.gpoaccess.gov/cgi/t/text/text-idx?c=ecfr&sid=7c6ebbb3acf53d253acbcf58ee31d425&rgn=div8&view=text&node=21:5.0.1.1.4.1.1.2&idno=21.

[8] See www.fda.gov/fdac/special/testtubetopatient/drugreview.html.

[9] See www.fda.gov/cder/pdufa/2008_rates.htm

[10] Public Law No. 110–85; see chapter 1 for an overview of this legislation.

was most recently reauthorized under the Food and Drug Administration Amendments Act of 2007.

Although these fees are high, the Secretary of Health and Human Services, Michael O. Leavitt, has committed to implement certain agency reforms, particularly speeding the review period by FDA. He has established new goals to reduce review times from 10 months to 6 months. In the future, he expects that 90% of all NDAs will be reviewed in this time frame. These reforms are supplementary to and do not invalidate the legal requirement that the agency take action within 180 days of receipt of a filed application.[11]

Applicants should be aware that there are laws and regulations that provide exceptions to those listed above. The Orphan Drug Act allows the FDA to grant special status to a drug intended to treat a rare disease or condition. To qualify for orphan status, the drug must be intended to treat a disease or condition that affects fewer that 200,000 people in the United States each year. With so few patients, it would be difficult for the applicant to recoup the development cost. Therefore, the Act provides incentives to applicants to develop these drugs. One incentive is a waiver of the PDUFA fee.

The regulations for accelerated approval of drugs for serious or life-threatening illnesses are codified in 21 CFR 314 Subpart H. Under these regulations, the FDA may grant marketing approval for a new drug product on the basis of adequate and well-controlled clinical trials establishing that the drug product has an effect on a surrogate endpoint that is reasonably likely to predict clinical benefit.[12] Accelerated approval of an NDA allows the applicant to market its drug while conducting confirmatory studies to establish clinical benefit.

Section 112 of the Food and Drug Administration Modernization Act of 1997 (FDAMA) "Expediting study and approval of fast track drugs" mandates the agency facilitate the development and expedite the review of drugs and biologics intended to treat serious or life-threatening conditions and that demonstrate the potential to address unmet medical needs. *Fast track* adds to existing programs, such as accelerated approval, the possibility of a "rolling submission" for the NDA. This allows sponsors to submit sections of the NDA as they are completed, expediting the review process. An important feature of *fast track* is that it emphasizes the critical nature of close early communication between the FDA and sponsor to improve the efficiency of product development.[13]

As you can see, use of the different laws and regulations can have a strategic impact on the development of the NDA. Therefore, applicants should identify which laws and regulations are applicable to their drug early in their development program.

---

[11] FDCA, Section 505(c)(1).

[12] 21 Code of Federal Regulations 314.510.

[13] See www.fda.gov/cber/inside/fastrk.htm.

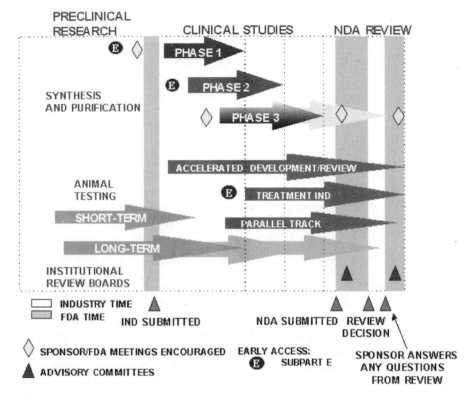

Figure 1 The new drug development process.

DEVELOPMENT OF THE NDA

As you can see in Figure 1,[14] the development program leading to the submission of an NDA is both time-consuming and costly. Therefore, an applicant cannot wait until the end of its pivotal studies to start thinking about the NDA submission. Instead, an approval pathway for the new drug should be outlined in a regulatory development plan (RDP) throughout the preclinical and clinical stages of the new drug development process.

The RDP is usually prepared by the regulatory affairs representative on the development team. In addition to knowing the regulations and contents of guidance documents, this individual should have an understanding of the disease or condition being investigated, the approved drugs available to patients with the disease, and the basis of approval for those drugs. In addition, this representative should have knowledge of the expectations of the reviewing division at the FDA.

---

[14] See www.fda.gov/cder/handbook/develop.htm.

This information can be found by searching the FDA Web site for approval summaries, transcripts of advisory committee meetings, and approved product labeling. Additionally, a PubMed search for articles written by members of the FDA review teams may provide insight that could help with the development program.

With this information, an RDP can be developed that provides input into the design and timing of nonclinical and clinical studies to support the NDA.

Of all the activities that take place prior to the submission of an NDA, meetings between the applicant and the review Division at the FDA are critical. Applicants should plan to meet with the FDA at each stage of clinical development to discuss issues and ensure that the evidence necessary to support a marketing approval will be developed.

Prior to submitting an NDA, the applicant should schedule a pre-NDA meeting with the FDA to discuss and reach agreement on critical issues such as the following:[15]

- Whether preliminary evidence of effectiveness was seen in the principal controlled trials intended to provide evidence of effectiveness
- Structure, content, and timing of submission of the Biologic License Application (BLA) or NDA
- Structure and content of any electronic submissions
- Structure, content, and timing of submission of portions of an application for marketing approval, if such submission is appropriate
- Readiness for, and proposed timing of, preapproval inspections
- Potential for, and proposed timing of, advisory committee presentation, if applicable

CONTENTS OF THE NDA

The required content of an NDA for submission in the United States is outlined in the Food, Drug and Cosmetic Act and Title 21 of the US Code of Federal Regulations Part 314. An NDA application must contain reports of all investigations of the drug product sponsored by the applicant and all other information about the drug pertinent to an evaluation of the application that is received or obtained by the applicant from any source.[16]

There are 20 different items that may be required for the submission; however, the actual required items of each NDA will be unique. The number of items and their contents can vary because of many factors such as the type of drug, the information available at the time of submission, or special requests for information from the FDA. This variability underscores the need for significant

---

[15] See http://www.fda.gov/cder/guidance/5645fnl.htm#_Toc77574464.

[16] Available at: http://ecfr.gpoaccess.gov/cgi/t/text/text-idx?c=ecfr&sid=7c6ebbb3acf53d253acbcf58 ee31d425&rgn=div8&view=text&node=21:5.0.1.1.4.2.1.1&idno=21.

planning throughout the NDA development process. In addition, applicants should discuss the contents of their NDA with the reviewing division at the FDA to assure that the contents of the application will be accepted for filing.

The following is a discussion of each item required in an NDA.

Administrative Items

The following may be considered administrative items that are required in an NDA. These items provide pertinent information about the application such as the identity of applicant, the drug and its intended use, the content of the submission, and certifications of Good Clinical Practice and legal compliance.

Application Form: [21 CFR 314.50(a)]

Each applicant is required to submit a signed Form FDA 356h,[17] reprinted here in Appendix A. This form is published by the FDA and updated periodically. The form contains information about the sponsor, the drug and the proposed indication, as well as a checklist of the items contained in the NDA. By signing the form, the responsible official or agent of the NDA certifies that all information in the application is true and accurate and, in addition, that the applicant will comply with a range of legal and regulatory requirements. If the applicant is not located in the United States, the form must name an agent with a U.S. address.

Patent Information: [21 CFR 314.50(h) and 314.53]

The law requires patent information to be submitted with the NDA. An applicant is required to disclose all patent information that is related to the drug for which the NDA is being filed and to verify that the sponsor has all rights necessary to legally manufacture, use, and sell the drug, if the NDA is approved. The patent inquiry is a broad one and covers drug substance (active ingredient) patents, drug product (formulation and composition) patents, and method-of-use patents. In all likelihood, it should be signed only after review by a qualified attorney or patent agent who can provide an opinion as to the truth and accuracy of the completed form. The signature on the form, called a "verification" reads, "The undersigned declares that this is an accurate and complete submission of patent information for the NDA, amendment or supplement pending under section 505 of the Federal Food, Drug, and Cosmetic Act. This time-sensitive patent information is submitted pursuant to 21 CFR 314.53. I attest that I am familiar with 21 CFR 314.53 and this submission complies with the requirements of the regulation. I verify under penalty of perjury that the foregoing is true and correct." In

---

[17] Form 356h is available at: www.fda.gov/opacom/morechoices/fdaforms/356Hes.pdf.

addition, applicants must maintain these patent statements and are required to submit updates before and after approval using Form FDA 3542(a) for each patent.[18]

We also note that there are "safe harbors" protecting a person from claims of patent infringement that apply expressly to drugs; this exemption essentially allows generic manufacturers or name-brand competitors to "jump start" the approval process by conducting required testing even though the original patent has not expired. The law reads: "It shall not be an act of [patent] infringement to make, use, offer to sell or sell within the United States or import into the United States a patented invention ... solely for uses reasonably related to the development and submission of information under a federal law which regulates the manufacture, use or sale of drugs or veterinary biological products."[19] Again, because patent infringement carries criminal penalties, consulting with a qualified patent attorney or agent is essential.

Patent Certification: [21 CFR 314.50(i) and 314.52]

If the new drug is covered by a patent or patents, which the applicant believe(s) to be invalid, a different procedure and format are used. Under this regulation, there is no specific form to file; there is a requirement to certify specific items, all as stated in the regulation. In this case, the patents must still be disclosed, but also, the applicant must certify under 21 CFR 314.50(i)(1)(i)(A)(4) that the patent is invalid, unenforceable, or will not be infringed, and further, the applicant is required to send a specific notice by registered or certified mail, return receipt requested to specified interested parties.[20] The purpose again is to prevent the agency from essentially wasting its time to review an application for a drug that cannot be legally manufactured.

Establishment Description: [21 CFR Part 600]

An establishment description is only applicable to certain biological drug products.

Debarment Certification [FDCA 306(k)(1)]

Section 306(k)(1) of the Food Drug and Cosmetic Act requires an NDA to contain a statement certifying that the applicant did not and will not use in *any* capacity the services of any person debarred by the FDA. The certification statement should not use conditional or qualifying language such as, "to the best

---

[18] The form can be found at http://www.fda.gov/opacom/morechoices/fdaforms/FDA-3542a.pdf.

[19] 35 USC Section 271(e)(1).

[20] See www.accessdata.fda.gov/scripts/cdrh/cfdocs/cfcfr/CFRSearch.cfm?fr=314.52.

of my knowledge." The following wording is considered the most acceptable form of certification by the FDA:[21]

> *[Name of the applicant] hereby certifies that it did not and will not use in any capacity the services of any person debarred under section 306 of the Federal Food, Drug, and Cosmetic Act in connection with this application.*

Field Copy Certification [21 CFR 314.50(d)(1)(v)]

The NDA must include a certification statement noting that the field copy, submitted to the local FDA office, is a true copy of the Chemistry Manufacturing and Controls section that was submitted in the archival and review copies of the application.

User Fee Cover Sheet (Form FDA-3397)

A User Fee Cover Sheet is to be completed and submitted with each new drug or biologic product NDA. The form provides a cross reference to the user fee paid by the applicant.

Financial Certification or Disclosure: [21 CFR 314.50(k)]

The NDA is required to contain information regarding all financial interests or arrangements between clinical investigators, their spouses and immediate family members, and the sponsor of the clinical trials that support the NDA. The applicant should submit an FDA Form 3454 to certify which investigators had no financial interests or arrangements. An FDA Form 3455 is submitted to disclose any financial interests or arrangements with an investigator that could affect the outcome of the study and a description of steps taken to minimize the potential bias of the study results.

An investigator who had financial interests to disclose is not disqualified from the application per se; a financially incented investigator should not enroll a majority of subjects nor be the principal investigator for the larger testing sites.

Other Information [21 CFR 314.50(g)]

The applicant can use this item to provide additional information as needed in the NDA, such as a request for a waiver from the requirement to conduct pediatric studies or an accurate and complete English translation of each part of the application not in English, including original literature publications.

---

[21] See http://www.fda.gov/cber/gdlns/debar.pdf.

Index [21 CFR 314.50(b)]

The NDA index is a comprehensive table of contents (TOC) that enables the reviewers to quickly find specific information in this massive document. It must show the location of every section in the archival NDA by volume and by page number. It should guide reviewers to data in the technical sections, the summary, and the supporting documents.

Labeling [21 CFR 314.50(e)]

The labeling section must include all draft labeling that is intended for use on the product container, cartons or packages, including the proposed package insert.

Application Summary [21 CFR 314.50(c)]

The application summary is an abbreviated version of the entire application. The summary should discuss all aspects of the application and synthesize the information into a well-structured and unified document. The summary should provide the reader with a good understanding of the application. The reader should "gain a good general understanding of the data and information in the application, including an understanding of the quantitative aspects of the data.... The summary should be written at approximately the level of detail required for publication in, and meet the editorial standards generally applied by, refereed scientific and medical journals.... To the extent possible, data in the summary should be presented in tabular and graphic forms."[22]

There are nine separate sections of the summary; the substantive sections are discussed in the following paragraphs.

Proposed Annotated Package Insert (Labeling)

The labeling requirements are very specific and detailed. Applicants must be familiar with all regulatory requirements, especially those under sections 21 CFR 201.56(d)(1) and 201.57.[23] The pertinent regulation at 201.56(d)(1) mandates that the labeling contain the specific information required under section 201.57(a), (b),

---

[22] 21 CFR Part 314.50(c).

[23] The authors note that product-labeling requirements have undergone substantial revision and that FDA is implementing these changes over a period of time. A full discussion of labeling is beyond the scope of this chapter; readers are directed to the recently revised regulations found at http://www.fda .gov/OHRMS/DOCKETS/98fr/06-545.pdf, titled "21 CFR Parts 201, 314, and 601. Requirements on Content and Format of Labeling for Human Prescription Drug and Biological Products and Draft Guidances and Two Guidances for Industry on the Content and Format of Labeling for Human Prescription Drug and Biological Products; Final Rule and Notices".

and (c) under the following headings and subheadings and in the following order:

Highlights of Prescribing Information
    Product Names, Other Required Information
    Boxed Warning
    Recent Major Changes
    Indications and Usage
    Dosage and Administration
    Dosage Forms and Strengths
    Contraindications
    Warnings and Precautions
    Adverse Reactions
    Drug Interactions
    Use in Specific Populations
Full Prescribing Information: Contents
Full Prescribing Information
Boxed Warning

  1 Indications and Usage
  2 Dosage and Administration
  3 Dosage Forms and Strengths
  4 Contraindications
  5 Warnings and Precautions
  6 Adverse Reactions
  7 Drug Interactions
  8 Use in Specific Populations
     8.1 Pregnancy
     8.2 Labor and delivery
     8.3 Nursing mothers
     8.4 Pediatric use
     8.5 Geriatric use
  9 Drug Abuse and Dependence
     9.1 Controlled substance
     9.2 Abuse
     9.3 Dependence
 10 Overdosage
 11 Description
 12 Clinical Pharmacology
     12.1 Mechanism of action
     12.2 Pharmacodynamics
     12.3 Pharmacokinetics
 13 Nonclinical Toxicology
     13.1 Carcinogenesis, mutagenesis, impairment of fertility
     13.2 Animal toxicology and/or pharmacology

14 Clinical Studies
15 References
16 How Supplied/Storage and Handling
17 Patient Counseling Information

Each section of the labeling must include annotations referencing the information in the summary and technical sections of the application that support the inclusion of each statement in the labeling with respect to animal pharmacology and/or animal toxicology, clinical studies, and Integrated Summary of Safety (ISS) and Integrated Summary of Effectiveness (ISE).

Pharmacologic Class, Scientific Rationale, Intended Use, Potential Clinical Benefits

This section contains the basic information about the drug product and is generally one to two pages long.

Foreign Marketing History

The summary must include a list of any countries in which the drug is or was marketed, along with the dates when it was marketed, if they are known. It must also include a list of any countries in which the drug has been withdrawn from marketing for any reason relating to safety or efficacy or in which an application has been rejected. The applicant is required to provide specific reasons for the withdrawal or the rejection of the application.

If any related form of the drug has been marketed in another country, its foreign marketing history is included as well.

Chemistry, Manufacturing and Controls Summary

This includes an abbreviated version of the Chemistry, Manufacturing, and Controls (CMC) information on the drug substance or drug product. The summary should include a tabular list of all formulations used in the important clinical studies.

Nonclinical Pharmacology And Toxicology Summary

This portion of the summary should include information on pharmacology, toxicology and pharmacokinetics (PK).

Human Pharmacokinetics And Bioavailability Summary

This section includes a tabular listing and brief description of each human pharmacokinetics and bioavailability (HPKB) study as well as an integrated summary including the drug product's pharmacokinetic characteristics. If pertinent, the applicant should compare the drug product's bioavailability with other dosage forms. This summary will also identify differences in PK in various subgroups, for example, age group or renal status. Finally, the applicant should include a brief discussion of the drug product's dissolution profile.

Microbiology Summary

A section on microbiology is only required for antibiotic drugs.

Clinical Data Summary and Results of Statistical Analysis

This summary must include

Clinical pharmacology. The applicant provides a table of clinical pharmacology studies, narrative results of each study, and an integrated conclusion.

Overview of clinical studies. The applicant provides an overview of clinical trials conducted, a summary of any important discussions of FDA interaction on major issues, and an explanation of clinical features such as duration, study design, and adverse events expected.

Controlled clinical studies. Following the same format as the clinical pharmacology section, the applicant includes a table of controlled clinical studies, narrative results of each study, and an integrated conclusion.

Uncontrolled clinical studies. Following the same format as the clinical pharmacology and controlled clinical studies sections, the applicant includes a table of uncontrolled clinical studies, narrative results of each study, and an integrated conclusion.

Other studies and information. The applicant provides a summary of information not covered under clinical pharmacology, controlled and uncontrolled clinical trials. This might include information on other studies, publications, and analyses of foreign marketing experience or epidemiologic data.

Safety summary (general safety conclusions). This addresses the extent of exposure and adverse reactions attributable to the drug. It includes tables of the most important adverse events (AEs), such as serious and/or frequent events. It provides a separate analysis of controlled and uncontrolled studies and also integrates the safety data for controlled and uncontrolled studies. The applicant should discuss differences related to dose, duration, age, and gender and provide an analysis of discontinuations.

Overdosage and drug abuse. This section provides information on treatment of overdose. If the drug product has potential for abuse, the applicant should provide a summary of studies performed and other relevant information. If the drug is not considered abusable, but belongs to a class of drugs with potential for abuse, the applicant should provide reasons why drug abuse studies were not performed.

Discussion of Benefit/Risk Relationship

The summary must include a brief benefit/risk assessment based on ISE to ISS and results of the clinical studies. It includes information on the toxicity and safety of the drug from both human and animal studies and presents the benefits and risks of alternative treatments for the population. Finally, the section should describe any postmarketing studies that the applicant proposes.

This section concludes the summary; an overview of the technical sections follows.

Chemistry, Manufacturing and Controls [21 CFR 314.50(d)(1)]

The first technical section of the NDA is the chemistry section. It includes information on the composition, manufacture, and specifications of the drug substance and the drug product. The three main elements are (*i*) CMC information; (*ii*) samples, and (*iii*) methods validation package. Deficiencies in this section are common.

Description of the Drug Substance

The CMC information must include a description of the drug substance, or active ingredient, including its stability and physical and chemical characteristics. The applicant is required to provide the *names/designations* of the drug substance, including

- generic/common name,
- chemical name (IUPAC/USAN/CAS), and
- code(s) (CAS/internal).

Note that deficiencies often arise when multiple internal code numbers do not correspond to codes used in the documents that accompany the submission.

In addition, the section provides a *structural overview*, including

- molecular structure,
- empirical formula,
- molecular weight, and
- elemental composition.

The applicant should be certain that chemical names and structure accurately convey stereochemistry/chirality.

The description of the drug substance's *physical and chemical characteristics* should include the following:

- Appearance, including color, crystalline form and odor
- Melting/boiling point
- Refractive index, viscosity and specific gravity
- Polymorphs, including modifications (forms) and relative kinetic/thermodynamic stabilities

Note that common deficiencies in the description of physical characteristics arise when temperatures are not precisely controlled and/or specified for temperature-dependent physical and chemical criteria. Solubility studies at different pH's that are not adequately designed to differentiate from counter-ion effects can also result in a deficiency.

The physical and chemical characteristics should also include solubility, ionization constants, and partition coefficients at various pHs. The applicant should discuss solubility in common organic solvents as well as in various aqueous media.

- Water
- 0.1 N HCl
- 0.02 N HCl
- SGF without pepsin
- Water buffered to various acidic/neutral/basic pHs

The solubility data in aqueous media must correlate with the drug product–dissolution characteristics. Inadequate correlation can result in a deficiency.

Other common deficiencies include partitioning studies that are not logically designed and inadequate physical or chemical data on alternative polymorphs and stereoisomer.

Additionally, this section should provide a *reference standard* to elucidate the drug substance's chemical structure, including preparation method, test methods, and test results as shown by a certificate of analysis. The applicant should be sure to include the specification for the reference standard and provide proof that the reference standard was adequately tested as well as characterize the spectra completely.

This section should provide structural elucidation using a reference standard as applicable. Measures might include the following:

- X-ray (in the case of absolute configuration or polymorphism)
- UV/visible spectrum
- FTIR spectrum
- ^{1}H NMR/^{13}C NMR spectrum
- Low-resolution/high-resolution mass spectrum
- Elemental analysis

- Other spectrums as appropriate (e.g., heteroatom nuclear magnetic resonance (NMR), fluorescence, raman, microwave)

The CMC information must also include the *names, addresses, and functions of each site where the drug substance is manufactured or tested.* Synthesis often takes place at more than one site. If this is the case, it must be adequately represented in the submission to avoid a deficiency.

Drug master file (DMF) authorization letters must be included; the applicant must ensure that these are current.

The description of the drug substance *manufacturing methods* must include the following:

- Synthesis scheme
- Synthesis description
- Typical executed manufacturing record
- Compilation of and analytical controls for starting materials; reagents, solvents and catalysts; and intermediates
- Suppliers for starting materials

Note that deficiencies commonly arise when synthesis descriptions are not precise, when the in-process testing for the reaction completion cited for various synthetic steps is insufficient or when reviewers deem that the explanation provided when multiple syntheses are involved is inadequate.

The applicant must provide a description of and specifications for the *container and closure components* used for the bulk drug substance. Common deficiencies in this section include providing inadequate specifications and using a container-closure system that does not exactly match the one used in stability studies.

The discussion of *drug substance analytical controls* should include the following:

- Specifications
- Methods
- Rationale for methods/specifications
- Method validations
- Batch analytical data (including impurity profiles cross-referenced with toxicology studies)
- Sampling plan

An NDA may be deficient if the specifications, methods, or method validations are inadequate.

To be considered adequate, specifications should reflect more than one identification test. They should be based on batch history and scientific justification, and individual and total impurity standards must be established properly. The specification should account for all possible stereoisomers and should include proper limits on particle size.

Methods will be found inadequate if (*i*) no reference standards are established for impurities when using an external standard approach for impurity testing; (*ii*) if the assay is performed by a nonspecific method, such as titration, with no correction for the impurities that are present; (*iii*) if the sampling plan does not have a statistical basis; or (*iv*) if there is insufficient system suitability.

Method validations are inadequate if the method validation is performed outside the specified range or if it does not support system suitability.

The applicant must provide information on *drug substance stability*, including

- ambient/accelerated stability data,
- retest dating, and
- Highly stressed (e.g., acid, base, reflux) data.

The application is deemed deficient if it offers insufficient or marginal data for filing; this is especially the case with Investigational New Drug (IND) filings. Another common deficiency is lack of proper control over conditions—such as temperature, humidity, or high-intensity light exposure—that affect stability. Finally, if the analytical methods used do not indicate stability, the information is deficient.

Description of the Drug Product

The CMC technical section also includes a description of the drug product. The description will include some of the same kinds of information required in the description of the drug substance.

Information on the *drug product components/composition* should include qualitative and quantitative listings of each drug product component used in the clinical formulation or formulations (when filing IND) and marketed formulation or formulations (when filing NDA). Deficiencies result when the quantitative composition does not match the composition listed in the batch record, when component ranges are given without proper validation, or when the component ranges provided actually are specifications.

The applicant must provide a listing of all *inactive ingredients*. For compendial [e.g., United States Pharmacopeia (USP)/National Formulary (NF)] inactive ingredients, the section should reference the appropriate current compendial monographs and provide more precise specifications as necessary. Applicants should be aware that misinterpretation of compendial monographs is a common deficiency.

For noncompendial ingredients that fall under 21 CFR, such as D&C and FD&C dyes, the applicant should reference the appropriate section of 21 CFR and provide any additional specifications.

For noncompendial items that are not regulated by 21 CFR, the applicant should provide appropriate analytical specifications and methods.

The section should include the names, addresses, and functions of each site where the *drug product is manufactured, tested, or packaged*; however, if too many sites are involved, reviewers may determine that the overall manufacturing scheme is too complex. This aspect should be addressed in the development strategy.

As noted above, DMF authorization letters must be included, and these must be current, that is, within the last two years.

The applicant should provide information on the following *drug product–manufacturing methods*:

- Summary and schematics of manufacturing procedure
- Master batch record for proposed marketed products, including actual operating conditions, type and size of equipment, and in-process controls and tests
- Executed batch record

Applications are often found deficient because the master and executed batch records that are submitted vary too much from one to another. The master batch record itself is deficient when the description of equipment is too limited or restrictive or when the in-process controls are inappropriate. Examples of the latter include controls that do not address key in-process criteria or that do not correlate with the finished process controls.

The section on *drug product packaging* must include the following:

- Summary of container/closure system(s)
- Listing of packaging components and component/resin suppliers
- Specifications for each packaging component
- DMF authorization letters
- Description of the packaging process
- Test methods (as appropriate)
- Developmental data that confirm the suitability of the packaging. This includes water vapor permeation data for plastic containers/closures, and compatibility testing for solutions, suspensions, emulsions, etc.

Applications are often found deficient because the product packaging does not exactly match the product packaging described in the application. The applicant should also be aware that certain complex packaging components, such as bottle liners, may create difficulties. For example, the use of certain vinyl polymers in bottle liners may necessitate a test for the corresponding vinyl monomer. Ideally, appropriate component identification testing should be performed upon receipt of packaging components.

The discussion of *drug product analytical controls* should include the same elements as the corresponding discussion of the drug substance:

- Specifications
- Methods
- Rationale for methods/specifications

- Method validations
- Batch analytical data (including impurity profiles)
- Sampling plan

As in the discussion of drug substance analytical controls, the information is deficient if the specifications, methods, or method validations are inadequate. In addition to those points noted above, common reasons for deficiencies in this section include use of frequently inferior methods of impurity/degradant analyses in lieu of frequently superior methods—for example, thin layer chromatography (TLC) instead of high-pressure liquid chromatography (HPLC) as well as interference from the excipient matrix, particularly if the specific method was developed using an earlier, and therefore different, formulation.

The *drug product stability* information will differ slightly from the drug substance stability information. For the drug product, the applicant should provide the following:

- Unstressed/stressed stability data
- Statistical analysis to establish consistency of data and expiration dating
- Expiration dating
- Postapproval stability commitment/protocol

Insufficient supporting stability data is a common deficiency as is an attempt to convert to a reduced stability protocol without a sufficient existing stability database. Another pitfall is overcommitment with regard to marketed stability studies.

For an NDA, the applicant should provide a list of all *drug product investigational formulations* used in clinical studies, along with the quantitative composition of each formulation. References to each pivotal clinical and bioavailability study and to the batch used should also be included.

Every NDA must contain either an environmental assessment (EA) or a claim for an exemption to the EA submission requirement. The regulation applies regardless of whether the product is manufactured in the United States or overseas. The EA, also called the environmental impact analysis report, includes an analysis of the manufacturing process and ultimate use of the drug product as well as a discussion of how the process and the drug product may affect the environment.

Under current regulations, the FDA grants categorical exclusions to most drugs and biologics as long as the application's approval will not increase the use of the active moiety, i.e., if the active moiety at the point of entry into the aquatic environment due to use at the fifth year of marketing will be below 1 part per billion (PPB).

Samples

In addition to the CMC information, the CMC technical section must include a commitment to submit samples to FDA laboratories for testing and validation of analytical methods. Actual samples are submitted only on FDA request. If samples are requested, the drug product, the drug substance, and the reference standards are all submitted.

Methods Validation Package

The final component of the CMC technical section is the methods validation package. The package must comprise the following:

- Specifications and test methods for each component used in the drug product
- Specifications and methods for the drug product
- Validation of test methods
- Names and addresses of component suppliers
- Names and addresses of the suppliers of the container closure system
- Names and addresses of contract facilities for manufacturing or testing

Nonclinical Pharmacology and Toxicology [21 CFR 314.50(d)(2)]

The second technical section of the NDA provides a description or summary of all animal and *in vitro* studies with the drug.

The *TOC* should clearly identify all studies not previously submitted with the IND.

This section includes a narrative *summary* of notable findings in all studies and a discussion of notable findings across the various studies. This discussion might include intra- and interspecies differences or similarities. A tabular display of data, and cross-references to individual study reports should be provided.

This section includes *individual study reports*, including pharmacology, toxicology, and ADME studies. For the pharmacology studies, the applicant should present data as follows:

1. Effects related to the therapeutic indication, such as the pharmacodynamic ED50 in dose-ranging studies and the mechanism of action (if known)
2. Secondary pharmacological actions in order of clinical importance as possible adverse effects or as ancillary therapeutic effects
3. Interactions with other drugs (or cross-reference the location of the information in any of the above subsections)

The toxicology information must include information on acute toxicity, multidose toxicity (including subchronic, chronic, and carcinogenicity) and special toxicity studies, as well as reproduction studies and mutagenicity studies.

This section presents toxicology data by intended route of administration in the following order:

1. Oral
2. Intravenous

3. Intramuscular
4. Interperitoneal
5. Subcutaneous
6. Inhalation
7. Topical
8. Other in vivo
9. In vitro

Data is provided first for males, followed by females, then groups.

For acute toxicity studies, the animal study data is presented in the following order:

1. Mouse
2. Rat
3. Hamster
4. Other rodent(s)
5. Rabbit
6. Dog
7. Monkey
8. Other nonrodent mammal(s)
9. Nonmammals

The ADME data is presented in the following order:

1. Absorption
2. Distribution (protein binding, tissue distribution, accumulation)
3. Metabolism (enzyme induction or inhibition)
4. Excretion (serum half-life)

When compiling the Nonclinical Pharmacology section, the applicant must identify the structural formula for all names by which the compound is referred. Similarly, all metabolites and reference compounds are identified by chemical name or structural formula. Batch or lot numbers of the test substance are included and all animal suppliers and animal strains used in the studies are specified. Reports of any studies used to determine safety should include good laboratory practice (GLP) statements per 21 CFR 314.50(d)(2)(v) and 21 CFR Part 58.

Human Pharmacokinetics and Bioavailability [21 CFR 314.50(d)(3)]

This technical section includes data from Phase I safety and tolerance studies in healthy volunteers and ADME studies.

The first element in this section is a *tabulated summary of studies* showing all in vivo biopharmaceutic studies performed; listed in descending order of importance.

This section includes a *summary of data and overall conclusions*. This summary addresses all bioavailability and pharmacokinetic data and conclusions. It should include a table of PK parameters, giving the values for the major parameters, such as the following:

- Peak concentration (Cmax)
- Area under the curve (AuC)
- Time to reach peak concentration (tmax)
- Elimination constant
- Distribution volume (Vd)
- Plasma and renal clearance
- Urinary excretion

Drug formulation information includes a list of all formulations used in clinical trials and *in vivo* bioavailability and PK studies. This section should also identify the studies in which each formulation was used. In addition, any significant manufacturing and formulation changes for the drug product that affected those batches used in bioavailability and PK studies should be noted.

This section also summarizes the *analytical methods* used in each *in vivo* biopharmaceutic study. It includes detailed information, such as sensitivity, linearity, specificity, and reproducibility of the analytical test methods used in each study.

This section should also provide *dissolution* data on each strength and dosage form for which an approval is sought. The applicant should include a comparative dissolution study with the lot in the in vivo biopharmaceutic study as well as a summary of the product's dissolution performance, dissolution method, and specifications.

This technical section must include *individual study reports* from any of five types of biopharmaceutic studies as described below.

Pilot or background studies are carried out in a small number of subjects to provide preliminary assessment of ADME information as a guide to the design of early clinical trials and definitive kinetic studies.

Bioavailability/bioequivalence studies include several types of studies. Bioavailability studies define the rate and extent of absorption relative to a reference dosage form, such as IV, solution or suspension. Bioequivalence studies compare pharmaceutical alternatives to establish equivalent extents and, where necessary, equivalent rates of absorption. Dosage strength equivalence studies show that equivalent doses of different dosage forms deliver the same amount of drug. For example, three doses of 100 mg is equivalent to a single 300-mg tablet.

Pharmacokinetic studies are designed to define the drug's time course and, where appropriate, major metabolite concentrations in the blood and other body compartments. With this type of study, it is critical to demonstrate the rate of drug absorption and delivery to systemic circulation and the rate of elimination of the drug through metabolic or excretory processes. Dose-dependent changes in kinetic parameters are of particular interest. Other information from PK studies may include the influence of demographic characteristics such as age, gender, or race; certain disease states (e.g., cirrhosis); or external factors such as meals or other drugs. The applicant should include information on studies that show drug binding to biological constituents such as plasma protein or red blood cells; studies performed in special patient populations (e.g., steroid-dependent patients), and studies performed under conditions of therapeutic use.

Other in vivo studies include any bioavailability studies that employ pharmacological or clinical measurements or endpoints in humans or animals. In addition, chemical analysis of body fluids in animals may be used when appropriate.

In vitro studies include studies designed to define the release rate of a drug substance from the dosage form. Such studies are conducted to characterize a dosage form and to assure consistent batch-to-batch behavior. Other *in vitro* studies may be conducted for further characterization of the drug moiety (e.g., protein binding). Batch analyses of testing of inactive ingredients and drug product are also included.

Microbiology [21 CFR 314.50(d)(4)]

The microbiology technical section is required only for anti-infective drug products.

Antimicrobial drugs differ from other classes of drugs in that they are designed to affect microbial physiology rather than patient physiology. *In vitro* and *in vivo* studies on the effects of the antimicrobial drug on the microorganism are critical in establishing the new drug's effectiveness, especially if the microorganism has the potential to develop, or has developed, resistance to other antimicrobial drugs. It is usually necessary to compare the microbiological testing of the new drug to other closely related antimicrobial products.

This section requires the following technical information and data:

1. A complete description of the biochemical basis of the drug's action on microbial physiology.
2. The drug's antimicrobial spectrum, which includes results of *in vitro* studies demonstrating the concentrations of the drug that are required for effective use.
3. A description of any known mechanisms of resistance to the drug with information or data of any known epidemiologic studies demonstrating prevalence to resistance factors.
4. Clinical microbiology laboratory methods, such as *in vitro* sensitivity discs, necessary to evaluate effective use of the drug.

Clinical Data [21 CFR 314.50(d)(5)]

This technical section of the NDA consists of 10 elements. The document's largest and most complex section, the clinical data and analyses are key to the FDA's understanding of the new drug's safety and effectiveness.

The first element in this section is a *list of investigators and list of INDs and NDAs*. The list of investigators should include all investigators who have used any dosage form. The list is alphabetized and notes each investigator's address, the type of study, the study identifier, and its location in the NDA. The section provides a list of all known INDs under which the drug, in any dosage form, has been studied. Any relevant NDA of which the applicant is aware is also included.

The next element is the *background/overview of clinical investigations*. This narrative should describe the general approach and rationale used in developing the clinical data. It should explain how information about the drug derived from clinical pharmacology studies led to critical features of the clinical studies. The narrative should support the basis for the design features of the clinical trials, such as number of patients, duration, selection criteria, and controls. The overview should provide references to FDA clinical guidelines, explaining any deviations from them, and reference any discussions between the FDA and the drug sponsor. The applicant should address the reason for selecting areas of special interest, such as demographics, gender, or drug interactions, and discuss any effectiveness or safety issues raised by other drugs in the same pharmacologic or therapeutic class. Finally, the applicant should answer any specific questions raised by the clinical trials for the study drug or by other similar drugs that were not answered in the clinical program.

The *clinical pharmacology* section should include ADME studies, pharmacodynamic dose range, and dose response studies, and any other studies of the drug's action. The format and order of presentation is as follows:

1. A table of all studies grouped by study type. The investigators, study numbers, start date, and location of the report in the NDA are provided.
2. For each group of studies, a brief synopsis of each study
3. An overall summary of the clinical pharmacology data

For the *controlled clinical trials* section, provide the following material in the order presented below:

1. A table of all studies
2. Full clinical trial reports of all controlled studies in the following order:
   i. Completed studies (U.S. studies followed by non-U.S. studies and any published trials)
   ii. Ongoing studies with interim results (same order as above)
   iii. Incomplete or discontinued studies (same order as above)

3. Full reports of dose-comparison concurrent control studies, followed by those for "no-treatment" concurrent control, active control studies, and historical control studies.

The above material may be followed by an optional summary of all of the controlled clinical studies, but it is preferable to include the results in the integrated summaries elsewhere at the end of the clinical data section.

Uncontrolled clinical trials generally do not contribute substantial evidence for the effectiveness of a drug. They may be used to provide support for controlled studies and to provide critical safety information. This section should include a table of all studies. Full reports of studies are grouped according to completeness and availability of Case Report Forms (CRFs). The summary of these studies is incorporated into the integrated summaries.

The *other studies and information* section should include a description and analysis of any additional information that the applicant has obtained from any source, foreign or domestic, that is relevant to evaluating the product's safety and effectiveness. It should include a table of all studies followed by reports of other controlled and uncontrolled studies. These should be followed by information on commercial marketing experience and foreign regulatory actions, including

- list of countries in which the drug has been approved;
- details of any rejected registrations;
- copies of approved labeling (package inserts) from major regions such as Europe, Canada, Australia, New Zealand, and Japan; and
- any other reports from the literature not provided elsewhere in the NDA.

Key sections of the NDA are the ISE and ISS, the integrated summary of effectiveness data, and the integrated summary of safety data, respectively. In response to the problems sponsors seem to have in submitting these sections, FDA has issued a proposed draft guidance to clarify agency thinking and expectations. As of this printing, the proposed guidance remains in draft form; however, it contains valuable insight:

> The word *summary* in the terms *integrated summary of effectiveness* and *integrated summary of safety* has caused confusion for companies submitting applications in the CTD format, as it suggests a reference to the abbreviated overview documents that are placed in Module 2 of an application in the CTD format. However, the ISE and ISS are not summaries but rather detailed integrated analyses of all relevant data from the clinical study reports that belong in Module 5.2 The FDA considers the ISE and ISS critical components of the clinical efficacy and safety portions of a marketing or licensing application. Therefore, the ISE and ISS are required in applications submitted to the FDA in accordance with the regulations for NDA submissions (21 CFR 314.50(d)(5)(v) and

21 CFR 314.50(d)(5)(vi)(a), respectively). Although there are no corresponding regulations requiring an ISE or ISS for BLA submissions, applicants are encouraged to provide these analyses.

The guidance then continues:

This guidance focuses on where to place ISE and ISS documents within the structure of the CTD or eCTD. It does not outline in detail the content for the ISE and ISS. The content will be addressed in future guidances.[24]

The purpose of the *Integrated Summary of Effectiveness* data is to demonstrate substantial evidence of effectiveness for each claimed indication. It should also include a "summary" of evidence supporting the dosage and administration section of the labeling, including the dosage and dose interval recommended, and evidence regarding individualization of dosing and any need for dosage modifications for specific subgroups. It should include a table of all studies.

The narrative should first identify the adequate and well-controlled studies. Next, it should compare and analyze the results of all controlled trials. Data should only be pooled across similar studies. If the studies do not support the anticipated conclusions, the discrepancy must be explained. Uncontrolled studies must be discussed to the extent that they contribute supportive evidence of effectiveness.

The applicant is to provide an integrated summary and analysis of all data relevant to the relationship of dose response or blood level response to effectiveness, including data from animal, pharmacokinetic, pharmacodynamic, controlled, and uncontrolled studies. The applicant must explain how this information comes to bear on dose selection, dose interval, starting and maximal dosing, method of dose titration, and any other instructions in the proposed labeling. The effectiveness summary should also include an analysis of responses in subsets of patients. The ISE addresses drug-demographic, drug-drug and drug-disease interactions and describes any evidence of long-term effectiveness, tolerance, and withdrawal effects.

The *Integrated Summary of Safety information* incorporates safety data from all sources, including pertinent animal data, clinical studies, and foreign marketing experience. The database from which every analysis is derived must be carefully defined.

This section requires a table of all studies and extent-of-exposure tables. The latter must include patient exposure by time period, by gender, by other subgroups, and by dose.

The applicant must also describe the demographics and other characteristics of the entire drug-exposed population and also of logical groups of studies.

The section also includes a narrative discussion of adverse events in all studies, supported with tabulations and analyses. Studies (i.e., controlled, similar

---

[24] See www.fda.gov/cder/guidance/7621dft.pdf [dated 07-2-2007].

duration, foreign/domestic) are grouped to determine event rates. Additionally, adverse events are grouped by body system. The section will analyze the adverse events to compare treatment and control rates, relationship to the study drug, dose, duration of treatment, cumulative dose, demographics, and other variables. The summary will also display and analyze deaths and dropouts due to adverse events and other serious events and evaluate them in terms of their relationship to the study drug.

The applicant presents an analysis of clinical laboratory data, evaluating clinically significant abnormalities. Adverse events and laboratory abnormalities from sources other than clinical trials are also reported.

The section includes a summary of any animal data pertinent to human safety, emphasizing carcinogenicity and reproductive toxicology results, and an integrated analysis of data from animal and human studies that show any relationship between dose response and adverse events.

The section includes a discussion of drug-drug interactions, including any potential interactions, from any source; any drug-demographic or drug-disease interactions are also summarized.

Any pharmacologic effects of the drug other than the property of principal interest must be discussed, as should long-term effects and data from any long-term studies. Summarize specific studies regarding any evidence of withdrawal effects.

Drug abuse and overdosage information is required if the drug has potential for abuse. In this section, the applicant should describe and analyze studies or information related to abuse of the drug and include a proposal for scheduling under the Controlled Substances Act.

Ordinarily the *integrated summary of benefits and risks of the drug* recapitulates the evidence for effectiveness and safety. This section can also include information on the presence of a particularly severe known or potential human toxicity as well as a positive, or possibly positive, carcinogenicity finding. It may include information that indicates marginal or inconsistent effectiveness. It may also point to a particularly limited database or the use of surrogate endpoints.

Safety Update Reports [21 CFR 314.50(d)(7)]

A pending application must be updated when new safety data become available that could affect any of the following:

- Statements in draft labeling
- Contraindications
- Warnings
- Precautions
- AEs

Safety update reports are not to be used to submit any new final reports that may impact FDA review time, unless the FDA agrees at the pre-NDA meeting that it will accept the reports in this manner.

Safety updates are submitted four months (120 days) after the initial application, following the receipt of an approval letter and at any other time that the FDA requests such an update.

Statistics [21 CFR 314.50(d)(6)]

This technical section includes descriptions and documentation of the statistical analyses performed to evaluate the controlled clinical trials and other safety information. It must include copies of

- all controlled clinical trial reports,
- integrated efficacy and safety summaries, and
- integrated summary of risks and benefits.

Pediatric Use [21 CFR 314.50(d)(7)]

The NDA should contain a section describing the investigation of the drug for use in pediatric populations. Applicants should include an integrated summary of clinical and non-clinical information that is relevant to the safety and effectiveness, and benefits and risks of the drug in pediatric populations.[*] Applicants may request a waiver from this requirement on the basis of the proposed indication or stage of the drug's development.

Case Report Form Tabulations [21 CFR 314.50(f)(1)]

This section must include complete tabulations for each patient from every adequately or well-controlled Phase II and Phase III efficacy study and from every Phase I clinical pharmacology study. It also must include tabulations of safety data from *all* clinical studies. Routine submission of data from uncontrolled studies is not required.

Note that data listings are most often placed with the final reports in each section rather than with the CRF tabulations.

Case Report Forms [21 CFR 314.50(f)(2)]

It is necessary to include the complete CRF for each patient who died during a clinical study and for any patients who were dropped from the study because of an AE, regardless of whether the AE is considered to be related to the study drug, even if the patient was receiving a placebo or comparative drug.

Additional CRFs must be provided at the request of the FDA.

---

[*] www.accessdata.fda.gov/scripts/cfdoes/cfcfr/CFRSearch.cfm.

FORMAT AND PREPARATION OF THE NDA

The presentation and organization of the NDA can be instrumental in gaining a positive approval decision from the FDA. As discussed in the previous section of this chapter, an NDA contains vast amounts of complex information and data that must be analyzed by the FDA before an approval decision can be made. By presenting the information and data in a clear and organized manner, an applicant can direct the reviewer to the required information that will support the claims contained in the proposed labeling and possibly decrease the time needed to review the application. Therefore, an applicant should use the pre-NDA meeting to concur with the reviewing division on the format and media that will be used to prepare the NDA.

There is no regulation that requires the submission of an NDA in any particular format. In the past, most NDAs were large paper submissions organized according to the sections described in the regulations. To help applicants prepare their submissions, the FDA published numerous guidance documents regarding the format, assembly, content, and submission of the NDA. These documents are located on the FDA Web site, http://www.fda.gov/cder/regulatory/applications/nda.htm#FDA%20Guidances. Applicants can still prepare and submit their NDA in this manner; however, the FDA now strongly recommends that an applicant prepare the NDA according to the format of the common technical document (CTD).

The Common Technical Document

The CTD is an agreed upon format for the preparation of a well organized application that will be submitted to regulatory authorities to support the registration of pharmaceuticals for human use. This format was developed and agreed upon by the parties involved with the International Conference on Harmonization of Technical Requirements for Registration of Pharmaceuticals for Human Use (ICH). The ICH is a joint initiative involving both regulators and research-based industry representatives of the European Union, Japan, and the United States in scientific and technical discussions of the testing procedures required to assess and ensure the safety, quality, and efficacy of medicines.[25]

The initial goal of the ICH initiative was to harmonize the technical requirements for the registration of pharmaceuticals. By establishing the CTD format, the organization of the technical requirement sections in the CTD has now been harmonized. It is important for applicants to understand that the CTD format provides guidance on the organization of the documents in the submission. The content of the CTD is determined by regulations and discussions with regional regulatory authorities. In our case, a sponsor may decide to use the CTD format, but the contents of the NDA are dictated by the regulations discussed earlier, especially 21 CFR Part 314.

---

[25] See http://www.ich.org/cache/compo/276-254-1.html.

The CTD Triangle

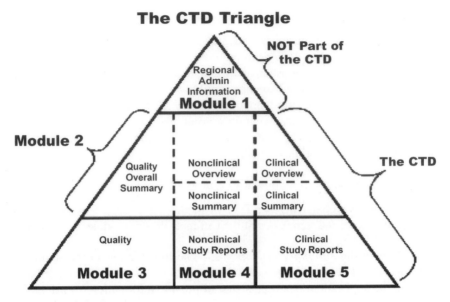

Figure 2 The CTD triangle.

The use of the CTD format assists applicants with the preparation of global submissions. By eliminating the need to prepare multiple region-specific submissions, applicants can save valuable resources and reduce costs. In addition, the use of the CTD format can prevent the omission of critical data or analyses that could cause the FDA to refuse to file the application. This common format also facilitates the exchange of regulatory information between regulatory authorities.

The CTD format and organization are outlined in the following four guidance documents that were issued by the FDA. M4: Organization of the CTD;[26] M4E: The CTD—Efficacy;[27] M4Q: the CTD—Quality;[28] and M4S: the CTD—Safety.[29]

The organization of the CTD format is depicted in Figure 2,[30] the CTD Triangle.

The CTD format organizes the NDA submission into five separate modules. Module 1 is not part of the CTD because it is not harmonized. The contents of this module differ because it contains region-specific information. Modules 2 through 5 are harmonized and contain the technical information required in a registration submission. The following is a brief discussion of each module.

---

[26] See www.fda.gov/cder/guidance/6673fnl.htm; December 2004, Rev. 3.

[27] See www.fda.gov/cder/guidance/4539E.htm.

[28] See www.fda.gov/cder/guidance/4539Q.htm.

[29] See www.fda.gov/cder/guidance/4539S.htm.

[30] See www.fda.gov/cder/present/DIA62002/molzon/sld006.htm.

Module 1: Administrative and Prescribing Information

For an NDA submission in the United States, this module contains all of the administrative and labeling documents required for the submission. This includes all application forms and administrative documents discussed earlier in this chapter. In addition, all of the proposed labeling would be included in this module such as the prescribing information, annotated labeling, and packaging labels for the drug. Module 1 should also contain a comprehensive TOC and the Index for the entire submission. The TOC should list all documents contained in the submission and their location.

Module 2 Common Technical Document Summaries

Module 2 contains a comprehensive TOC of modules 2 through 5 as well as the following overviews and summaries of the technical data in modules 3 through 5.

Introduction to the summary documents. The introduction to the summary documents should be a one page general introduction about the pharmaceutical product in the application. Applicants should provide information regarding the pharmacologic class, mode of action, and proposed clinical use of the drug.

Quality overall summary. The quality overall summary should provide the reviewer with an overview of the CMC information contained in module 3. The summary should not restate the detailed CMC information contained in module 3. Instead, the summary should address key parameters of the product and discuss how the CMC information in module 3 relates to the other modules in the submission.[31]

Nonclinical overview. The nonclinical overview should provide an interpretation of the data, the clinical relevance of the findings cross-linked to the quality aspects of the pharmaceutical, and the implications of the nonclinical findings for the safe use of the pharmaceutical.[32]

Nonclinical written and tabulated summaries. The nonclinical written and tabulated summaries should provide a comprehensive, factual synopsis of the nonclinical data.[32]

Clinical overview. The clinical overview should provide a succinct discussion and interpretation of the clinical findings that support the application together with any other relevant information such as pertinent animal data or product quality issues that may have clinical implications.[33]

---

[31] Guidance for Industry M4Q: The CTD—Quality.

[32] Guidance for Industry M4Q: The CTD—Safety.

[33] Guidance for Industry M4Q: The CTD—Efficacy.

Clinical summary The clinical summary should provide a detailed factual summarization of the clinical information in the application.[34]

Module 3 Quality

Module 3 contains the detailed technical information regarding CMC information. This module contains a TOC for module 3 only, detailed information regarding the drug substance and drug product, and literature references.

Module 4 Nonclinical Study Reports

Module 4 contains a TOC for module 4 only, nonclinical study reports contained in the application, and literature references.

Module 5 Clinical Study Reports

Module 5 contains a TOC for module 5 only and a tabular listing of all clinical studies, clinical study reports, and literature references.

Mapping the Content of the NDA to the CTD Format

The required content of an NDA, as determined by U.S. regulations, can be easily mapped to the CTD format. Table 1 lists the location of regulatory requirements for an NDA in relationship to the CTD modules.[35]

Electronic Submissions

The preparation of an NDA in electronic format provides many advantages to the applicant as well as the review team at the FDA. An electronic file can be stored and sent to the FDA on compact discs, magnetic tapes, or via a web interface. More importantly, an electronic NDA can decrease the amount of time required to review an application because the information is hyperlinked throughout the application, and data sets can be analyzed using software at the FDA. With the implementation of mandatory review timelines by PDUFA, it is obvious why the agency would prefer the submission of an NDA as an electronic file that follows the format of the CTD.

In addition to harmonizing the CTD format, the ICH initiative has developed specifications for the electronic common technical document (eCTD). The eCTD is defined as an interface for industry-to-agency transfer of regulatory information while at the same time taking into consideration the facilitation of the creation, review, life-cycle management, and archival of the electronic submission.[36] The

---

[34] ibid.

[35] Guidance for Industry: Submitting Marketing Applications According to the ICH-CTD Format— General Considerations.

[36] ICH M2 EWG: Electronic common technical document specification.

Table 1 Location of NDA Requirements in Relation to the CTD Modules[37]

NDA requirement per 21 CFR 314.50	CTD module
(a) application form	Module 1
(c)(2)(i) annotated text of proposed labeling	
(d)(1)(v) statement of field copy	
(e) samples and labeling	
(h) patent information	
(i) patent certification	
(j) claimed exclusivity	
(k) financial certification or disclosure	
(b) comprehensive TOC	Module 2
(c) summaries	
(d)(5)(vii) abuse potential	
(d)(1) CMC	Module 3
(d)(2) nonclinical pharmtox	Module 4
(d)(3) human pharmacokinetics	Module 5
(d)(4) microbiology	
(d)(5) clinical data	
(d)(6) statistical section	
(d)(7) pediatric use	
(f) CRF and CRT	

Abbreviations: TOC, table of content; CMC, chemistry, manufacturing, and controls; CRF, case report forms; CRT, case report tabulations.

specifications incorporate the use of Extensible Markup Language (XML) technology and document type definitions to define the overall structure of the document. The use of the XML backbone for the submission constitutes a comprehensive TOC and provides corresponding navigation aids. In addition, the technology manages the metadata for the entire submission and each document. The use of this technology allows the FDA to manage the life cycle of the NDA over long periods of time by replacing documents or modules within the NDA.

As of January 2008, an applicant who plans to submit an electronic CTD to the FDA must submit the application according to the specifications outlined in the ICH M2 EWG, electronic common technical document specification. It is essential that the applicant discuss the preparation of an electronic file with the FDA prior to submission, preferably during the pre-NDA meeting.

SUBMISSION AND REVIEW OF THE NDA

Once the NDA is complete, the applicant needs to prepare archival, review, and field copies of the application for submission to the FDA.

[37] See www.fda.gov/CBER/gdlns/mrktapich.htm Appendix B.

The *archival copy* contains all sections of the NDA, including the cover letter, Form FDA-356h, the administrative sections, a comprehensive NDA index, and all technical sections. It must contain four copies of the Labeling section. It must contain three additional copies of the CMC and Methods Validation Package in a separate binder. The archival copy is the only copy that contains the Case Report Tabulation and Case Report Forms.

The *review copy* contains the technical sections of NDA, each packaged for reviewers in the corresponding technical disciplines. In addition to the appropriate technical section, each review copy also includes the cover letter, Form FDA-356h, the administrative sections, and the comprehensive NDA index as well as an individual TOC, the labeling section and the application summary.

The *field copy* has been required since 1993 for use by FDA inspectors during preapproval facilities inspections. It includes the cover letter and Form FDA-356h, the administrative sections, and the comprehensive NDA index as well as an individual TOC, the Labeling section, the Application Summary, and the CMC and Methods Validation Package.

An applicant that submits an NDA electronically may only need to submit the archival copy since the reviewers and the local FDA office will have access to the electronic file. Applicants should address this question with their project manager at the FDA prior to submitting their NDA.

PDUFA Fee

While the archival, review, and field copies of the application are being prepared, the applicant should arrange to make payment of the PDUFA user fee. The applicant initiates this process by completing and submitting a Form FDA 3397 online at the FDA Web site. This form gathers the minimum information about the applicant and the content of the NDA. This information is used to track the payment of the NDA submission and determine the amount of the user fee. Once submitted, the system provides the applicant with a completed Form FDA 3397 for inclusion in the NDA. The form will list the amount of the user fee and a user fee payment identification number. This identification number should be referenced on the cover letter of the NDA submission and with the payment of the user fee. It is important for applicants to coordinate payment of the user fee with the submission of the NDA because the FDA cannot begin its review of the NDA unless the user fee has been paid.

With the user fee paid and the submission copies complete, the applicant is ready to submit the NDA to the FDA for review. The application is sent to the controlled document room for processing and recording. Once the application is received by the controlled document room, the review clock, as mandated by PDUFA, begins.

Review of the NDA

As discussed earlier in the chapter, once the review clock is initiated for the NDA, the FDA has 60 days to decide whether or not to "file" it for review. The

controlled document room sends the NDA to the reviewing Division for evaluation. The Division will send the applicant a letter acknowledging the receipt of
the NDA. The letter will contain the NDA number, the project manager's contact
information, and the receipt date of the NDA. The project manager will perform
a preliminary review of the application to ensure that it is complete. If deficiencies are found, the Division can issue a refusal to file letter notifying the
applicant of the deficiencies. The Division may request the applicant to correct
minor deficiencies while the review of the application continues.

If the NDA passes this preliminary review, the project manager will forward the appropriate sections of the NDA to the different members of the review
team. This team may include clinicians, pharmacokineticists, pharmacologists,
toxicologists, statisticians, microbiologists, and chemists. Each member will
review his technical section to ensure that the correct information has been
included in the NDA. If a reviewer determines that the application is incomplete,
for example, some required studies may be missing,[38] the Division can refuse to
file the application. The purpose of this second review, which usually occurs
within 45 days of receiving the NDA, is meant to justify formal review of the
application. The Division will notify the applicant within 60 days of receiving
the NDA if it will issue a refusal to file letter or accept the NDA for formal
review.

During the formal review of the NDA, the review team attempts to confirm
and validate the sponsor's conclusion that a drug is safe and effective for its
proposed use.[39] In addition, the reviewing Division will schedule preapproval
inspections of drug manufacturing sites and clinical trial sites as needed. These
inspections are needed to verify the information contained in the NDA and to
evaluate compliance with Good Manufacturing Practices and Good Clinical
Practices. Deficiencies found during an inspection can delay approval of the
NDA or have negative impact on the approval decision.

In order to support the review and inspection activities of the FDA, the
applicant should assemble a response team that can respond to agency questions
and requests for additional information. Quick responses by the applicant will
facilitate the review of the application. This team would also be available to meet
with the reviewing Division as requested. The Division may schedule a post-
NDA meeting which provides the applicant with the opportunity to present the
NDA to the review staff while answering any outstanding questions.

Once the technical review of the application is complete, each member of
the review team will prepare a written evaluation of their section of the NDA. At
this time, the reviewers can begin to evaluate the text in the proposed labeling
as this text must be justified by the data and information submitted in the NDA.
If the reviewing Division has an issue with the proposed labeling, it will
negotiate revised text for the label with the applicant.

---

[38] See www.fda.gov/fdac/special/testtubetopatient/drugreview.html.

[39] See www.fda.gov/cder/handbook/acceprvi.htm.

Once the written evaluations of the NDA, the site inspections, and the product label negotiations are complete, the reviewers and their supervisors will make one of the following recommendations regarding the NDA. A recommendation for "approval" means that the drug is ready to be marketed, under the provisions of the Food, Drug, and Cosmetic Act. If the recommendation is "approvable," the applicant may need to resolve additional issues before it can market the drug. If the recommendation is nonapprovable, then the drug cannot be marketed, and the review team will need to justify this recommendation.

All of the review information and a draft action letter, noting the recommendation by the review team, are sent to the Division Director for review. The Division Director will make the final decision regarding approval of the application and issue an action letter to the applicant regarding the decision.

MAINTENANCE OF THE NDA

After an NDA receives approval, the applicant must conduct extensive post-marketing surveillance of the drug to monitor safety. Applicants are required to review all of the adverse drug experience (ADE) information that they receive about their drug from any source such as postmarketing clinical investigations, commercial marketing experience, postmarketing epidemiological/surveillance studies or reports in scientific papers.

Postmarketing 15-Day Alert Reports

For reports of ADEs that are both serious and unexpected, the applicant must report the ADE to the FDA within 15 days of receiving the information. The report is sent to the FDA electronically or on paper using a FDA Form 3500A, also known as a MedWatch form.

An ADE is serious if it results in any of the following outcomes: death, a life-threatening ADE, inpatient hospitalization or prolongation of existing hospitalization, a persistent or significant disability/incapacity, or a congenital anomaly/birth defect. These events can occur at any dose. An ADE is unexpected if it is not listed in the current labeling of the product.

Postmarketing 15-Day Alert Reports Follow-up

Applicants are required investigate the ADEs that are the subject of a 15-day report and provide follow-up information to the FDA within 15 days of receiving the new information.

Periodic Adverse Drug Experience Reports

Following the approval of an NDA application, an applicant is required to submit a periodic ADE report. This report is submitted quarterly for the first three years after approval and then at annual intervals. This report contains all ADEs not reported as a 15-day alert report during the reporting period. Periodic reporting does not apply to reports from postmarketing studies, reports in scientific literature, or reports from foreign marketing experience.

NDA Annual Report

Within 60 days of the anniversary of the NDA approval, the applicant is required to submit an NDA annual report. The content of this report is defined in 21 CFR 314.81. The purpose of the report is to provide the FDA with an update of any new information about the drug, the status of clinical and nonclinical development, and product labeling changes, thereby preserving the marketing approval.

CONCLUSION

The NDA is the capstone of drug development. It is a process that deserves intense scrutiny; it balances the need for drugs whose benefits outweigh the risks of their side effects. The public hopes that the agency "gets it right"; but ultimately, the decisions are reflective of the science, the data, and the uncertainties presented by the human condition.

As new discoveries and technologies permit new therapies and approaches to curing, mitigating, and diagnosing disease and the public demand for even more rapid access to safe medications, increases, we can anticipate that the rules and regulations governing the agency will continue to evolve.

DEPARTMENT OF HEALTH AND HUMAN SERVICES
FOOD AND DRUG ADMINISTRATION

APPLICATION TO MARKET A NEW DRUG, BIOLOGIC, OR AN ANTIBIOTIC DRUG FOR HUMAN USE
(Title 21, Code of Federal Regulations, Parts 314 & 601)

Form Approved: OMB No. 0910-0338
Expiration Date: September 30, 2008
See OMB Statement on page 2.

FOR FDA USE ONLY

APPLICATION NUMBER

APPLICANT INFORMATION

NAME OF APPLICANT	DATE OF SUBMISSION
TELEPHONE NO. (Include Area Code)	FACSIMILE (FAX) Number (Include Area Code)
APPLICANT ADDRESS (Number, Street, City, State, Country, ZIP Code or Mail Code, and U.S. License number if previously issued):	AUTHORIZED U.S. AGENT NAME & ADDRESS (Number, Street, City, State, ZIP Code, telephone & FAX number) IF APPLICABLE

PRODUCT DESCRIPTION

NEW DRUG OR ANTIBIOTIC APPLICATION NUMBER, OR BIOLOGICS LICENSE APPLICATION NUMBER (If previously issued)

ESTABLISHED NAME (e.g., Proper name, USP/USAN name)	PROPRIETARY NAME (trade name) IF ANY
CHEMICAL/BIOCHEMICAL/BLOOD PRODUCT NAME (if any)	CODE NAME (if any)
DOSAGE FORM: / STRENGTHS:	ROUTE OF ADMINISTRATION:

(PROPOSED) INDICATION(S) FOR USE:

APPLICATION DESCRIPTION

APPLICATION TYPE *(check one)* ☐ NEW DRUG APPLICATION (NDA, 21 CFR 314.50) ☐ ABBREVIATED NEW DRUG APPLICATION (ANDA, 21 CFR 314.94)
☐ BIOLOGICS LICENSE APPLICATION (BLA, 21 CFR Part 601)

IF AN NDA, IDENTIFY THE APPROPRIATE TYPE ☐ 505 (b)(1) ☐ 505 (b)(2)

IF AN ANDA, OR 505(b)(2), IDENTIFY THE REFERENCE LISTED DRUG PRODUCT THAT IS THE BASIS FOR THE SUBMISSION

Name of Drug _____ Holder of Approved Application _____

TYPE OF SUBMISSION (check one) ☐ ORIGINAL APPLICATION ☐ AMENDMENT TO A PENDING APPLICATION ☐ RESUBMISSION
☐ PRESUBMISSION ☐ ANNUAL REPORT ☐ ESTABLISHMENT DESCRIPTION SUPPLEMENT ☐ EFFICACY SUPPLEMENT
☐ LABELING SUPPLEMENT ☐ CHEMISTRY MANUFACTURING AND CONTROLS SUPPLEMENT ☐ OTHER

IF A SUBMISSION OF PARTIAL APPLICATION, PROVIDE LETTER DATE OF AGREEMENT TO PARTIAL SUBMISSION: _____

IF A SUPPLEMENT, IDENTIFY THE APPROPRIATE CATEGORY ☐ CBE ☐ CBE-30 ☐ Prior Approval (PA)

REASON FOR SUBMISSION

PROPOSED MARKETING STATUS (check one) ☐ PRESCRIPTION PRODUCT (Rx) ☐ OVER THE COUNTER PRODUCT (OTC)

NUMBER OF VOLUMES SUBMITTED THIS APPLICATION IS ☐ PAPER ☐ PAPER AND ELECTRONIC ☐ ELECTRONIC

ESTABLISHMENT INFORMATION (Full establishment information should be provided in the body of the Application.)
Provide locations of all manufacturing, packaging and control sites for drug substance and drug product (continuation sheets may be used if necessary). Include name, address, contact, telephone number, registration number (CFN), DMF number, and manufacturing steps and/or type of testing (e.g. Final dosage form, Stability testing) conducted at the site. Please indicate whether the site is ready for inspection or, if not, when it will be ready.

Cross References (list related License Applications, INDs, NDAs, PMAs, 510(k)s, IDEs, BMFs, and DMFs referenced in the current application)

This application contains the following items: *(Check all that apply)*

- ☐ 1. Index
- ☐ 2. Labeling *(check one)* ☐ Draft Labeling ☐ Final Printed Labeling
- ☐ 3. Summary (21 CFR 314.50 (c))
- ☐ 4. Chemistry section
- ☐   A. Chemistry, manufacturing, and controls information (e.g., 21 CFR 314.50(d)(1); 21 CFR 601.2)
- ☐   B. Samples (21 CFR 314.50 (e)(1); 21 CFR 601.2 (a)) (Submit only upon FDA's request)
- ☐   C. Methods validation package (e.g., 21 CFR 314.50(e)(2)(i); 21 CFR 601.2)
- ☐ 5. Nonclinical pharmacology and toxicology section (e.g., 21 CFR 314.50(d)(2); 21 CFR 601.2)
- ☐ 6. Human pharmacokinetics and bioavailability section (e.g., 21 CFR 314.50(d)(3); 21 CFR 601.2)
- ☐ 7. Clinical Microbiology (e.g., 21 CFR 314.50(d)(4))
- ☐ 8. Clinical data section (e.g., 21 CFR 314.50(d)(5); 21 CFR 601.2)
- ☐ 9. Safety update report (e.g., 21 CFR 314.50(d)(5)(vi)(b); 21 CFR 601.2)
- ☐ 10. Statistical section (e.g., 21 CFR 314.50(d)(6); 21 CFR 601.2)
- ☐ 11. Case report tabulations (e.g., 21 CFR 314.50(f)(1); 21 CFR 601.2)
- ☐ 12. Case report forms (e.g., 21 CFR 314.50 (f)(2); 21 CFR 601.2)
- ☐ 13. Patent information on any patent which claims the drug (21 U.S.C. 355(b) or (c))
- ☐ 14. A patent certification with respect to any patent which claims the drug (21 U.S.C. 355 (b)(2) or (j)(2)(A))
- ☐ 15. Establishment description (21 CFR Part 600, if applicable)
- ☐ 16. Debarment certification (FD&C Act 306 (k)(1))
- ☐ 17. Field copy certification (21 CFR 314.50 (l)(3))
- ☐ 18. User Fee Cover Sheet (Form FDA 3397)
- ☐ 19. Financial Information (21 CFR Part 54)
- ☐ 20. OTHER *(Specify)*

CERTIFICATION

I agree to update this application with new safety information about the product that may reasonably affect the statement of contraindications, warnings, precautions, or adverse reactions in the draft labeling. I agree to submit safety update reports as provided for by regulation or as requested by FDA. If this application is approved, I agree to comply with all applicable laws and regulations that apply to approved applications, including, but not limited to the following:

1. Good manufacturing practice regulations in 21 CFR Parts 210, 211 or applicable regulations, Parts 606, and/or 820.
2. Biological establishment standards in 21 CFR Part 600.
3. Labeling regulations in 21 CFR Parts 201, 606, 610, 660, and/or 809.
4. In the case of a prescription drug or biological product, prescription drug advertising regulations in 21 CFR Part 202.
5. Regulations on making changes in application in FD&C Act section 506A, 21 CFR 314.71, 314.72, 314.97, 314.99, and 601.12.
6. Regulations on Reports in 21 CFR 314.80, 314.81, 600.80, and 600.81.
7. Local, state and Federal environmental impact laws.

If this application applies to a drug product that FDA has proposed for scheduling under the Controlled Substances Act, I agree not to market the product until the Drug Enforcement Administration makes a final scheduling decision.
The data and information in this submission have been reviewed and, to the best of my knowledge are certified to be true and accurate.
Warning: A willfully false statement is a criminal offense, U.S. Code, title 18, section 1001.

SIGNATURE OF RESPONSIBLE OFFICIAL OR AGENT	TYPED NAME AND TITLE	DATE:

ADDRESS *(Street, City, State, and ZIP Code)*	Telephone Number ( )

Public reporting burden for this collection of information is estimated to average 24 hours per response, including the time for reviewing instructions, searching existing data sources, gathering and maintaining the data needed, and completing and reviewing the collection of information. Send comments regarding this burden estimate or any other aspect of this collection of information, including suggestions for reducing this burden to:

Department of Health and Human Services
Food and Drug Administration
Center for Drug Evaluation and Research
Central Document Room
5901-B Ammendale Road
Belleville, MD 20705-1266

Department of Health and Human Services
Food and Drug Administration
Center for Biologics Evaluation and Research (HFM-99)
1401 Rockville Pike
Rockville, MD 20852-1448

An agency may not conduct or sponsor, and a person is not required to respond to, a collection of information unless it displays a currently valid OMB control number.

4

Meeting with the FDA

Alberto Grignolo
PAREXEL Consulting, Lowell, Massachusetts, U.S.A.

INTRODUCTION

Face-to-face meetings with the Food and Drug Administration (FDA) are a critical component of the regulatory review and approval process for new prescription drugs, biologics, and medical devices. These direct exchanges between agency personnel and company scientists provide a forum for the sharing of information that is essential to demonstrating the safety, efficacy, and quality of a product to the "FDA's satisfaction." The purpose of this chapter is to illustrate the types and objectives of various meetings with the FDA and to highlight some of the critical success factors and pitfalls associated with Agency interactions. While the main focus of the chapter is on drugs, the principles apply broadly to all meetings with the FDA.

Successful meetings with the FDA depend on three key factors: good science and good medicine, regulatory knowledge, and sound management of the meeting process. While a pharmaceutical product's approval is ultimately determined by the strength and adequacy of its scientific data, the way a sponsor interacts with the FDA throughout the lengthy drug development and regulatory review process can spell the difference between a relatively smooth, timely approval and a costly delay or rejection of an application. A product's chances for approval can be substantially increased if the sponsor manages the meeting process in a way that presents the scientific data effectively and facilitates reaching consensus on key issues.

If handled properly, these meetings can actually reduce the approval time for a new product. A study by the Tufts Center for the Study of Drug Development indicated that companies that hold effective pre-IND and end-of-phase II meetings with the FDA achieve shorter clinical development times.[1] This is a significant finding for the highly competitive pharmaceutical industry, where time to market is a crucial success factor. By employing the right resources and the right approach—and avoiding some common pitfalls—sponsors can take full advantage of the opportunities presented by FDA meetings to expedite the review process and help their products reach the market more quickly.

TYPES OF FDA MEETINGS

The purpose of meeting with the FDA and its review divisions is to present proposals, provide answers, and resolve scientific and technical issues that arise concerning the development of a pharmaceutical product at various stages of the regulatory review process. These meetings also mark major development milestones, helping to determine if a product will be able to move forward to the next stage. The most important types of FDA meetings are:

Pre-IND Meetings

In these meetings, a sponsor presents characterization, manufacturing and non-clinical test data, and other information and discusses the initial plan and protocols for human clinical trials. The goal of these meetings is to receive the FDA feedback on the proposed studies and to reach agreement on what information the sponsor needs to submit in the IND application so that it is likely to be placed on active status by the FDA (rather than being placed "on hold" because of safety concerns on the part of the Agency). While the agency (in particular the review division) will not commit to not placing the IND on hold until the IND is submitted by the sponsor, it may be willing to state that at the time of the pre-IND Meeting there appear to be no issues that would require a hold.

End-of-Phase II Meetings

These are, perhaps, the most critical regulatory meetings during the development process. The sponsor is expected to provide "proof of concept" for the product through early efficacy data and other information demonstrating that the drug is performing a desired function. Equally important, phase III trial designs are discussed during these meetings, including the types of information on

---

[1] DiMasi JA, Manocchia M. Initiatives to speed new drug development and regulatory review: the impact of FDA-sponsor conferences. Drug Inf J 1997; 31:771–788.

indications, dosing, safety, and manufacturing that the FDA would expect to see in a "strong" new drug application (NDA) or biologics license application (BLA).

Special Protocol and Ad Hoc Technical Meetings

These are held to discuss and resolve specific technical issues that arise during drug development, including detailed review of key clinical protocols, discussion of challenging manufacturing issues, or review of carcinogenicity study protocols.

Pre-NDA/BLA Meetings

In these meetings, a sponsor and the FDA typically discuss process-oriented issues concerning an upcoming application—how the data will be presented and how the application will be organized.

Advisory Committee Meetings

These meetings, which take place as a public forum after an NDA/BLA submission, are conducted for certain products when the FDA wants to obtain the advice of academic, medical, and other external experts about the approvability of an application. Essentially, the FDA convenes a panel of experts to hold public meetings and receive the recommendations of key opinion leaders on whether and under what conditions a marketing application might be approved by the Agency. Advisory committees are not empowered to approve or reject an application.

Labeling Meetings

In these meetings, the negotiations take place between the FDA and the sponsor on the specific language of the product labeling, or prescribing information. These meetings are held after an NDA/BLA is submitted and are the final and critical stages in drug development prior to the FDA approval of a drug.

There are some variations among the three FDA centers focused on drugs, biologics, and medical devices for human use—Center for Drug Evaluation and Research (CDER), Center for Biologics Evaluation and Research (CBER), and Center for Devices and Radiological Health (CDRH)—concerning the different types of meetings as well as differences among the divisions within each center. A guidance document—"Guidance for Industry: Formal Meetings with Sponsors and Applicants for PDUFA Products"—is available from the FDA that details the regulations covering these meetings. Meeting guidelines are also published by each of the centers (see Table 1).

In addition, meetings with the FDA are classified as one of three different types—type A, type B, or type C—for the purpose of setting priorities and

Table 1 How to Obtain Meeting Guidance Information from the FDA

Guidance document	Web site address
Guidance for Industry: Formal Meetings With Sponsors and Applicants for PDUFA Products	http://www.fda.gov/cder/guidance/2125fnl.pdf
Formal Meetings Between CDER and CDER's External Constituents	http://www.fda.gov/cder/mapp/4512-l.pdf
Guidance for Industry: IND Meetings for Human Drugs and Biologies; Chemistry, Manufacturing and Controls Information	http://www.fda.gov/cber/gdlns/ind052501.pdf
Disclosure of materials provided to advisory committees in connection with open advisory committee meetings convened by the center for drug evaluation and research beginning on January 1, 2000	http://www.fda.gov/cder/guidance/3431fnl.pdf
Draft Guidance for Industry: Disclosing Information Provided to Advisory Committees in Connection with Open Advisory Committee Meetings Related to the Testing or Approval of Biologic Products and Convened by the Center for Biologics Evaluation and Research	http://www.fda.gov/cber/gdlns/advguid0201.htm
Early collaboration meetings under the FDAMA, final guidance for industry and CDRH staff	http://www.fda.gov/cdrh/ode/guidance/310.htm
Special Protocol Assessment	http://www.fda.gov/cder/guidance/3764fnl.pdf

Abbreviations: FDA, Food and Drug administration; PDUFA, Prescription Drug User Fee Act; CDER, Center for Drug Evaluation and Research; IND, investigational new drug; FDAMA, FDA Modernization Act; CDRH, Center for Devices and Radiological Health.

timelines for action on the basis of their urgency. A type A meeting is one that is immediately necessary to resolve an issue that is preventing a drug development program from moving forward—a high priority or "critical path" meeting. An example is a phase III study in which the dosage specified in the trial protocol is not effective, requiring a new study design or protocol. It is vitally important to the sponsor to discuss and agree with the FDA on the new proposed design. Type B meetings are those with normal priorities, including pre-IND, end-of-phase II, and pre-NDA meetings. Type C meetings, with the lowest priority, encompass any other type of meeting. Meetings involving issues with a submitted NDA/BLA take priority over other meetings because of the performance targets established by Prescription Drug User Fee Act (PDUFA) for FDA for processing submissions. A meeting's classification determines its scheduling: Type A meetings should occur within 30 calendar days of the FDA receiving the request; type B, within 60 days; and type C, within 75 days. While the sponsor makes the request for a certain meeting classification, it is the FDA that makes the final classification and determination of a meeting's priority.

FDA EXPECTATIONS

In addition to the FDA's formal regulations covering these different types of meetings, an informal "FDA Meetings Way" has evolved over time with common criteria and characteristics about how the Agency generally expects its interactions with the pharmaceutical industry to be conducted in any type of meeting. Understanding and abiding by these expectations is just as important as following the formal regulations.

The most important characteristic to remember is that all the FDA meetings are *serious and formal.* The main order of business in every meeting is a discussion of science and medicine, and the orientation of that discussion is scientist-to-scientist. A typical FDA meeting might be compared with a scientific "summit," with chief negotiators, numerous people in attendance, a limited time frame, a very specific agenda, and minute-takers. Consistent with their scientific orientation, the emphasis at the FDA meetings is on building consensus [on the] basis of sound scientific data. That also means that the attendees representing the sponsor should mostly be scientists who are prepared to discuss the relevant data. Financial and product promotional discussions are seldom, if ever, appropriate at the FDA meetings.

What does the FDA expect from a sponsor during these meetings? First and foremost, the agency expects a data-driven discussion of a product with the strong support of good science and good medicine. All meetings should be focused on scientific or medical issues that directly relate to the product and the FDA regulations. Every meeting should also have a clear purpose. Sponsors must know what they want to accomplish, develop a meeting agenda that helps answer the key questions, then adhere to that agenda. In addition, the sponsor is expected to be well prepared—to bring the right people who understand the issues involved. Sponsors must be knowledgeable about the applicable regulations and guidelines for their products as well, so that they are speaking the same language as the FDA. A sponsor should also be careful to schedule meetings with the FDA at the appropriate times, when useful discussions are possible and the company is genuinely seeking Agency input.

Another important characteristic of FDA meetings is that sponsors are expected to present positions for discussion, rather than ask the agency open-ended questions about what the sponsor should do. The FDA is not in the business of developing drugs or designing sponsors' drug development plans. What the agency will do is comment on a sponsor's plans, provide input, voice objections, and give advice on the basis of its broad experience with other sponsors and drugs (within the bounds of maintaining confidentiality on sponsor-proprietary information, of course). Instead of asking the FDA personnel to suggest a course of action, a sponsor should tell them about the company's plans, provide full data-driven justification for those plans, and then seek the Agency's scientific input and concurrence.

PREPARING FOR FDA MEETINGS

Because preparation is essential for a successful FDA meeting, sponsors should allow plenty of time in advance of any meeting to strategize, organize materials, select attendees, and rehearse key discussions. This preparation begins with scheduling the meetings. As discussed above, every meeting is classified as type A, B, or type C, and each classification carries its own timeline for scheduling and the pre-meeting submission of documentation. If a type A meeting is requested, the FDA will expect the sponsor to provide justification for the claimed high priority and will make the final decision about the classification. It is also important to request the meeting through the proper person in the Review Division (usually the Project Manager assigned to the product or sometimes a Meeting Coordinator) to avoid confusion or delay.

The sponsor requests the meeting by sending to the applicable FDA Review Division a Meeting Request Letter in accordance with a specific FDA-recommended format.

1. Product name and application number (if applicable)
2. Chemical name and structure
3. Proposed indication(s)
4. The type of meeting being requested (i.e., type A, type B, or type C)
5. A brief statement of the purpose of the meeting
6. A list of the specific objectives/outcomes expected from the meeting
7. A preliminary proposed agenda, including estimated time needed for each agenda item and designated speaker(s)
8. A draft list of specific questions, grouped by discipline
9. A list of all individuals (including titles) who will attend the proposed meeting from the sponsor's or applicant's organization and consultants
10. A list of agency staff requested by the sponsor or applicant to participate in the proposed meeting
11. The approximate date on which supporting documentation (i.e., the information package) will be sent to the review division
12. Suggested dates and times (i.e., morning or afternoon) for the meeting

It is strongly recommended that the sponsor give considerable thought to all elements of the Meeting Request letter, and especially to the questions (item 8). The FDA will likely grant or decline the meeting primarily on the basis of the detailed nature and specificity of the questions.

Once a meeting has been granted and scheduled by the Review Division, the sponsor must submit supporting documentation at least two weeks in advance of Type A and Type C meetings, and at least one month in advance of a Type B meeting. This documentation, variously called a Briefing Package or Information Package or Briefing Document, is the most critical part of the pre-meeting preparations, because it sets the agenda for the meeting and defines the issues to be discussed. To have a successful meeting, it is essential for the sponsor to provide a strong, focused Briefing Document that clearly states the purpose of the meeting and the issues upon which the sponsor seeks consensus. The documents must also provide sufficient background information on the drug (including Chemistry, Manufacturing, Nonclinical and Clinical Summaries, and data tables) to orient the FDA attendees to those issues.

Once again, the FDA recommends a specific structure for the briefing document.

1. Product name and application number (if applicable)
2. Chemical name and structure
3. Proposed indication(s)
4. Dosage form, route of administration, and dosing regimen (frequency and duration)
5. A brief statement of the purpose of the meeting
6. A list of the specific objectives/outcomes expected from the meeting
7. A proposed agenda, including estimated time needed for each agenda item and designated speaker(s)
8. A list of specific questions grouped by discipline
9. Clinical data summary (as appropriate)
10. Preclinical data summary (as appropriate)
11. Chemistry, manufacturing, and controls (CMC) information (as appropriate)

In recent years, the Briefing Document has completely replaced the sponsor's opening presentations at meetings with the FDA. Meetings now begin with an immediate discussion of the issues raised in the Briefing Document, which the FDA personnel have read and analyzed in advance of the meeting. In that context, a sponsor presentation of the same information is superfluous and a poor use of the limited time made available by the FDA for the meeting (usually 1 hour).

An important innovation has occurred in recent years. Many Review Divisions have adopted the habit of providing to the sponsor written detailed responses to all the questions in the Briefing Document 24 to 48 hours (and sometimes even 7 days) prior to the meeting. These responses have often been 8 to 12 pages in length and extremely thorough and informative. The clear benefit to both the sponsor and the FDA is that these "advance responses" have removed the guesswork surrounding the Agency's opinion of the questions and issues, have allowed the sponsor to prepare counter-responses, and have enabled the face-to-face meetings with the FDA to be more relaxed, productive, and mutually satisfying. In effect, this innovation has dramatically increased the efficiency of the interaction and provided for far better substance and style of sponsor-FDA communication.

When planning a meeting with the FDA, the sponsor will be faced with the important decision of selecting the right people to attend the meeting. This decision can present significant internal challenges for the sponsor when dealing with corporate politics, organizational issues, and egos. However, the selection criteria should always be focused on choosing those who can contribute to the *scientific and technical* discussions, because that is what matters in the end. Depending on the stage of product development, a sponsor might draw on internal (or external consultant) expertise in areas such as pharmacology, toxicology, pharmacokinetics, chemistry, manufacturing, clinical development, and biostatistics, as well as regulatory affairs.

While marketing personnel are always interested in the timelines for drug approval, they should be "silent partners" at most FDA meetings (if they attend at all) except when the negotiation of the final product labeling occurs. Because the sponsor's marketing and promotional activities will be directly affected by the FDA-approved language of the product labeling, it is appropriate for marketing personnel to participate in the labeling negotiation process.

In general, company lawyers and chief executive officers (CEOs) should not attend typical FDA meetings unless there are legal issues to be discussed (which would be unusual at scientific meetings with the agency) or unless the CEO is also the sponsor's chief scientist, with intimate knowledge of the science behind the drug. Expert consultants can play a role if they can help a sponsor articulate particular scientific or regulatory positions.

In preparing for an FDA meeting, it is also important to recognize the decision-making authority of the people who will be attending for the Agency, so that the issues being debated are commensurate with the authority of the attendees. For example, technical commitments can only be made by a therapeutic area Division Director or higher, not by the Division Project Manager, who is the sponsor's usual day-to-day contact. Drug approval decisions can only be made by Division Directors and Office Directors. Policy decisions can only come from a Center Director or the FDA Commissioner's office. It is not appropriate for the sponsor to discuss high-level FDA policy (e.g., "Why do INDs exist?") with a Division Director.

Rehearsals are the final ingredient in good meeting preparation. A team leader should be appointed to coordinate the company's responses during the meeting with the FDA. The role of each team member at the meeting should be discussed and decided in advance, and all attendees should practice what they are going to say—although formal presentations are not typically made. Emphasis should be placed on keeping all attendees focused on the crucial issues to be discussed at the meeting and the outcomes desired by the sponsor. It is often useful to ask the regulatory affairs professional on the team to "role play" the FDA during rehearsals—asking tough questions and challenging the sponsor's positions to help the team members think through their answers carefully and thoroughly.

Now that many Review Divisions provide "advance responses" to the Briefing Document, sponsor rehearsals do not focus on anticipating possible FDA comments, but are instead devoted to preparing counterproposals to the known FDA objections, if any. And it is quite customary to focus only on the issues where the FDA and the sponsor disagree, leaving the agreed issues off the table. Finally, it is not uncommon for sponsors to actually cancel the face-to-face meeting with the FDA if the "advance responses" received as late as the day before the meeting reflect FDA concurrence with the sponsor positions. Why waste precious time for a meeting?

CONDUCT AT FDA MEETINGS

How should attendees conduct themselves during an FDA meeting? The most important thing to remember is to *listen*. Introductory remarks should be brief and confined to introducing the sponsor team and stating briefly the purpose of the meeting from the sponsor's point of view. Also, the sponsor's team should not plan to make a formal presentation to convey the company's case—although it is always a good idea to have back-up material (e.g., in the form of transparencies) ready to present in case questions arise. A properly prepared Briefing Document will present the company's case in advance and spell out the issues to be discussed during the meeting.

In fact, most FDA meetings now begin with the Agency reminding the sponsor that "advance responses" were provided and that it is up to the sponsor to "run the meeting" and drive the agenda. Sponsors then typically discuss the issues where there is disagreement with the FDA, and the meeting focuses on those issues primarily or exclusively. Attendees should listen carefully to what the FDA reviewers say, take extensive notes, and, most important, *should not interrupt*. Once the discussions begin, let the sponsor team leader orchestrate the team's responses to FDA questions and statements and stay focused on the agenda and objectives of the meeting. It is essential that the sponsor's team avoid being aggressive, arrogant, condescending, or confrontational. Keep in mind that the goal of every FDA meeting—both for the sponsor and for the agency—is to seek consensus and resolve all issues professionally and scientifically so that the drug development effort can proceed. At the end of the meeting, be sure there is a clear understanding about any decisions that have been made, as well as any actions that need to be taken—and by whom. If there are action items to be addressed after the meeting, be sure to follow up promptly with the FDA.

According to its own guidelines, the Agency is expected to provide the official minutes of the meeting within four weeks. Delays are common, but the

Agency is trying to improve its performance in this regard. A sponsor can request changes to the minutes but should not expect to make wholesale alterations. The sponsor can also provide the company's own minutes of the meeting, which should be delivered to the FDA within two to three days to maximize the possibility that the sponsor's input will be considered in the FDA's minutes. It must be remembered that the FDA will consider its own minutes to be the only official record of the meeting.

AVOIDING THE PITFALLS

By understanding the FDA's expectations and following the above guidelines for a successful meeting, most sponsors should be able to avoid the common pitfalls that can slow the regulatory approval process and delay a product's progress toward the market. But because these mistakes continue to occur regularly, it is worthwhile to reiterate some of the more frequent slips that sponsors make during their encounters with the Agency.

One of the most common errors is to present the Agency with open-ended questions rather than reasoned proposals based on science. Following are some examples that illustrate the difference.

Open-Ended Questions

1. The Phase II trials showed that several different dosages were effective for this condition. What would you recommend as the dosage for the Phase III trials?
2. How many patients should be included in the Phase III trials?
3. This drug has shown efficacy against several diseases. Which one should be selected for development first?

Reasoned Proposals

1. Several dosages were tried, and the 5- and 10-mg doses seem to be the most promising for the Phase III trials (as shown in the briefing document). Do you agree?
2. A statistical power calculation shows that a Phase III study with 1000 patients will provide valid results. Do you agree that 1000 will be sufficient?
3. This drug has shown efficacy against several diseases. Condition X has been chosen for the first Phase III studies because there is no therapeutic alternative and enrollment can be completed rapidly. Do you concur?

Remember that it is not the FDA's role to make scientific, marketing, or drug development decisions for sponsors, but to provide insight and guidance on the basis of the regulations and the Agency's expertise.

Here are some other important "Dos" and "Don'ts" for FDA meetings.

Do	Don't
Be prepared	Waste time
Be polite	Be aggressive or rude
Reach consensus	Argue or be confrontational
Meet at the appropriate time	Meet when discussion is not useful
Discuss key product issues	Socialize or make a sales pitch
Focus on the agenda	Bring up side issues or complaints
Bring scientists and technical experts	Bring lawyers and CEOs
Present strong data	Try to rely on charm or hype
Be open and truthful	Lie or stonewall
Be clear	Obfuscate
Know key contacts	Go "blind" into the meeting
Rely on the data	Rely on political clout
Be reliable	Fail to follow through on commitments

Avoiding these meeting pitfalls can spell the difference between a successful, productive relationship with the FDA and a contentious relationship that slows the regulatory process for everyone.

SPECIFIC MEETING OBJECTIVES

In addition to understanding the characteristics and approaches that are common to all FDA meetings, it is worthwhile to note the specific purposes and objectives of the major FDA meeting categories mentioned earlier in this chapter. It is also important to keep in mind that, while most are not mandatory, these meetings play a significant role in the successful development of any new drug.

Pre-IND Meetings

The pre-IND meeting has several important purposes—all of which are designed to prepare the FDA for the submission of the IND application for a new drug. If the sponsor is a small company or one that is not well known to the FDA, the pre-IND meeting presents an opportunity to discuss the company's background and qualifications. The most important objective of these meetings is to introduce the new drug to the FDA, including the presentation and discussion of the entity's characterization, manufacturing process, and other nonclinical data collected in the laboratory.

At this meeting, the sponsor will typically present the overall clinical investigational plan for the drug and relate that plan to the targeted labeling or prescribing information or even the Target Product Profile (TPP; http://www.fda. gov/cder/guidance/6910dft.pdf). The initial clinical protocol might also be discussed, and there could be agreement on some of the details of the protocol. If the sponsor is aware of any critical scientific or technical issues concerning the drug (e.g., nonclinical safety data showing slight liver enzyme elevations in an animal species), they would be introduced—and sometimes even resolved—in this meeting. The ultimate goal of the pre-IND meeting is for the sponsor to reach an agreement with the FDA so that an IND can be submitted. It should be noted, however, that a successful pre-IND meeting does not guarantee that the FDA will activate the IND application after it is reviewed in detail. The agreement only means that there is no compelling reason why the IND should not be submitted for review.

End-of-Phase II Meetings

Sponsors should *always* have an end-of-Phase II meeting before beginning Phase III clinical trials. The end-of-Phase II meeting is an indispensable step in the drug development process. With the pivotal importance—and significant cost—of Phase III trials for new drugs, the end-of-Phase II meeting is a vital opportunity to obtain the FDA's commitment on Phase III study designs and key trial end points. This meeting also gives the sponsor a chance to solicit the FDA input on the final development plan, which can help "fine-tune" the approaches for CMC, toxicology, and other key data, as well as help shape the anticipated labeling language and claims.

When should an end-of-Phase II meeting be held? It should be scheduled once the Phase II trials have produced the key data needed to support expanded trials. This means that an effective dose has been established, and the pharmacokinetic/pharmacodynamic understanding of the drug is well advanced. It also means that the earlier trials have produced the information needed to solidify the proposed labeling and that the design for the Phase III trials is essentially complete. As the name implies, it should be held *before* the sponsor has made a commitment to the significant financial investment required for Phase III trials.

The briefing document for these meetings must be thorough and informative in order to solicit the most helpful feedback from the FDA, with detailed discussions of pertinent clinical and nonclinical data. The best way for a sponsor to ensure a successful end-of-Phase II meeting—in addition to having strong scientific data—is to present all of the relevant information about the drug openly and completely. Sponsors should state their positions about the compound and the trials clearly and present a strong, well-designed Phase III development plan. There should be no attempt to hide any shortcomings of the early clinical data or to postpone difficult decisions. Any issues or problems will be even more difficult—and costly—if they are brought to the surface later in the development process. The sponsor's credibility can also be significantly damaged. Being forthright and working together with the FDA in a spirit of teamwork to resolve any issues will greatly increase the likelihood that this vital part of the regulatory process will reach a satisfactory conclusion. A fundamental requirement of end-of-Phase II meeting is to lay a firm foundation for Phase III. It is not uncommon for the FDA to object that a sponsor has not provided an adequate justification for the Phase III study dose(s) and that additional Phase II studies are therefore necessary. Sponsors are forewarned to expect this objection and to be prepared to address it with relevant and persuasive data.

Special Protocol Meetings

This is a fairly new category of meetings, which the FDA grants in connection with three specific aspects of the drug development process: carcinogenicity studies, stability studies, and Phase III trials that will support an efficacy claim. The FDA grants these meetings because regulators understand that these types of studies are costly and time consuming. The meetings allow both parties to agree on study designs and end points in advance, with the agreement being documented by a binding written document.

Sponsors do not always submit their Phase III studies to the Special Protocol Assessment process (SPA; http://www.fda.gov/cder/guidance/3764fnl.pdf), which takes 45 days or more. Some are not willing to delay phase 3 start, others are skeptical that the SPA agreement is truly binding. But careful consideration should be given to the advantage of the FDA's in-depth and documented review of a study protocol, which is a benefit to the sponsor and could pave the way for a readier acceptance of the resulting data in the NDA.

Pre-NDA Meetings

Before submitting an NDA, sponsors should *always* schedule a pre-NDA meeting with the FDA. These meetings will uncover any unresolved issues that might delay the review of the submission, orient the reviewers about the content and format of the NDA, and help sponsors understand key FDA expectations about the NDA contents—such as identifying critical studies and discussing proposed analyses.

From the FDA's point of view, the pre-NDA meeting provides an important opportunity to review the NDA plan and understand its content, which will facilitate the Agency's processing of the document. The FDA will want to review any issues that were raised at the end-of-Phase II meeting to ensure that they have been addressed. The actual submission process will also be discussed, including its timing, format (electronic vs. paper, the organization of tables, etc.), and, increasingly, agreement on the common technical document (CTD) or e-CTD format of the NDA. A successful pre-NDA meeting will produce a consensus that makes it likely the FDA will accept the NDA for review if the agreements reached at the meeting have been satisfied.

Advisory Committee Meetings

In some cases, the FDA may want to obtain outside expert opinions about an NDA and the approvability of a new drug. In those circumstances, the Agency has the authority to convene an official Advisory Committee to review the NDA and hold public meetings about whether the product should be approved for sale. The FDA maintains a number of standing Advisory Committees, each with a specific therapeutic focus (for the list of standing Advisory Committees, visit www.fda.gov/oc/advisory/default.htm). These Advisory Committee meetings are unique to the FDA (compared with its counterpart agencies in other countries) and also uniquely stressful for the sponsor—primarily because they are open to the public, including competitors, financial analysts, the media, patients, patient advocates, and other consumers. Regulations require that the sponsor's presentation materials to the Advisory Committee be made available to the public no later than one day before the meeting. At these meetings, the sponsor and the FDA have the opportunity to present key findings about the safety and efficacy of the product to the Committee. The Advisory Committee members offer their own views, discuss the benefits and risk of the drug, and at the end of the meeting, take a vote on whether to recommend it for FDA approval. The FDA is not obligated to follow the recommendations of its Advisory Committees, but it usually does.

Advisory Committee meetings are recorded on audio and videotape, transcribed, and broadcast on the Web. This unusual public forum is particularly risky for the sponsor because years of development and investment are at stake. Extensive preparation by the sponsor is essential to ensure that the company's position is presented thoroughly, concisely, and professionally. Many sponsors utilize both in-house and external consultant resources and prepare hundreds or even thousands of backup slides that can be used to respond to detailed questions by Advisory Committee members. It is not uncommon for sponsors to hold 6 to 10 rehearsals in the weeks leading up to an Advisory Committee presentation. The main goal of the sponsor is to present the "case for approval" by demonstrating a favorable benefit-risk profile of the drug on the basis of clinical and nonclinical data. Advisory Committee meetings have been convened by the FDA for other purposes as well—such as discussion of draft therapeutic drug guidelines, Rx-to-OTC switches, or assessment of drug safety in an era where this has become a "hot topic" in the public arena. Advisory Committee deliberations and votes receive coverage in the business and lay media and are commonly regarded as directly relevant to the public health.

Labeling Meetings

Labeling meetings are the final link in the long chain of drug development. They occur at the end of the NDA review process, when the FDA and the sponsor meet to negotiate the formal language that describes to physicians what specific indications a product has been approved for, the recommended dosages, the side effects, and other specific information that physicians and patients need to know about a new prescription drug. This prescribing information is known as the product labeling.

All the effort that goes into developing a new drug begins with the goal to achieve a certain target labeling, because it is this prescribing information that determines how the product will be used and, ultimately, how successful it will be on the market. This approach is commonly known as "beginning with the end in mind," and it helps sponsors focus on specific, achievable objectives for a drug at an early stage of the development process.

With so much riding on the outcome, labeling meetings can sometimes involve very difficult negotiations to reach agreement on the final language. Several rounds of meetings may be required, and extensive internal consultations within the sponsor organization (e.g., with the marketing department) occur. It is increasingly common to hold labeling meetings via teleconference; this enables both the Agency and the sponsor to put the conversation on "mute" and work out their respective positions in private before resuming negotiations. While this removes the advantage of observing each other's body language, it usually accelerates the negotiation process. The importance of the outcome makes it even more vital to maintain a spirit of cooperation and consensus during this process. The fundamental goal of both the FDA and the sponsor is to bring a useful new medicine to the market; finding labeling language that satisfies both parties benefits everyone. Once the final language has been approved, the product can be launched.

CONCLUSION

While the information in this chapter should provide some guidance about the best way to approach meetings with the FDA, it also illustrates how complex and demanding the regulatory review process can be. How the sponsor works with the FDA throughout the approval process can have a substantial impact on the approval time for a new product. The best way to approach this process is to assemble the right resources with the knowledge and experience to manage your meeting strategy efficiently—allowing the scientific data to be presented effectively and promoting consensus on key product issues. By applying sufficient resources with the proper background to manage FDA meetings, a sponsor can substantially increase a product's chances for approval and significantly reduce time to market.

Fundamentally, meetings with the FDA are opportunities for the sponsor to build FDA trust in the development plan, the regulatory strategy, the data, and the sponsor itself. With trust, communication is more effective and efficient, product approval is more likely, and crisis management becomes a joint sponsor-FDA team effort. Building trust depends in good measure on not "surprising" the Agency with unwelcome news, premature claims, and unreasonable demands, and it is primarily the sponsor's responsibility.

5

FDA Medical Device Regulation

Barry Sall
PAREXEL Consulting, Waltham, Massachusetts, U.S.A.

INTRODUCTION

Since the technological advances of the 1950s and 1960s, the rate of innovation in the medical device industry has greatly accelerated. These innovations have led to very substantial therapeutic, monitoring, and diagnostic benefits in all areas of medicine. Often, these innovative devices were selected and used by health care professionals who received their basic scientific training before these technologies were developed. By the early 1970s, many medical devices were becoming so complex that medical professionals were no longer able to fully assess their attributes. Device developers and manufacturers were also encountering situations where devices interacted with the body in unanticipated ways or deficiencies in the production process led to patient injuries and deaths. In the United States, this history was the driving force behind the 1976 Medical Device Amendments to the Food, Drug, and Cosmetic Act of 1938. By 1978, when the regulations required by this new law came into full effect, the production and clinical testing of medical devices were subject to the Food and Drug Administration (FDA) review. Many new devices entering the U.S. market had to undergo the FDA review, either through the 510(k) premarket notification process, or the PMA, premarket approval process. The 1976 Amendments have been modified several times over the years and now also cover the device development process. This chapter provides an introduction to medical device classification, the preparation of premarket submissions, medical device clinical research, and manufacturing regulations.

The regulations developed as a result of the 1976 Medical Device Amendments sharing a common goal with the existing pharmaceutical regulations. They both strive to protect the public health; however, they approach this goal in different ways. The device regulations recognize differences between medical devices and pharmaceuticals and between the medical device industry and the pharmaceutical industry. In general, therapeutic medical devices exert their effects locally by cutting tissue, covering a wound, or propping open a clogged artery; therefore, both preclinical and clinical testing can be simplified as compared with the pharmaceutical approach. Many diagnostic devices do not even contact the patient; so, in these cases, pharmaceutical safety testing is entirely inappropriate. Differences in the structure of the medical device industry as compared with the pharmaceutical industry do not have a direct effect on regulation, but they do affect the pace of innovation. There are a relatively small number of very large pharmaceutical companies with large experienced regulatory staffs. There are a large number of very small medical device companies with few or no dedicated regulatory staff. In addition, the product life cycle time for a medical device might be as short as two or three years, or approximately one-tenth the time for a pharmaceutical product. In general, many 510(k)s and PMA supplements are submitted for incremental changes in medical devices. All of these factors make it essential that medical device professionals have an adequate understanding of both the technology underlying their company's products and of the applicable regulations. Development timelines in this industry are very short, and inappropriate strategic decisions can generate substantial delays or even preclude the introduction of a potentially lifesaving technology.

The objective of this chapter is to provide the reader with a step-by-step introduction to the regulatory issues associated with the medical device development process in the United States This information will enable the reader to identify the major steps in that process. References are provided, throughout the text, for more detailed information.

IS IT A DEVICE?

Product Jurisdiction

When preparing the regulatory strategy for a product or technology, it is important to first determine which regulations apply. Is the product a device? A drug? A biologic? Two factors must be considered to make this determination. First, the indication for use of the product must be determined by management and clearly stated. Then the primary mode of action for the product should be identified. And only then can the developer determine if that action is achieved through chemical action and metabolism (a drug) or by a physical action (device). If an alginate wound dressing contains an antibacterial agent, it is regulated as a device, so long as its primary intended purpose is to act as a (physical) barrier between the wound and the environment and the antibacterial agent only functions to enhance that device function. On the other hand, if the indication for use is to deliver the antibacterial agent (chemical) to the wound to treat an existing infection, then the alginate dressing might be considered as an inactive component of a drug product. In order to make this determination, one must carefully review the definition of a medical device contained in the 1976 Medical Device Amendments of the Food, Drug, and Cosmetic Act.

"an instrument, apparatus, implement, machine, contrivance, implant, in vitro reagent, or other similar or related article, including any component, part or accessory, which is —

(1) recognized in the official National Formulary, or the USP, or any supplement to them,
(2) intended for use in the diagnosis of disease or other conditions, or in the cure, mitigation, treatment, or prevention of disease, in man or other animals, or
(3) intended to affect the structure or any function of the body of man or other animals, and which does not achieve its primary intended purposes through chemical action within or on the body of man or other animals and which is not dependent upon being metabolized for the achievement of any of its principal intended purposes"

In addition to this definition, there are also intercenter agreements[1] between Center for Devices and Radiological Health (CDRH), Center for Drug Evaluation and Research (CDER), and Center for Biologics Evaluation and Research (CBER) that discuss jurisdictional issues. The Medical Device User Fee Act of 2002 (MDUFA02) established the Office of Combination Products. This office is an excellent source of information on these issues. See: http:// www.fda.gov/oc/combination/default.htm for more information on the Office of Combination Products and its functions. The FDA Office of Combination Products defined the primary mode of action in an August 25, 2005, federal register notice (available at: http://www.fda.gov/OHRMS/DOCKETS/98fr/ 05-16527.pdf). If a sponsor requires an official product jurisdiction determination, he/she can file a request for designation with the Office of Combination Products. Assuming that the product is regulated as a medical device, we can consider the type of device and level of regulation.

---

[1] Food and Drug Administration, Intercenter Agreements, October 1991. Available at: http://www .fda.gov/oc/combination/intercenter.html.

Table 1 Medical Device Types

Function	Form
Therapeutic	Durable
Monitoring	Implantable
Diagnostic	Disposable

Types of Medical Devices

There are a wide variety of medical devices in use today. They range from room-sized imaging systems that weigh several tons to ophthalmic implants that are less than 2-mm long and weigh only a few grams. Most in vitro diagnostic products (blood and urine tests) are also regulated as medical devices. The table above describes most devices using two of their characteristics (Table 1).

Using this table, one can easily characterize most medical devices by determining the function of the device from the left column, then its form from the right column. For instance, a lithotriptor that uses sound waves to break up kidney stones would be considered a durable therapeutic device, a pacemaker would be considered an implantable therapeutic device, and so on. Issues such as reuse, shelf life, and device tracking impact different types of devices in different ways.

MEDICAL DEVICE CLASSIFICATION

Once a determination has been made that a product is a medical device, the next issue that must be addressed is medical device classification. In simpler terms, "What kind of submission do I need to commercialize this device? Is it exempt from 510(k) notification requirements, subject to those requirements, or must we file a PMA application?" In order to answer this question, we need to know the class of the device.

There are three classes of medical devices. Class I devices are the simplest devices, posing the fewest risks and subject to general controls. Most of them are exempt from premarket notification requirements [510(k)], and some are also exempt from compliance with the Quality System Regulation (QSR). Examples of class I devices include toothbrushes, oxygen masks, and irrigating syringes. The FDA estimates that approximately half of the medical devices it regulates are class I devices.

Class II devices include many moderate risk devices. In order to market a class II device in the United States, the manufacturer must obtain clearance of a 510(k) premarket notification prior to commercialization. The purpose of this notification is to demonstrate that the new device is *substantially equivalent* to another device that has already gone through the 510(k) process or to a device that was on the market before the Medical Device Amendments were signed on May 28, 1976. Class II devices are subject to special controls, that is, Office of

Device Evaluation (ODE) guidance documents, FDA-accepted international standards, and the QSR. Ultrasound imaging systems, Holter cardiac monitors, pregnancy test kits, and central line catheters are all class II devices. The FDA estimates that slightly less than half of the medical devices it regulates are class II devices. Approximately 3200 class II devices are cleared on to the U.S. market each year.[2]

Most class III devices require PMA approval prior to marketing in the United States. These are devices that are not substantially equivalent to any class II device. They are usually technologically innovative devices. There are a small number of class III preamendments 510(k) devices; however, the FDA has been working diligently to either downclassify them to class II, or if their risk profile does not justify downclassification, call for PMAs. There were 39 PMAs approved in 2006.[3]

Determining Device Classification

If the product in development is similar to other medical devices already on the U.S. market with respect to its indication for use and its technological characteristics, then our classification determination becomes a search of the regulations. 21 Code of Federal Regulations (CFR) 862–892 contains descriptions of a wide variety of medical devices arranged by medical practice area. The classifications and exemptions from 510(k) or QSR, if any, are listed in this section of the regulations. The classification database in the CDRH Web site can also be a useful tool for determining device classification (Table 2) (Fig. 1).

If a description in the CFR is consistent with the characteristics of the new device, then the device classification listed in that section of the CFR should apply. Precedents can be identified in another manner as well. If one is aware of other competing devices that are already on the market, one can search the 510(k)[4] or PMA[5] databases, within the CDRH Web site, for those products and determine how they were classified. Figure 5 illustrates the process one can follow to identify possible predicate devices when only the name of a competitor is known.

When there is no obvious precedent to follow, it can be difficult to determine the appropriate device classification. The question can be explored informally via telephone calls with the appropriate branch chief within the ODE, but no binding decision will result from such discussions. Device developers can

---

[2] Food and Drug Administration, 510(k) database. Available at: http://www.accessdata.fda.gov/scripts/cdrh/cfdocs/cfPMN/pmn.cfm.

[3] Food and Drug Administration, PMA database.

[4] Food and Drug Administration, available at: http://www.accessdata.fda.gov/scripts/cdrh/cfdocs/cfPMN/pmn.cfm.

[5] Food and Drug Administration, available at: http://www.accessdata.fda.gov/scripts/cdrh/cfdocs/cfPMA/pma.cfm.

Table 2 Medical Device Classification

Device classification panel or specialty group	21 CFR part
Anesthesiology	868
Cardiovascular	870
Clinical chemistry and clinical toxicology	862
Dental	872
Ear, nose, and throat	874
Hematology and pathology	864
Immunology and microbiology	866
Gastroenterology and urology	876
General and plastic surgery	878
General hospital and personal use	880
Neurology	882
Obstetrical and gynecological	884
Ophthalmic	886
Orthopedic	888
Physical medicine	890
Radiology	892

Abbreviation: CFR, Code of Federal Regulations.

obtain a formal classification decision using the 513(g) request for classification process. The sponsor submits a brief document to the ODE describing the device, how it works, materials used, and similar devices, if any. The indication for use and draft labeling is also included along with a suggested classification and supporting rationale. There is a user fee of $2498 for a 513(g). In 60 days, the sponsor will receive a letter from the ODE, either confirming the sponsor's classification rationale or stating an alternate classification.

Reclassification

Once the FDA determines that a device is a class III PMA device, that type of device will always be a class III device, no matter how many other competitors follow with similar products. All the competitors that develop similar products will have to follow the PMA process to market their devices in the United States. The only way that situation can change is if the FDA approves a reclassification petition and downclassifies the device to class II. This type of reexamination can be initiated by either the FDA or the industry. In recent years, the FDA has examined many device types, their overall risk, and actual frequency of problems in the field and downclassified significant numbers of devices either from class III to II or from class II to I. These actions enable the FDA to focus more of its resources on the higher risk products. Industry groups have also submitted their own reclassification petitions and succeeded in downclassifying devices.

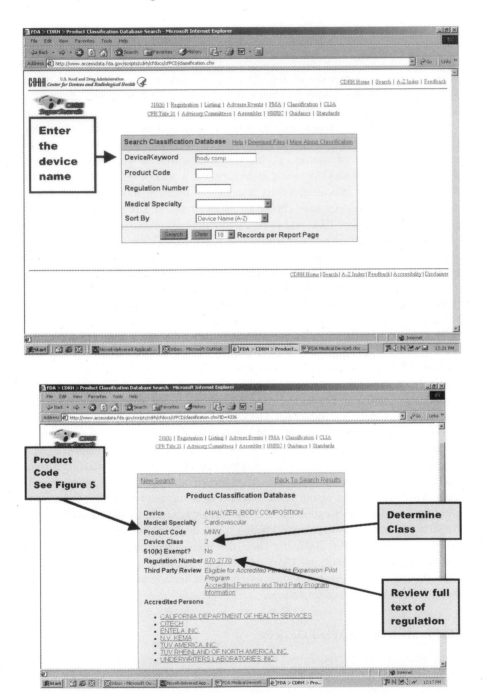

Figure 1 Device classification database search.

AN INTRODUCTION TO THE MEDICAL DEVICE APPROVAL PROCESS

Strategic Choices

Now that the classification of the device is known, we can now identify an appropriate regulatory pathway. Unlike the pharmaceutical regulatory process, a medical device developer is frequently presented with more than one regulatory path to the U.S. market. A device such as software that analyzes magnetic resonance imaging (MRI) images is designated as a class II 510(k) product if it only measures the size or volume of anatomical structures. However, if the software detects abnormalities or provides diagnostic information, it would be considered a class III PMA device, so the indication for use is critical to determination of the regulatory path. A device developer may choose to "start small" and begin the FDA inter-actions with a simpler 510(k) and then, after gaining experience, move to the more challenging PMA once a revenue stream is established. Generally, both the industry and the FDA would prefer to review medical devices as 510(k)s. This process provides the industry with timely reviews and conserves reviewing resources for the FDA. So, when speed to market is the prime consideration, one always attempts to follow the 510(k) path. Even within the 510(k) pathway, there are branches. If the FDA-recognized standards apply to the new device, the sponsor may choose to submit an abbreviated 510(k) or a traditional 510(k). The review time is the same, but instead of containing the complete testing reports, an abbreviated 510(k) will contain a list of the recognized standards followed during device testing and a summary of the test results. This results in a smaller submission. Of course, a sponsor may choose an alternate test method, in which case the test protocol would need to be included in a traditional 510(k). In some cases, device developers may choose to propose a more complex PMA indication for use, or in a situation where the device classification is not clear, suggest the more complicated class III PMA designation. This can make sense when the developer may not have a strong intellectual property position but does have sufficient resources to conduct clinical trials. This strategy can result in the erection of a regulatory barrier of entry for other, less well-funded organizations. This strategy is often called creation of a "regulatory patent." Another consideration when deciding on a regulatory path is user fees. Since October 2002, the ODE has been authorized to charge fees for reviewing 510(k)s, PMAs, and PMA supplements (Table 3) (Fig. 2).

All the submission types mentioned in this section are discussed in more detail in later sections of this chapter.

Modification of Marketed Devices

Many changes can be made to 510(k) devices by following the design control provisions of the QSR, rather than submission of a new 510(k). Even when a new 510(k) is necessary, in many cases, a sponsor can choose to submit a special 510(k). The review period for a special 510(k) is 30 days. Changes to PMA products follow a more rigid process. Most changes require advance approval via the PMA

Table 3 Selected MDUFA02 Standard User Fees Fiscal Year 2008

Application type	Fee
PMA	$185,000
Panel track PMA supplement	$138,750
180-days PMA supplement	$27,750
Real-time PMA supplement	$12,950
30-days notices	$2960
513(g)s	$2498
510(k)—all types	$3404
IDEs	No charge

Abbreviations: MDUFA, Medical Device User Fee Act of 2002; PMA, premarket approval; IDE, investigational device exemption.

supplement process. There are several types of PMA supplements with approval times ranging from 180 days to 30 days. The sponsor must also submit PMA annual reports that update ODE on all device changes and any new clinical data. Both the premarket and postmarket obligations must be considered when determining the preferred route to market. More information on postmarketing issues can be found in the section "Postmarketing Issues." The ease of modifying devices and other postmarket considerations also factor into the strategic regulatory planning process. It is far easier to update a 510(k) device than a PMA device.

DESIGN CONTROLS

Once the product definition and regulatory strategy have been prepared, class II and III device developers must work to comply with the design control provisions of the QSR (21 CFR 820) as the device development process moves forward. The QSR is the medical device equivalent of the pharmaceutical current good manufacturing practices (cGMPs). The QSR, unlike cGMPs, also regulates the device development process via its design control provisions (21 CFR 820.30). This section describes the device developer's obligations under the design control provisions of QSR. Other sections of the QSR are discussed in the section "The Quality System Regulation."

The Difference Between Research and Development

The preamble to the QSR[6] states that research activities are not regulated by the QSR, but development activities are regulated. The regulation does not provide guidance for distinguishing between the two activities; however, the preamble does add, "The design control requirements are not intended to apply to the development of concepts and feasibility studies. However, once it decides that a

---

[6] Food and Drug Administration. Final Rule. Medical Devices; Current Good Manufacturing Practice (CGMP). Final Rule; Quality System Regulation. Federal Register 1996; 61:195,52602–52662.

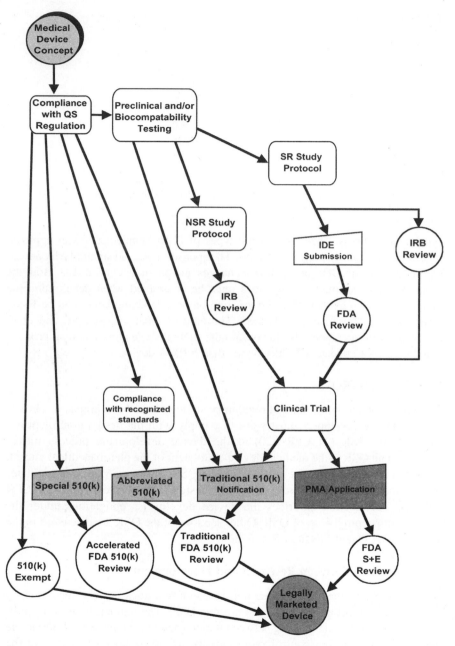

Figure 2   Selected pathways for marketing medical devices in the United States.

design will be developed, a plan must be established... ." Most device developers categorize investigations of a general technology as research and application of that technology to a particular product's development. For example, if a device developer creates a new laser technology, that effort would be considered research. Once the developer begins to apply that technology to a particular device with specific indications for use and user requirements, then they have begun the development phase and design controls must be applied. A device developer's design control standard operating procedures (SOPs) should clearly describe the point in the development process when design controls apply, and that definition should be consistently followed for all design projects.

Design Control Components

There are eight components of design controls that stretch from planning for the development effort through design transfer (from development to manufacturing) and maintenance of existing designs. These controls apply to all class II and III medical devices and a small number of class I devices. The purpose of these controls is to ensure that devices are developed in a rational manner, in compliance with the firm's existing design control SOPs. Table 4 summarizes these components. If a company is just starting to develop a medical device for the

Table 4   Design Control Components

Design activity	Personnel involved	Examples of issues
Design and development planning	Development, marketing, management	• Determine timing for design reviews • Determine documentation requirements and departmental documentation responsibilities • Determine overall project timelines and budget
Design input	Development, management, sales and marketing, quality, regulatory	• Identify users of the new device • Specify where the new device will be used • Describe the operating environment for the device • Document how long the new device will be used • Determine and meet the user/patients requirements • Meet regulations and standards • Develop specifications for the device • Develop, select, and evaluate components and suppliers • Develop and approve labels and user instructions • Develop packaging

(Continued)

Table 4 Design Control Components (*Continued*)

Design activity	Personnel involved	Examples of issues
		• Document the processes and details of the device design • If applicable, develop a service program
Design output	Development	The design is executed
Design review	Development, management, and others, as needed, including one person not directly involved in the design effort	• Determine if the design meets customer needs • Confirm that manufacturability and reliability issues are adequately addressed • Establish that human factors' issues are adequately addressed
Design verification	Development	Confirm that the design outputs meet the design input requirements by reviewing data from tests, inspections, and analysis
Design validation	Development, management, and clinical	• Performed under defined operating conditions on initial production units, or equivalent • Include software validation and risk analysis, where appropriate • Ensure that devices conform to defined user needs and intended uses • Include testing under actual or simulated use conditions • Validation plans, methods, reports, and review must be conducted according to approved SOPs
Design transfer	Development, management, quality, and manufacturing	• Prepare a plan for the transfer of all the design components to manufacturing • Develop manufacturing facilities and utilities • Develop and validate manufacturing processes • Assure that all affected personnel are adequately trained • Assure that all manufacturing and quality systems function according to specifications
Design changes	Development, management	• Assure that design changes are tracked, verified and validated • Assure that corrective actions are completed • Assure that the DHF is kept current and includes all design revisions

first time, the design control process must be fully described in SOPs and fully implemented before the development planning begins. Design controls are closely linked to many other QSR components and the entire system must work together to produce good product. Refer to the section "The Quality System Regulation" for discussion of the other components of the QSR.

The design control regulation sets requirements for the development process. Firms must prepare and follow SOPs that comply with the regulations and that fully describe how the firm will meet all relevant regulatory requirements. All the relevant activities must be fully documented in the firm's design history file (DHF). For example, the regulation requires device developers to prepare a list of design inputs. Like just about every other design control–related document, this list cannot be considered a static document. As the design process progresses, inputs are modified, added, or subtracted. The design input file must be maintained as a current document throughout the development process. Another important design control function is the design review. At least once during the design process, and more frequently for a complex design effort, the design must be reviewed to ensure that the design satisfies the design input requirements for the intended use of the device and the needs of the user. All other sources of design information, including design output reports, design verification documentation, and even actual prototypes should be part of this review. Most importantly, for regulatory compliance, a report must document all the design review activities and their results and list the individuals that participated in the review. The regulation requires that at least one member of the review team be an independent reviewer who has not been directly involved with the design effort.

MEDICAL DEVICE CLINICAL RESEARCH

Once the regulatory pathway has been determined and development is underway, clinical data may be necessary. Keep in mind that the vast majority of 510(k) notifications do not contain clinical data. Figure 3 graphically depicts the pathways for medical device clinical research. Unlike the pharmaceutical model, there are three levels of regulation of medical device clinical research. Some research is exempted from the investigational device exemption (IDE) regulation, some is subject to just some sections of the IDE regulation, and other types of research is subject to all sections of the IDE regulation. More information on risk determinations can be found at: http://www.fda.gov/cdrh/d861.html.

Exempted Studies

Most exempted studies involve either previously cleared or approved devices or investigational in vitro diagnostic devices. If a sponsor wishes to conduct a study that, for example, compares the performance of their own previously cleared device with the performance of their competitor's previously cleared device, that study would be exempt from the IDE regulations, so long as both devices are used for their cleared indications. No prior FDA review or approval of the study is necessary.

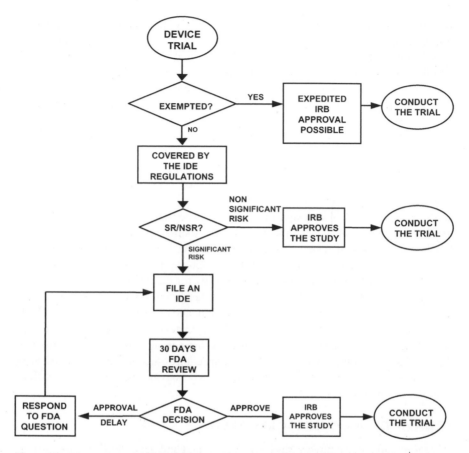

Figure 3 Regulatory paths for medical device clinical research.

Of course, due to privacy concerns and institutional regulations, any human clinical trial should use an informed consent form and be reviewed and approved by the appropriate institutional review board (IRB). Most in vitro diagnostic field trials are also exempt, so long as invasive means are not used to collect samples and the data obtained from the investigational assay are not used to make treatment decisions. Also, in some cases when archived de-identified samples are used for in vitro diagnostic field trials, informed consent may not be necessary. See http://www.fda. gov/cdrh/oivd/guidance/1588.pdf for more information. Animal studies and custom device studies are also exempt from the IDE regulation.

Nonsignificant Risk Studies

Many studies that do not involve highly invasive devices; risky procedures and/ or frail patients can be conducted under the nonsignificant risk (NSR) provisions of the IDE regulation. See http://www.fda.gov/cdrh/d861.html. These provisions provide an intermediate level of control for the study without requiring the study sponsor to prepare and file an IDE. See Table 5 for a comparison of sponsor and investigator responsibilities. Areas where the requirements for NSR and significant risk studies differ are shaded. When a sponsor determines that a study is NSR, no FDA involvement is required, although many sponsors will consult with the FDA to confirm that the study is indeed NSR and that its design is consistent with the FDA expectations. Each IRB that reviews an NSR study must document three conclusions. First, that they concur with the sponsor's NSR determination; next, that the study protocol is approved; and last, that the consent form is approved. If just one IRB formally determines that a study is not NSR, then the sponsor must report this to the ODE. If all IRBs approve the study, it may proceed. In this case, the local IRBs monitor the progress of the study according to their own SOPs, and the FDA is not in the process (Table 5).

Significant Risk Studies

Significant risk studies require an approved IDE to treat patients in the United States. Typical significant risk studies involved implantable devices or devices that introduce significant quantities of energy into the body. Studies with devices that sustain or support life are nearly always considered significant risk. If a study sponsor is unsure of the risk status of a study, consultation with the appropriate branch within the ODE should be considered.

The Investigational Device Exemption (IDE)

The IDE serves the same function for a significant risk medical device clinical trial as the IND, described in Chapter 3, does for pharmaceutical clinical trials. The submission contains data that are similar in many respects to data contained in an IND. There are, however, some significant differences between the two submissions types due to the differences in regulatory requirements between devices and drugs. First, although preclinical testing data are included in both submissions, the data in an IDE conforms to the ISO 10993 biocompatability testing standard as modified by the FDA (see http://www.fda.gov/cdrh/g951. html), rather than the International Conference on Harmonization (ICH) guidance. Relevant FDA guidance documents (special controls) may also list additional data expectations. The IDE regulation requires an investigational plan, but does not specify an investigator brochure. The international ISO 14155 medical device clinical research standard does include an investigator brochure. The IDE regulation also requires that the sponsor include a clinical monitoring SOP in the submission. Under the cost recovery provision of the IDE regulation, the sponsor may charge for the investigational device, so long as only research and development and manufacturing costs are recovered. An investigator agreement serves the function of the FDA form 1572, used for pharmaceutical studies. More detailed information regarding IDEs can be found at http://www.fda.gov/cdrh/devadvice/ide/index.shtml.

Table 5 NSR/SR Comparison Chart

Item	NSR		SR	
	Sponsor	P.I.	Sponsor	P.I.
Submit an IDE to the FDA	−	−	+	−
Report ADEs to sponsor	−	+	−	+
Report ADEs to reviewing IRBs	+	+	+	+
Report ADEs to the FDA	+	−	+	−
Report withdrawal of IRB approval to sponsor	−	+	−	+
Submit progress reports to sponsor, monitor, and reviewing IRB	−	+	−	+
Report deviations from the investigational plan to sponsor and reviewing IRB	−	−[a]	−	+
Obtain and document informed consent from all study subjects prior to use of the investigational device	−	+	−	+
Maintain informed consent records	−	+	−	+
Report any use of the device without prior informed consent to sponsor and reviewing IRB	−	+	−	+
Compile records of all anticipated and unanticipated ADEs and complaints	+	−	+	−
Maintain correspondence with PIs, IRBs, monitors, and the FDA	−[a]	−[a]	+	+
Maintain shipment, use, and disposal records for the investigational device	−[a]	−[a]	+	+
Document date and time of day for each use of the IDE device	−	−	−	+
Maintain signed investigator agreements for each PI	−[a]	−	+	+
Provide a current investigator list to the FDA every 6 mo	−	−	+	−
Submit progress reports to the IRB, at least yearly	+	−	+	−
Submit a progress report to the FDA, at least yearly	−	−	+	−
Submit final study report to the FDA	−	−	+	−
Submit final study report to all reviewing IRBs	+	−	+	−
Monitor the study and secure compliance with the protocol	+	−	+	−
Notify the FDA and all reviewing IRBs if an investigational device has been recalled	+	−	+	−
Comply with IDE advertising, promotion, and sale regulations	+	+	+	+
Comply with IDE-labeling regulations	+	+	+	+

[a]Compliance with IDE regulations is recommended.

Abbreviations: NSR, nonsignificant risk; SR, significant risk; IDE, investigational device exemption; FDA, Food and Drug Administration; ADEs, adverse drug events; IRB, Institutional Review Board; PI, principal investigator.

Unique Aspects of Medical Device Studies

The informed consent, financial disclosure, and IRB regulations described in Chapter 9 apply equally for medical device studies. Provisions of the IND regulation and ICH guidelines do not apply to medical device studies. This section describes some of the unique features of medical device studies. Before we consider the regulatory differences between pharmaceutical and device studies, we need to review the procedural differences. Test article administration is frequently a prime concern in trials of therapeutic devices. In most drug trials, IV, IM, or PO administration of the test article is a trivial concern that is hardly discussed. The manner in which a surgical device is used or the technique by which an implantable device is placed in the body can mean the difference between success and failure in the trial. Because of this, investigator training is a critical aspect of many device trials. Protocol compliance while using the device and while recording data is also a critical issue. In addition, the clinical research associate (CRA) is called upon to transmit technical data between the technical development staff and investigators. Another global issue involves overall study design. Unlike most pharmaceutical studies that are both masked and randomized, the vast majority of device studies are not masked. Most of the time, it is not possible or ethical to mask the device, especially if the device is an implant or a surgical device. Often it is possible to mask a patient assessor to reduce bias. There are also several key regulatory differences between pharmaceutical clinical trials and medical device clinical trials. First, the ICH guidelines only apply to pharmaceutical studies, not to medical device studies. The greatest effect is seen on adverse device effects analysis and reporting. Refer to Figure 4 on the following page. The IDE regulations permit an investigator to analyze a potential adverse device effect for 10 days before reporting it to the local IRB and the sponsor (most sponsors impose a 24-hour reporting period). The sponsor then has another 10 days to evaluate the event to determine if it should be reported to the ODE, all reviewing IRBs, and all participating investigators. The IDE regulations do require the sponsor to directly communicate this information to the IRBs. This responsibility cannot be delegated to the investigators. While ICH guidances do not apply, some, such as those that describe format and contents of clinical study reports, may offer device companies good suggestions for organizing their study reports. The IDE regulation also does not require the preparation of an investigator brochure. In some cases, especially for multinational studies, a sponsor may choose to prepare such a document, even though it is not required. The FDA form 1572 is another inapplicable document. It requires the investigator to comply with key provisions of the IND regulation, so it is not relevant to device studies. In its place we have the investigator agreement. It serves roughly the same purpose as the form 1572. Its contents are specified in 21 CFR 812.43(c). Although not required by the regulation, many sponsors ask that the principal investigator list the subinvestigators in the agreement, as this list will simplify the gathering of financial disclosure information. There is usually a second investigator agreement, not subject to the FDA review, that covers financial compensation, publishing priorities, and

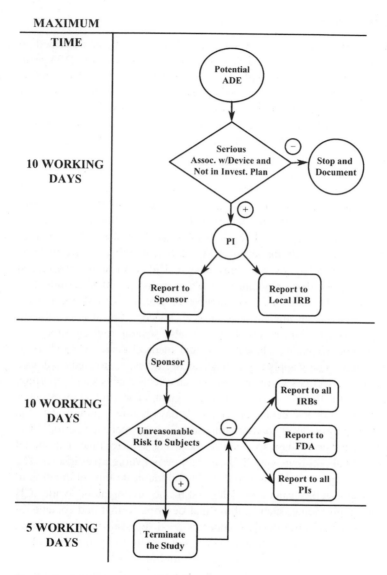

Figure 4 Adverse device effect reporting.

other unregulated activities. Lastly, the cost recovery provision of the IDE regulation [21 CFR 812.20(b)(8)] permits the sponsor to charge for the device. The
sponsor can charge enough to recover research and development costs. This provision cannot be used to commercialize an investigational device.

THE 510(K) PREMARKET NOTIFICATION

More than 3000 medical devices are cleared on to the U.S. market every year through the 510(k) premarket notification process. This represents approximately half the new devices that appear in the U.S. market in a given year. The 510(k) process is relatively rapid, flexible, and adaptable to many different device types and risk levels.

The goal of the 510(k) process is

> Demonstration of substantial equivalence to a device that was on the U.S. market prior to May 28, 1976 or to a device that has *already gone through the 510(k) clearance process.*

Devices that have successfully gone through the 510(k) process are described as "510(k) cleared." A distinction is made between those devices that have been reviewed according to the substantial equivalence standard from those that have been reviewed according to the PMA application, safety, and effectiveness standard. PMA devices are "approved."

The previously cleared device included for comparison purposes in a 510(k) is called the predicate device. A 510(k) may contain multiple predicate devices that address various features of the device. The device designers should be able to provide regulatory personnel with assistance, identifying key technological characteristics that demonstrate substantial equivalence. These data should already be part of the design inputs required as part of design controls. Generally, little manufacturing data are included in a 510(k). Sterile devices will include information on the sterilization process, including sterilization process validation activities and the sterilization assurance level. In vitro diagnostic products will frequently include data on the production of key reagents such as antibodies or nucleic acid probes. The other part of substantial equivalence relates to the indication for use. Frequently, one medical device can be used for many indications in a variety of medical specialties. When new indications are added, those indications must be cleared in a traditional or abbreviated 510(k). The 510(k) must cite a predicate device with the same indication for use.

When searching for potential predicate devices, several information sources are useful. Two FDA databases, the 510(k) database[7], and the classification database[8] can be very helpful. The 510(k) database is especially useful when one knows either the name of potential predicate devices or the manufacturer of the device. The classification database can be used to identify a

---

[7] Food and Drug Administration, available at: http://www.accessdata.fda.gov/scripts/cdrh/cfdocs/cfPMN/pmn.cfm.

[8] Food and Drug Administration, available at: http://www.accessdata.fda.gov/scripts/cdrh/cfdocs/cfPCD/classification.cfm.

particular device type and its corresponding product code. One can then transfer the product code to the 510(k) database and generate a listing of all similar devices. Sales and marketing staffs and competitor Web sites are also excellent sources of predicate device information (Fig. 5).

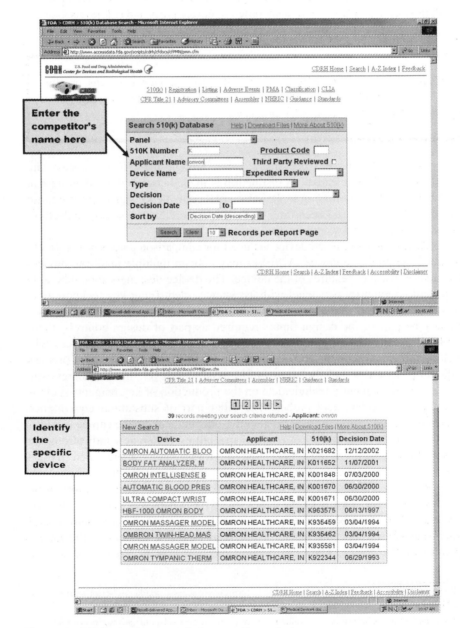

Figure 5 510(k) database search for a predicate device.

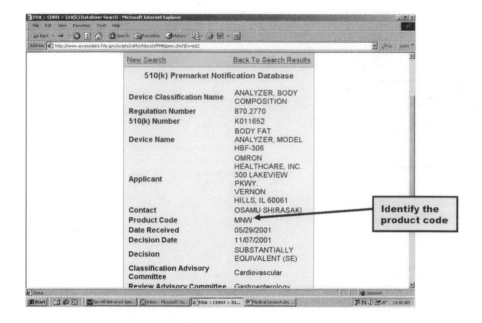

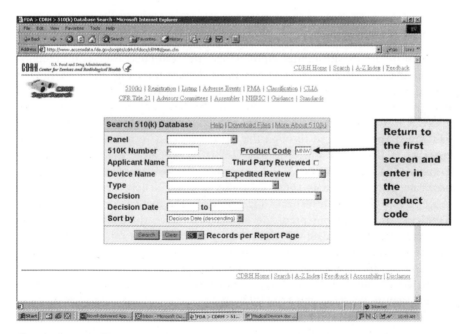

Figure 5 (*Continued on page 146 as well*)

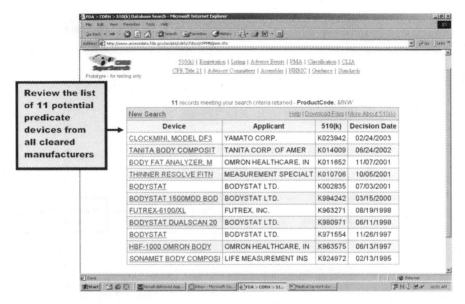

Figure 5 (*Continued*)

Substantial Equivalence

The two pillars of substantial equivalence are "intended use" and "technological characteristics." The sponsor must demonstrate that the new device has an intended use that is substantially equivalent to a predicate device and that the technological characteristics of the new device are substantially equivalent to a predicate device. The predicate device must be a device that has already been cleared through the 510(k) process or a device that was in commercial distribution prior to May 28, 1976, when the FDA was first able to regulate medical devices. A PMA-approved device cannot serve as a 510(k) predicate device. There is some flexibility in ODE's approach to the 510(k) process, especially with respect to technology. The devices do not have to be identical. An acceptable predicate device can have different technological characteristics from the new device, so long as they do not raise new questions of safety and effectiveness and the sponsor demonstrates that the device is as safe and as effective as the legally marketed device. Different technological characteristics might include changes in materials, control mechanisms, overall design, energy sources, and principles of operation. Safety and effectiveness can be demonstrated through engineering analysis, bench or animal testing, or human clinical testing. If it is not possible to identify a suitable predicate device, or devices, the sponsor may have to consider filing a PMA or a de novo 510(k), if appropriate.

Types of 510(k)s

There are four types of 510(k) premarket notifications. They are briefly described below. The following figure describes the decision process used to determine which type of 510(k) should be submitted. Each type of 510(k) is briefly described in the following sections. For more information on these types of 510(k)s see http://www.fda.gov/cdrh/ode/parad510.pdf (Fig. 6).

Traditional 510(k)

The traditional 510(k) is filed when the sponsor has developed a device that they believe is substantially equivalent to a device that has already been cleared through the 510(k) process, or was already on the market before the 1976 Medical Device Amendments were signed on May 26, 1976. In addition, the subject device is not a modification of one of the manufacturer's cleared devices nor does the application contain any declarations of conformance with the FDA-recognized standards.[9] Once this 510(k) is submitted, the ODE has 90 days to review the document.

Abbreviated 510(k)

This 510(k) is similar to the traditional 510(k) in function. A sponsor can choose to comply with the FDA-accepted standards during the testing process. A declaration of conformance is included in the 510(k), stating that the device meets the specifications in the referenced standards. Unlike a traditional 510(k), entire test reports do not need to be included. This simplifies both the 510(k) preparation and review processes. Once this 510(k) is submitted, ODE has 90 days to review the document. More information on the format for both traditional and abbreviated 510(k)s can be found at: Format for Traditional and Abbreviated 510(k)s—Guidance for Industry and FDA Staff http://www.fda.gov/cdrh/ode/guidance/1567.pdf.

Special 510(k)

A special 510(k) is submitted when a sponsor has modified his/her own device, has not added a new indication for use, and has not altered the fundamental scientific technology of the device. Design controls, including a risk analysis must be conducted. Reviews for special 510(k)s are processed within 30 days.

De Novo 510(k)

The de novo 510(k) is a 510(k) without a predicate device. It is not a commonly used path (4 clearances in 2006), but in some circumstances it is appropriate:

---

[9] Food and Drug Administration, available at: http://www.accessdata.fda.gov/scripts/cdrh/cfdocs/cfStandards/search.cfm.

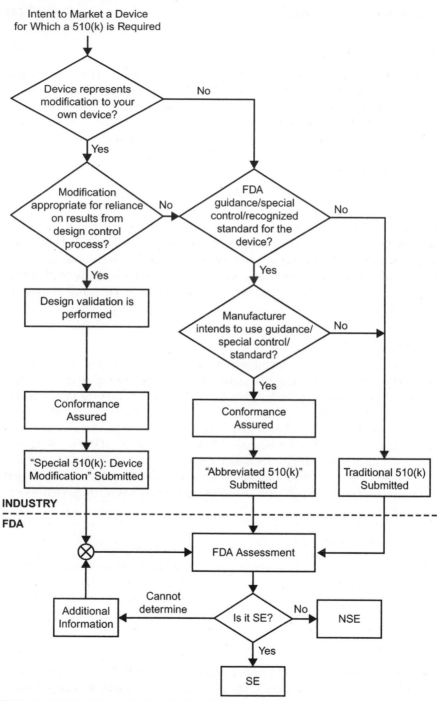

This flowchart should only be considered in conjunction with the accompanying proposed text.

Figure 6 The New 510(k) paradigm. *Source*: From "A New 510(k) Paradigm—Alternate Approaches to Demonstrating Substantial Equivalence in Premarket Notifications." U.S. Food and Drug Administration.

where the sponsor can demonstrate that the product has few risks and the extensive PMA safety and effectiveness review is not warranted. The device should be discussed with ODE in advance, before embarking on this path.

510(k) Components

The most common sections of a traditional 510(k) are described below. Many of these sections are also present in the other types of 510(k)s.

The Cover Sheet (FDA Form 3514)

This five-page form provides the ODE with general information related to the submission in a standardized format. Completion of this document is not mandatory. Only relevant data fields should be completed. The applicant signature is not required. Indications should be taken word for word from the body of the 510(k). A sample cover sheet can be found at http://www.fda.gov/opacom/morechoices/fdaforms/FDA-3514.doc.

The Cover Letter

This letter should be no more than one or two pages long and identify the device, very briefly summarize the contents of the application, and provide the name, address, telephone, and fax numbers of the contact person. The type of 510(k) should also be specified.

The Table of Contents

This section helps to create a "reviewer friendly" document by making it easy for the reviewer to locate each key section. Although it is not specifically required in the regulations, it is an expected component of any 510(k). Key sections of the 510(k) should be listed in the order they appear in the 510(k) along with the page number of the section. Index tabs, used selectively, can also aid the reviewer during the review process. All pages of the 510(k) should be numbered consecutively. This numbering facilitates communication between the reviewer and the sponsor during the review process.

User Fee Information

A copy of the completed medical device user fee cover sheet (available at: http://www.fda.gov/oc/mdufma/coversheet.html) must be included in this section. The unique payment identification number present in this form enables the ODE to confirm that the user fee payment has been received. The actual user fee payment is not included in the 510(k). The information at the preceding URL describes the user fee payment process in detail. The FY08 user fee for all types of 510(k)s is $3404.

Statement of Substantial Equivalence

This optional section can "sell" the 510(k) to the ODE by providing a well-reasoned rationale for a substantial equivalence determination. This section may not be necessary when there is a very simple comparison between a single predicate device and the new device. When a traditional or abbreviated 510(k) involves multiple predicate devices and complex technological comparisons, this type of statement can help communicate the sponsor's rationale. It contains a brief summary of device background information, along with a list of the predicate device(s), and most importantly, a narrative description of the sponsor's substantial equivalence claim. If appropriate, cross-references to other sections of the 510(k) may be included.

Labeling

This section must provide the ODE with all printed material associated with the device, including printing fixed to the outside of the device, its packaging, operator's manual or in the case of software-controlled devices, programmed into the electronics for display. Frequently, information displayed on video display screens is also reproduced in the operator's manual; so it does not have to be included twice. Patient information brochures, if used, should also be included.

Advertising and Promotional Material

If provided, the ODE will review the documentation and inform the sponsor of areas of noncompliance. This is optional information. If included, material should be clearly copied. Copies of actual brochures, especially if they are not on standard-size paper or include foldouts, are difficult for ODE document control personnel to handle. Advertising copy must be consistent with the indications for use mentioned in the 510(k).

Comparative Information

This is the heart of the 510(k). This section must contain data that demonstrate that the 510(k) device is "substantially equivalent" to the predicate device(s). Careful selection of comparative parameters is essential. Comparison charts listing parameters and values for the predicate device and the 510(k) device are common. Bench and clinical testing data may also be included. Advertising for the predicate device may also be included to support statements describing the predicate device. This section must clearly demonstrate that the new device is substantially equivalent to one or more predicate devices with respect to indication for use and technological features such as materials used and operating principle.

Biocompatability Assessment (If Necessary)

Medical devices contain a wide variety of materials, from stainless steel and titanium in orthopedic implants to plastics in catheters or even living cells in wound care products.[10] The data in this section must demonstrate that the device materials do not cause toxicity. Toxicity can occur through direct contact between the device and the body, such as a wound care product or an implantable device. Toxicity can also occur if materials such as plasticizers or mold-release agents leach from polymers, such as the tubing and components of a heart-lung bypass circuit, which carry blood out of and back into the body. Adverse effects are often localized, but can be systemic, or even carcinogenic effects can occur; so the standard requires more extensive testing when the device is implanted, rather than contacting intact skin and for permanent implants, as opposed to devices that contact the body for less than 24 hours.

An FDA-modified version of the international standard ISO 10993 is used to determine testing appropriate for a specific device. For more information on the use of ISO 10993 see http://www.fda.gov/cdrh/g951.html. The FDA document includes a testing matrix that uses the length of exposure and type of exposure to determine which tests are appropriate. Before conducting recommended testing, it is advisable to confirm the testing plan with the ODE, as requirements may vary for some devices.

Full reports of each required test are included in a traditional 510(k), especially if the test protocols have been modified from those specified in ISO 10993. A summary table of all biocompatibility testing and summary of results are often useful. If the medical device does not contact the patient, biocompatibility data are generally not necessary.

Truthful and Accurate Statement

This statement identifies a person who takes legal responsibility for the accuracy of the 510(k). It follows the requirements of 21 CFR 807.87(j).

> I certify that, in my capacity as (*the position held in company*) of (*company name*), I believe to the best of my knowledge, that all data and information submitted in the premarket notification are truthful and accurate and that no material fact has been omitted.

The statement must be signed and dated by a responsible person at the submitting company. A consultant cannot sign it.

---

[10] Helmus MN, ed. Biomaterials in the Design and Reliability of Medical Devices. New York: Kluwer Academic/Plenum Publishers, 2003.

Clinical Data

ODE may request clinical data to demonstrate substantial equivalence to a predicate device. It may also be necessary when, as described in the section "Substantial Equivalence," the sponsor must demonstrate that the new device does not raise new questions of safety and effectiveness. At some point, ODE reviewers will become more familiar with the device and indication and will only require engineering data. This often occurs once the first three or four 510(k)s for that generic type of device have successfully gone through the review process. Clinical data requirements for other 510(k) devices are specified in guidance documents and do not change over time. Generally, 510(k) clinical trials are smaller and simpler than most PMA clinical trials. Depending on the risk level of the trial, an approved IDE may be necessary to conduct the trial.

Shelf Life (If Necessary)

Stability of device components and packaging integrity (for sterile devices) must be demonstrated. The "Shelf Life of Medical Devices" guidance document (http://www.fda.gov/cdrh/ode/415.pdf) offers general advice. The useful life of in vitro diagnostic products must be determined. Accelerated data are acceptable in most cases although sponsors should also initiate real-time studies at the same time that they begin accelerated studies. A full report of real-time or, where appropriate, accelerated aging studies must be included.

Indication for Use Form

This form clarifies, for any interested party, the device's cleared indication(s) for use. The sponsor lists the indications for use on an ODE form. If the sponsor wishes to promote the device for a new indication, another traditional or abbreviated 510(k) must be cleared. Once a 510(k) is cleared, this form, the clearance letter, and the 510(k) summary are available from the FDA via its Web site.

510(k) Summary

Summaries are released to the public via the FDA's Web site. They provide interested parties with a brief description of the device and some of the data included in the 510(k).

The content of the summary is described in 21 CFR 807.92. All relevant items must be present, or the ODE will request clarification, potentially delaying 510(k) clearance. When preparing summaries, regulatory professionals have to balance the regulatory requirements that mandate the inclusion of a wide variety of data describing the device and the development process with the business needs to limit disclosure of information that may benefit a competitor.

Practical Aspects for 510(k)s

It is important to conduct research early in the 510(k) process and become aware of the cleared indications and technologies for competitive products. It is possible to request a competitor's 510(k) under the Freedom of Information Act although processing times can often exceed 12 months, so this is not usually a practical option. For older 510(k)s, commercial information brokers may offer considerably faster response times.

Once a 510(k) is filed, ODE will mail the sponsor a letter acknowledging receipt of the submission and including the "K" number used for internal tracking. It is important to keep a copy of every document sent to or received from the FDA. Sponsors should also designate one company FDA contact person. That individual should document all phone conversations with reviewers. The FDA contact people should keep in mind that when ODE reviewers call with questions, they should listen carefully, but not leap to unsupported conclusions. If an ODE reviewer asks for specific data, confirm the data with experts in your company if you have any doubts. In most circumstances, a delay of a day or two will not be significant compared with the risk of misstatement. Increasingly, communications with reviewers occur via e-mail. Additional data can be officially submitted via fax or e-mail if the reviewer concurs. Once the reviewer's questions have all been answered, the reviewer's conclusions are reviewed prior to generating a clearance letter. A copy of the clearance letter is usually faxed to the sponsor shortly after it is signed. Commercial distribution can then begin. The official copy of the letter is mailed to the sponsor.

Postsubmission Considerations for 510(k)s

Manufacturers must comply with the QSR with respect to device modifications, production, and quality operations. Injuries or deaths (to patients or medical personnel) must also be reported to the FDA in accordance with the medical device reporting (MDR) regulation (21 CFR 803). Manufacturers are subject to inspection by the FDA investigators who review the QSR and the MDR compliance. Manufacturers must also register and list with the FDA. Refer to the section "Postmarketing Issues" for a more detailed discussion of postmarketing responsibilities.

THE PREMARKET APPROVAL APPLICATION

Introduction to the PMA

PMAs are necessary when the device developer wishes to market an innovative device in the United States That is not substantially equivalent to any other device that has been cleared through the 510(k) process. The PMA must demonstrate that the device is safe and effective. The PMA process is considerably more complex than the 510(k) process. Typical review times are approximately one year. Unlike most 510(k)s, a detailed manufacturing section describing the methods for building and testing the device must be included. Prior to final approval of the PMA, the CDRH office of compliance must review and approve the results of a preapproval inspection of the device manufacturing and development facilities. The sponsor of the clinical trial and two or three of the clinical investigation sites are also often subject to CDRH bioresearch monitoring (BIMO) inspections to confirm compliance with relevant sections of 21 CFR 812. Lastly, the postmarket requirements of a PMA are considerably more complex than those related to a 510(k). Specifically, a PMA annual report must be filed with the ODE each year and changes in labeling, materials, manufacturing, and quality methods, and specifications as well as changes in manufacturing location must all be reported to, and approved by, the ODE, in advance. This is done through the PMA supplement process.

The PMA Process

PMAs are large and complex documents, often greater than 2000 pages. It can frequently take several years to obtain all the preclinical, clinical, and manufacturing data necessary for the PMA. It is essential that the PMA preparation effort be well planned, with good coordination between all functional areas involved in the development process. Advance research before a regulatory strategy is prepared should include a wide variety of sources. Shortly after a PMA device is approved, the approval letter, summary of safety and effectiveness, and official labeling are placed on the CDRH Web site. These documents provide greater technical and regulatory detail than a 510(k) summary. The PMA submission itself is not available via the Freedom of Information process.

Once the indication for use and the device description have been established, it is important to confirm the key elements of the development plan with the appropriate reviewing branch within the ODE. The device developer may choose to obtain this information via an informal telephone call, an informal pre-IDE meeting, a formal designation meeting or a formal agreement meeting. See http://www.fda.gov/cdrh/ode/guidance/310.pdf for a more detailed description of these meetings. Generally, the more formal the meeting, the less interactive the discussion. Less formal meetings, while not generating binding agreements, can encourage very productive technical exchanges. The choice of meeting type involves balancing business, regulatory, and clinical needs.

Once a PMA development plan has been established and reviewed by the ODE, it is time to execute it. Generally, multiple activities such as manufacturing development and validation, preclinical functional and biocompatibility testing, and clinical testing proceed along parallel, often simultaneous tracks. In some cases, it may be clear during the planning phase that some data, such as manufacturing process information or preclinical testing data, may be available long before the clinical trial has ended. In these cases, it may be advantageous to submit the pieces of the PMA to the ODE as they are completed, rather than send all the data at the very end. This process is called a modular PMA. If a PMA sponsor chooses to submit a modular PMA, a PMA shell or outline of the PMA must be prepared and approved by the ODE. The shell describes the contents of each module. As the modules are submitted, the ODE reviews them independently. Once review of a module has been successfully completed, the ODE sends the sponsor a letter stating that the module is "locked" and will not be reopened unless some portion of data already submitted changes in later stages of the development process. When the last module is submitted, the ODE considers the PMA complete.

Advisory Panels

When a PMA device raises questions that the ODE reviewers have not previously addressed, they may choose to refer those questions to one of the advisory panels maintained for this purpose. Advisory panels are made up of experts in the field, who are not FDA employees or from the industry. Many panel members are in academic medicine. The panel has one nonvoting industry representative and one nonvoting consumer representative. An executive secretary, usually a senior ODE reviewer, coordinates administrative details. The conclusions of the advisor panel are not binding on the FDA although they are almost always followed. Transcripts of advisory panel meetings are available via the CDRH Web site. Videotapes of these meetings are also available from private sources. If competitive products have gone through the panel process, these meeting minutes can provide a great deal of valuable information on the types of data and analysis expected. If such a panel meeting occurs during your development process, it is very helpful if regulatory, medical, and technical development personnel attend in person. This can make preparation for your own panel meeting easier. More information on these panels can be found at: http://www.fda.gov/cdrh/panel/index.html.

Clinical Data

According to Section 515 of the Food, Drug, and Cosmetic Act, a PMA must provide valid scientific evidence that there is a "reasonable assurance" that a device is both safe and effective. 21 CFR 860.7(c)(2) states that this evidence can come from

- well-controlled investigations,
- partially controlled investigations,
- objective trials without matched controls,
- well-documented case histories conducted by qualified experts, and
- reports of significant human experience with a marketed device from which it can fairly and responsibly be concluded by qualified experts that there is reasonable assurance of safety and effectiveness of a device under its conditions of use.

In practice, the vast majority of PMA studies are designed as well-controlled studies where patients are randomized to either a treatment or a control group. Less frequently, studies can be designed to compare the investigational device to a historical control group, provided that the historical control group accurately reflects current U.S. medical practice and the demographics of the U.S. population. Data from other types of studies must always be reported to the ODE; however, they generally cannot stand as the sole source of performance data.

Use of International Data

Due to the international nature of the medial device industry, human clinical data may be available from ex-U.S. studies before U.S. development efforts have begun. How should these data be treated? Can they be used to support the PMA? Does the FDA require U.S. clinical data?

There are no FDA requirements that a PMA must contain U.S. clinical data. Good, credible, and ethical data will be accepted from any location. The ODE suggests that sponsors planning to submit international data in a PMA discuss their plans with them early in the development process. As with any clinical study, it is critical to assure that the study meets the ODE's expectations regarding medical and scientific issues such as the endpoints selected and the comparators used. If all of these parameters are consistent with ODE expectations, then there is one last set of tests before the data can be accepted. According to 21 CFR 814.15, the study must

- be conducted in accordance with the Declaration of Helsinki or local ethical procedures, whichever is stricter;
- use a patient population similar to the U.S. patient population;
- use a standard of care and medical practice similar to that in the United States;
- be performed by competent investigators; and
- generate data, including source documentation, that are available for audit by the FDA.

Sponsors must be especially careful that study patients are not treated with drugs or procedures that are not available in the United States.

Components of the PMA

The PMA regulation (21 CFR 814) contains a description of the components of a PMA. ODE has produced numerous guidance documents that describe various PMA sections. Many of these guidance documents are product specific. Two of the more generic guidance documents can be found at: http://www.fda.gov/cdrh/manual/pmamanul.pdf and http://www.fda.gov/cdrh/blbkmem.html#pma.

The items listed below include the major sections of a PMA. The length and complexity of each section will vary according to the technical details and regulatory issues associated with the product.

- Cover page
- Table of contents

- Summary of safety and effectiveness
- Device description and manufacturing data
- Performance standards referenced
- Technical data (nonclinical and clinical)
- Justification for a single investigator
- Bibliography
- Device sample (if requested)
- Labeling
- Environmental assessment (if necessary)

THE QUALITY SYSTEM REGULATION

The QSR regulates both the device development and the manufacturing process for all class II and class III devices from the beginning of the development phase until the device is no longer supported by the manufacturer. It also covers the manufacturing process for many class I devices. It does not cover the research process for any medical devices. The goal of the QSR is to create a self-correcting system that reliably produces robust device designs and production methods, ensuring that devices perform in a manner consistent with their intended use. In many ways, the QSR has evolved into the glue that holds the medical device regulatory process together from development through end of use. As discussed earlier, the existence of the QSR makes the special 510(k) possible. Once a device is marketed, the corrective and preventive action (CAPA) provisions of the QSR are closely related to compliance with the MDR regulation. An additional advantage of the QSR is that it follows the philosophy of the international medical device standard, ISO 13485, which helps to enable device companies that sell their product internationally to maintain common systems for most design- and production-related activities. In most cases, the QSR requires more extensive documentation than ISO 13485.[11] The system works by requiring specific activities and documentation beginning during the development process. The manufacturing and quality processes also require specific evaluations and procedures, all of which must be documented. Frequently, the FDA field investigators will follow the quality system inspection techniques (QSIT) approach[12] when inspecting a device facility. This process breaks QSR compliance into four main modules and four satellite modules, some of which may not be applicable to all device firms. The FDA investigator will choose a subset of those modules and determine the firm's compliance with QSR. This means that not every system is reviewed during a QSIT inspection;

---

[11] Trautman K. The FDA and Worldwide Quality System Requirements Guidebook for Medical Devices. Milwaukee, WI: ASQC Quality Press, 1997.

[12] Food and Drug Administration, Guide To Inspections of Quality Systems. Washington, DC, August 1999.

however, this process does yield a general assessment of the QSR compliance. Many firms consider the QSR requirements to be only a beginning and build on them, adding various customer-oriented feedback loops and financial accountability to the process. These integrated business systems can generate significant returns on the investment by reducing time to market, reducing the number of field corrections and recalls, and increasing customer satisfaction and device safety. The remaining portions of this section describe some of the provisions of the QSR. Design controls were already discussed in the section "An Introduction to the Medical Device Approval Process." Although these sections of the QSR are discussed separately, the figure below graphically demonstrates how these functions are connected to each other. Readers should refer to the regulation[13] for complete information (Fig. 7).

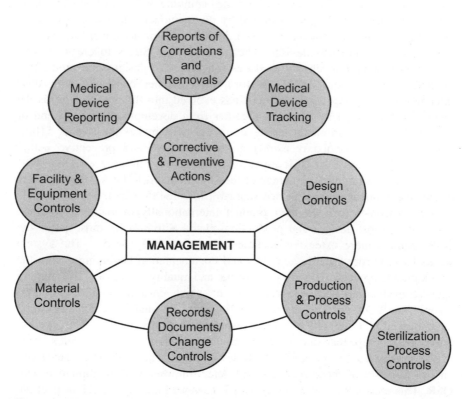

Figure 7 The seven primary QSR subsystems. *Abbreviation*: QSR, Quality System Regulation. *Source*: From FDA guide to inspections of quality systems, August 1999.

---

[13] Code of Federal Regulations Title 21 Section 820.

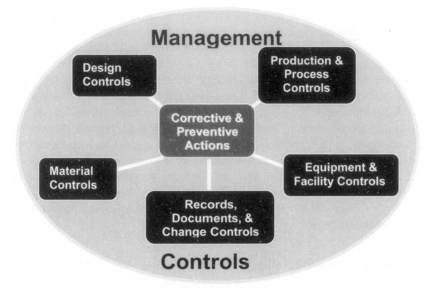

Figure 8 CAPA diagram. *Abbreviation*: CAPA, corrective and preventive action. *Source*: From the FDA QSIT workshop presentation.

Management Controls

Device firms need to demonstrate that they have management systems in place that can adequately control all the processes that take place in the life cycle of their products from the development phase onwards. As Figure 8 illustrates, management is at the center of the quality system. The QSR holds "management with executive responsibility" ultimately responsible for the tasks specified in the regulation. Clearly, a device manufacturer with six employees will have less complex systems than a manufacturer with 600 employees. One SOP or a single organizational structure would not be appropriate for all device manufacturers.

One key provision of the QSR involves the controls that management places on the regulated system. First, there must be a quality policy in place, implemented and understood by all levels of employees. A quality plan and quality system procedures must also be in place. Next, management has the responsibility to assure that there are adequate resources and organizational structures to carry out all the activities specified in the regulation. A management representative must be formally appointed, must be actively involved in maintaining the quality system, and must regularly report those efforts to management with executive responsibility. Part of maintaining the quality system involves testing the system with prescheduled audits conducted by company staff that is not directly involved in the function audited. These audits must be conducted according to an SOP and recorded in an audit log and audit results documented. (FDA investigators do not generally have the authority to request copies of these audit reports.) The function of these audits is for the company itself to identify and then correct any quality system problems detected in the audits. Management reviews of a wide variety of quality data must be conducted at regular intervals and documented. These data include, but are not limited to, audit reports. Other sources of quality data include rework records from the manufacturing floor, incoming quality control (QC) testing summaries, service records, customer complaints and inquiries, and final inspection records. All of these data sources combine to paint a picture of the status of the company's products. It is critically important that the firm can demonstrate that action is taken as a result of these data. Identification of quality issues is important, but correction of problems and confirmation of the effectiveness of such corrections must also be documented.

Corrective and Preventive Action

The CAPA portion of the regulation makes the firm's quality system self-correcting and self-improving. The five functional areas depicted in the boxes in Figure 9 feed information in the CAPA system. Under the supervision of the management, these data are processed and initiatives developed and executed that are intended to identify the causes of the problems and correct them. Data sources for the CAPA system include internal audits; incoming, in-process, and final QC testing results; service and repair records; and customer feedback. A variety of statistical tools may be used to better evaluate these data. Failure investigations should be conducted, according to a predetermined SOP, to determine the root cause of device failures. Once this has been done, a corrective action plan must be prepared and the corrective actions verified, or in appropriate instances, validated.

Production and Process Controls

Production and process controls are the systems at the heart of the manufacturing process. Documentation is a major part of the control process. The device master record (DMR), a compilation of records containing the procedures and specifications for a finished device, is a key document for this functional area. Rather than existing as a discrete document, it is frequently an index that directs the reader to other documents where the necessary information is located. The device history record (DHR) is a compilation of records containing the production history of a finished device or a production-run of devices. It usually contains manufacturing documentation, testing results, labeling documentation, and release/approval documentation. A single DHR may be generated for a large expensive durable medical device, while another DHR may describe a production run of 10,000 disposable devices. Validation documentation, when necessary, is also a key part of production

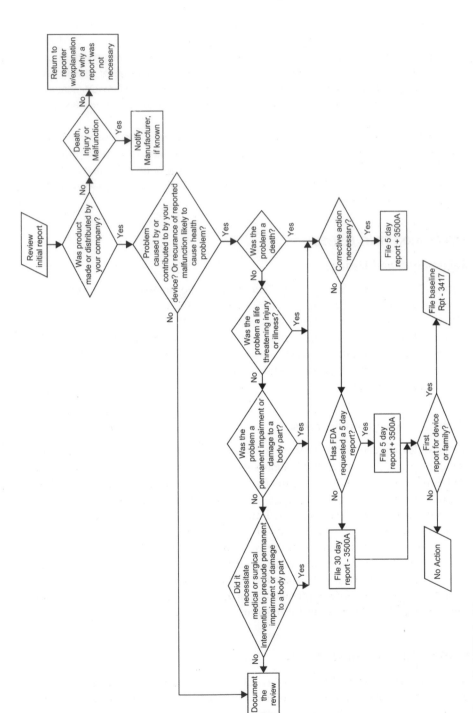

Figure 9 MDR decision tree.

and process controls. Any production process whose output cannot be 100% checked once it is completed must be validated to establish, by objective evidence, that a process consistently produces a result or product meeting its predetermined specifications. Typically, processes such as sterilization or molding of plastic parts are validated. Other activities such as calibration, servicing and maintenance of production and testing equipment, and cleaning and maintenance of buildings must also be documented.

The goal of the QSR is to weave a web of systems that closely monitor development efforts to assure that a high-quality design is created, that the production of that device occurs in a controlled and predictable manner, and that various streams of quality data are appropriately analyzed and used to effect CAPA, when necessary.

POSTMARKETING ISSUES

Registration and Listing

Within 30 days of placing a medical device into interstate commerce, the manufacturer must register and list with the FDA. The device registration fee in FY08 is $1706 per year. All device manufacturers, U.S. and international, must register. The purpose of registration and listing is to inform the FDA of the existence of the manufacturer. At some point after registration, the FDA may choose to inspect the device development and manufacturing facilities to ensure compliance with the QSR.

Medical Device Modifications

Medical device technology evolves at a very rapid rate. Often the version of the device that receives initial PMA approval is a version or two older than the one sold outside the United States or sold by their competitors at the time of the PMA approval. 510(k) devices also change quickly. In both cases, sponsors need to understand how the FDA process will affect their product upgrade timelines and budgets. Modifications for all class II and III devices must be developed in accordance with the design control provisions of the QSR. Design controls have added enough extraconfidence to the system so that, since 1998, the FDA has created new processes such as special 510(k)s and 30-day notices for PMAs that permit sponsors to rapidly implement some device modifications, as long as they comply with the design control provisions of the QSR.

Modifications to 510(k) Devices

There are three main classifications of 510(k) device modifications. They include those that require a documented review and a determination by the company that a new 510(k) is not needed, those that require a special 510(k), and

Table 6 Modifications to 510(k) Devices

Regulatory action	Examples of modifications
Review document in a memo to the file	Redesigning the external case of a durable medical device so that it consists of few pieces to reduce production costs.
File a special 510(k)	[a]Adding a feature that has already been incorporated in another device of the same type
File a traditional or abbreviated 510(k)	Adding a new indication, significant change in technology

[a]Modification to firm's own device and no change in intended use or fundamental scientific technology.

Table 7 PMA Supplement Types

PMA supplement type	Examples of modifications
180-days supplement	A major change in the design of the device or in manufacturing or QC methods
180-days panel track supplement	Adding a new indication for use where clinical data are required to support the application
[a]Special PMA supplement changes being effected	A change enhances the safety of a device, such as labeling changes that add or strengthen a contraindication, warning, precaution, or information about an adverse reaction.
[a]30-days notice	A change of the type of process used (e.g., machining a part to injection molding the part)
[b]Real-time supplement	Minor design modifications that would otherwise require a 180-days supplement
Annual report	Update the microprocessor for the device when equivalence test has previously been approved by the ODE.

[a]The sponsor may choose either submission type.
[b]With the prior approval of the responsible ODE branch chief.
Abbreviations: PMA, premarket approval; QC, quality control; ODE, Office of Device Evaluation.

those that require a traditional or abbreviated 510(k). A useful source of more detailed information on changes to 510(k) devices can be found at: http://www.fda.gov/cdrh/ode/510kmod.pdf. There are no annual reports required for 510(k) products (Table 6).

Modifications to PMA Devices

Modifications to PMA devices are more closely controlled than modifications to 510(k) devices. The table below briefly summarizes the various types of PMA supplements. See http://www.fda.gov/cdrh/ode/pumasupp.pdf (Table 7).

PMA sponsors must also submit a PMA annual report to ODE and pay a $6475 filing fee every year. This report contains updates on ongoing clinical trials, device modifications, adverse device effects, and MDR reports. More information on PMA annual reports can be found at: http://www.fda.gov/cdrh/ devadvice/pma/postapproval.html#annual.

Medical Device Reporting

Significant problems with marketed medical devices must be reported to the FDA, using the FDA form 3500A (MedWatch). While this same form is used to report pharmaceutical adverse events, section D, suspect medical device; section F, four use by user facility/distributor devices only; and section H, device manufacturers only are specific to devices. The process for evaluating and reporting device incidents is described in 21 CFR 803 and is not related to the ICH procedures employed for pharmaceuticals. The MDR regulation was originally implemented in 1984, and the final regulation was published in December 1995 and effective from July 31, 1996. An MDR SOP must be in place for every device manufacturer, regardless of device class. This applies even if the firm has never made an MDR report. MDR reports are available on the CDRH Web site at: http://www.fda.gov/cdrh/mdr/mdr-file-general.html. A flowchart that summarizes the MDR process is included (Figure 9).

MDR reporting time frames. The manufacturer must report incidents to the FDA five working days after becoming aware of events requiring remedial action to prevent an unreasonable risk of substantial harm or events for which the FDA has required five days of reporting. This type of notification commonly occurs when a recall or field correction is necessary. The manufacturer must report incidents to the FDA 30 working days after becoming aware of the information that reasonably suggests that a device may have caused or contributed to a death or serious injury or if the device malfunctions in a manner likely to cause or contribute to death or serious injury. It is important to note that the regulation does not differentiate between injuries to patients, medical professionals, or family members. An injury to anyone that is caused by the device can be reportable.

Key MDR definitions. Serious injury: life threatening, permanent impairment, or damage, or medical/surgical intervention necessary to preclude such damage. Cosmetic or trivial irreversible damage is not serious.

Malfunction: the failure of the device to meet its performance specifications or otherwise perform as intended.

"Becomes aware": when *any* employee, at any level of the company becomes aware of a reportable event.

"Reasonably suggests": a professional medical opinion relating to the causal relationship between the adverse event and the medical device. If a physician, working for the manufacturer, concludes that an event is not related to the device, no report is necessary. This decision must be documented.

"Caused or contributed to": causation can be attributed to device failures or malfunctions due to improper design, manufacturing methods, labeling, or operator error. Remedial action: any action that is not routine maintenance, routine servicing, and is intended to prevent the recurrence of the event.

Other MDR requirements. Manufacturers must retain all MDR records for two years or for the expected life of the device, whichever is longer. The types of records that must be retained include all MDR-related forms submitted to the FDA, explanations why reports were not submitted for specific events that were not reported, and documentation relating to all events investigated. Written procedures must be present for identification and evaluation of events, a standardized review process to determine reportability, and for procedures to assure that adequate reports are submitted to the FDA in a timely manner. Additional information on the MDR regulation can be found at: http://www.fda. gov/cdrh/mdr/.

Advertising and Promotion

Unlike pharmaceuticals, no preclearance of advertising copy is required for medical devices, even PMA devices. Promotional material must conform with cleared or approved indications for use. If a device is cleared for a general indication, more specific indications cannot be promoted, unless they are specifically cleared.

6

The Development of Orphan Drugs

Tan T. Nguyen

Food and Drug Administration, Center for Devices and Radiological Health, Rockville, Maryland, U.S.A.

INTRODUCTION

Approximately 25 million Americans and many more throughout the world suffer from more than 6000 rare diseases. Some of these diseases are well-recognized, such as Lou Gehrig's disease or cystic fibrosis, but little is known about many others, such as Adams-Oliver syndrome or Norrie disease. Almost all of them are serious, life-threatening, or fatal diseases. Despite the urgent need for safe and effective treatments, the small patient populations of these rare diseases often do not present sufficiently viable markets for drug sponsors to recover the high costs of therapeutic research and development, much less to expect profit. After investing resources to develop the drugs, the sponsors may not be protected from competitors since the potential uses of many drugs in rare diseases—often discovered during the course of study for other diseases and generally already in the public domain—may not be patentable.[1] Thus, even after being discovered, many of these drugs are not commercially pursued or "adopted." Hence, they come to be known as "orphan" drugs.

---

[1] A patent cannot be granted "if the invention was known or used by others in this country, or patented or described in a printed publication in this or a foreign country, before the invention thereof by the applicant for patent." 35 USC Section 102; 1994.

THE ORPHAN DRUG ACT OF 1983 AND ITS AMENDMENTS

Prompted by the urging of a small grassroots coalition of patient advocacy groups galvanized by Abbey Meyers and public sentiment stirred by Jack Klugman of the hit television series *Quincy, M.E.*, Congress passed the Orphan Drug Act ("the Act") in late December 1982.[2] On January 4, 1983, President Ronald Reagan signed it into law.

The Act as amended established financial and regulatory incentives to encourage the development of potentially promising orphan drugs.[3] The main incentives include: (*i*) regulatory assistance from the Food and Drug Administration (FDA) in the form of written recommendations for non-clinical and clinical investigations for marketing approval purposes; (*ii*) a tax credit covering 50% of the clinical drug testing expenses; (*iii*) federal funding of grants and contracts to help defray such expenses; and (*iv*) a seven-year exclusive marketing rights to the sponsor of the innovator drug after approval.[4]

To qualify for these benefits, the sponsor would need to request an orphan-drug designation from the FDA. As originally enacted, the FDA would grant such request if the disease or condition in question occurred so infrequently in the United States that there was no reasonable expectation the costs of developing and making the drug available would be recovered from its sales in the United States.[5] As such, all sponsors were required to provide to the FDA detailed financial information to demonstrate the anticipated lack of profitability, regardless of how rare a drug's target population would be. The response to the Act was less than enthusiastic, given the reluctance of sponsors to open their books to the FDA, and the difficulties with quantifying development costs and anticipated sales. Furthermore, the FDA did not have the necessary expertise to evaluate this information. To lessen this burden, Congress amended the Act in 1984 to alternatively allow a drug to receive orphan designation if the proposed

---

[2] See Public Law No. 97–414 of 1983 codified as amended at 21 US C Section 360aa–ee (1983). The Act added four sections—525, 526, 527, and 528—to the Federal Food, Drug, and Cosmetic Act: section 525 (21 USC Section 360aa) concerned written recommendations for nonclinical and clinical investigations of orphan drugs; section 526 (Section 360bb) concerned orphan-drug designation; section 527 (Section 360cc) concerned orphan-drug marketing exclusivity; and section 528 (Section 360dd) concerned treatment use ("open protocols") of experimental orphan drugs.

[3] The word "drug" will be used in this chapter to refer to a chemical drug or a biological product.

[4] Through the Food and Drug Administration Modernization Act of 1997, Congress created an additional incentive—exempting orphan drugs from the marketing application user fee (See discussion under "Exemption of Marketing Application Fee").

[5] It was thought at the time that setting an actual numerical prevalence threshold for rare diseases would be unwise since such a figure had not been generally defined. See 97th Cong. Rec., 1st Sess., S7877 (daily ed. July 17, 1981) (statement of Sen. Kassebaum).

disease or condition affects less than 200,000 persons in the United States.[6] A drug intended for a disease or condition exceeding this prevalence threshold would still be eligible for orphan designation, if the sponsor could satisfy the original financial criteria of the Act.

The Act initially allowed only designated orphan drugs "for which a United States Letter of Patent may not be issued" to qualify for the seven-year marketing exclusivity.[7] In 1985, the Act was amended to make all drugs eligible for this incentive, regardless of their patentability.[8] In addition, the amendment clarified that antibiotics would also be eligible for orphan drug incentives.

In 1988, Congress again amended the Act to require that the request for orphan-drug designation be filed prior to the submission of the application for marketing approval of the drug for the orphan indication.[9,10] Prior to this, a designation request could be filed anytime prior to marketing approval by the FDA.

To implement the Act, the FDA was charged with promulgating standards and procedures for determining eligibility criteria for orphan-drug incentives. In 1991, the FDA issued a notice of proposed rule making entitled "Orphan Drug Regulations."[11] After reviewing public comments, the FDA finalized the Orphan Drug Regulations in 1992.[12]

INCENTIVES FOR ORPHAN DRUG DEVELOPMENT

Orphan-Drug Marketing Exclusivity

The most significant incentive provided by the Act to ensure the innovator sponsor a predictable, often significant, revenue from sales is the seven-year

---

[6] See Public Law No. 98–551 (1984). The prevalence threshold of 200,000 persons was adopted as a surrogate for nonprofitability. Some have raised concerns that this fixed numerical threshold would not address growing patient populations. Subsequent orphan drug legislations elsewhere dealt with this issue differently. In Japan, the prevalence threshold for a rare disease was set at 50,000 persons (1993), and in Australia, at 2000 persons (1997). The European Union, however, adopted a prevalence rate of no more than five persons per 10,000 population (1999).

[7] It was assumed early on that most biological products ("biotech drugs"), being naturally occurring substances, would have difficulties in obtaining patents. Later it became clear that this assumption was not always correct since many biological products could be protected by process patents.

[8] See Public Law No. 99–91 (1985).

[9] See Public Law No. 100–290 (1988).

[10] A sponsor must file a new drug application (NDA) with the FDA to apply for permission to market a new drug, or a biological licensing application (BLA) for certain biological products such as vaccines, recombinant proteins, or blood-derived products. An NDA is approved under section 505(b) of the FDCA (21 USC Section 355(b)), and a BLA is licensed under section 351 of the Public Health Service Act (42 USC Section 262). Unless otherwise stated, the term *marketing application* used in this chapter refers to both NDA and BLA.

[11] See 56 Federal Register 3338 (1991).

[12] Code of Federal Regulations Title 21 Part 316 (57 Federal Register 62,076) (1992).

period of exclusive rights to market its orphan drug.[13,14] This means that after approving the sponsor's marketing application for the designated orphan drug, the FDA will not approve another sponsor's marketing application of the same drug for the same use for the next seven years, unless the exclusivity holder consents to such approval. If the sponsor fails to assure adequate supply of the drug to meet the needs of patients, however, the FDA may withdraw the exclusivity, whether or not there are alternative sources of drug supply. Since the needs of patients are the primary concern, the decision by the FDA to withdraw exclusivity under this circumstance cannot be appealed. The exclusivity will also be suspended if the sponsor's orphan-drug designation is revoked (see discussion under "Granting, Revocation, and Amendment of Orphan-Drug Designation").[15] The withdrawal of exclusivity in either case does not affect the marketing approval status of the drug. The sponsor must also notify the FDA at least one year in advance of any discontinuation of drug production after the drug is approved for marketing.[16] This requirement is necessary for the FDA to attempt to find another sponsor in time to keep the drug available on the market.

The scope of orphan-drug marketing exclusivity is restricted to the approved indication for use of the drug. During the period of exclusivity, another sponsor may receive marketing approval of the same drug for any use other than the "protected" use. For example, if the drug is approved for use in only a particular subset of patients with a rare disease, the accompanying exclusivity would not bar another sponsor from seeking and obtaining marketing approval of the same drug for use in a different subset or in the remaining patient population.

Tax Credit

As provided by the Act, the sponsor of a designated orphan drug may claim an orphan-drug credit equal to 50% of the expenses incurred by clinical testing of the drug for the rare disease or condition against the Federal taxes owed by the sponsor.[17]

---

[13] See section 527 of the FDCA (21 USC Section 360cc) and Code of Federal Regulations Title 21 Section 316.31.

[14] In accordance with section 111 of the Food and Drug Administration Modernization Act of 1997 (Public Law No. 105–115), the orphan-drug marketing exclusivity may be lengthened by the *pediatric exclusivity* for an additional six months, if the sponsor fulfils its commitments to conduct pediatric studies with the drug per the FDA's request. The six-month pediatric exclusivity provision was extended to 2007 by the Best Pharmaceuticals for Children Act (Public Law No. 107–109) (2002). Subsequently, Title V of the FDA Amendments Act of 2007 (Public Law No. 110–85) reauthorized FDA to extend the pediatric exclusivity for five more years.

[15] Code of Federal Regulations Title 21 Section 316.219(b).

[16] See section 526 of the FDCA (21 USC Section 360bb).

[17] The tax provisions are administered by the Internal Revenue Service (26 USC Section 45C and Code of Federal Regulations Title 26 Section 1.28–1). Public Law No. 104–188 (1996) created carry-back and carry-forward provisions for unused tax credit. Public Law No. 105–34 (1997) made the tax credit provision permanent as of May 31, 1997 (previously, these provisions required reauthorization by Congress each year).

Administered by the Internal Revenue Service, the tax credit is applicable only to clinical testing conducted between the date of the drug's designation and the date of its marketing approval. The clinical testing must be conducted under an approved investigational new drug application (IND). The tax credit is also allowed for clinical testing costs outside the United States, if the sponsor can show that there is an insufficient testing population in this country. The sponsor, however, cannot claim the tax credit for any expenditure funded by a grant, contract, or by a government entity. Presently, the unused tax credit is now a component of the general business credit that can be carried back one year and then forward 20 years.

Orphan Product Grants

The Orphan Product Grants Program is administered by the Office of Orphan Products Development (OOPD) in the FDA. The statutory provision for orphan product grants originated as section 5 of the Orphan Drug Act.[18] Initially, these grants were intended for defraying the clinical testing costs incurred in connection to the development of only orphan drugs. In 1988, the provision was amended to also qualify sponsors of medical devices and medical foods for rare diseases or conditions for orphan product grants.[19]

The objective of this program is to fund clinical investigations on the safety and effectiveness of experimental products to diagnose, treat, or prevent rare diseases or conditions in the United States. Grants are available to foreign or domestic, public or private, for-profit or nonprofit entities, state and local units of government, and federal agencies not part of the Department of Health and Human Services. To announce the availability of funds, OOPD publishes a request for applications (RFA) in the *Federal Register*. The RFA can also be accessed directly from the OOPD Web site.[20] The annual funds appropriated to the Orphan Product Grants Program over the past several years have remained unchanged at about $14 million.[21]

Grant applications are first administratively reviewed by OOPD for responsiveness to the program criteria set forth in the RFA. OOPD then convenes ad hoc panels of experts in the respective diseases or conditions to review the

---

[18] This statutory provision was not enacted as part of the FDCA. The FDA has administered its Orphan Product Grants Program under the authority of title III, section 301, of the Public Health Service Act (Public Law No. 78-410, as amended) (42 USC Section 241).

[19] With respect to medical devices and medical foods, a rare disease or condition is statutorily defined in section 5 of the Act (21 USC Section 360ee) as "any disease or condition that occurs so infrequently in the United States that there is no reasonable expectation that a medical device (or medical food) for such disease or condition will be developed without assistance. . . . " There is no numerical prevalence threshold for these products.

[20] See http://www.fda.gov/orphan/grants/index.htm (accessed October 2007).

[21] The unchanged annual appropriations at $14 million over the last several years represent a loss in the "buying power" to the Orphan Product Grants Program if one factors in the inflation rates and other economic adjustments.

responsive applications for scientific and technical merits, and to assign each a priority review score. The experts are from outside the FDA, although members of the FDA review divisions may be available to assist them with regulatory issues. These applications are next reviewed by the National Cancer Advisory Board at the National Cancer Institute for concurrence with the recommendations made by the review panels. Funding decisions are made by the FDA Commissioner or his designee.

Grants are awarded on a competitive basis based on the ranking of the priority review scores. At present, grants of up to $200,000 in total (direct plus indirect) costs per year are made to any phase 1, 2, or 3 clinical investigations for up to three years.[22] Phase 2 or 3 clinical investigations, however, may qualify for grants up to $400,000 per year, for up to four years. Clinical studies supported by the Orphan Product Grants program must be conducted under an approved IND (for drugs) or an approved Investigational Device Exemption (for medical devices).[23] They must also comply with applicable human research subject protection regulations and good clinical practice guidelines.[24,25]

Between 2000 and 2006, OOPD received about 70 grant applications annually and, on average funded 17 each year.[26] The majority of grant recipients (81%) were affiliated with academic/research institutions and medical centers; the remaining grantees (19%) were pharmaceutical companies. Approximately 64% of grants were for clinical studies of chemical drugs, 30% for biological products, and 6% for medical devices. A total of 475 orphan product grants have been awarded between the inception of the program in 1983 and June 2007. To date, they have supported marketing approval of 34 orphan drugs, six orphan medical devices, and numerous publications on the potential uses of experimental orphan products.

---

[22] The clinical drug development process is often described in terms of four temporal phases. Phase 1 starts with the initial administration of an experimental drug into humans (healthy volunteers or patients) to preliminarily determine its safety, tolerability, pharmacodynamic/pharmacokinetic properties, and, if possible, early activity. Phase 2 starts with the initiation of studies to explore the drug's efficacy profile. The objectives of Phase 2 are to determine the appropriate study design, dosage, target population, and endpoints for Phase 3 investigation. Phase 3 begins with the initiation of "pivotal" studies to demonstrate or confirm the drug's clinical benefit. They are intended to provide adequate safety and effectiveness data as bases for marketing approval. Phase 4 studies are performed after drug approval to optimize the drug's use. See also "E8 General Considerations for Clinical Trials" (1997) available at: http://www.fda.gov/cder/guidance/1857fnl.pdf (accessed October 2007).

[23] There is no comparable regulatory requirement for clinical trials of medical foods supported by orphan product grants.

[24] Relevant regulations related to human research subject protection (Code of Federal Regulations Title 45 Part 46) can be found at http://www.hhs.gov/ohrp/ (accessed October 2007).

[25] See "E6 Good Clinical Practice: Consolidated Guidance" (1996) available at: http://www.fda.gov/cder/guidance/959fnl.pdf (accessed October 2007).

[26] See http://www.fda.gov/orphan/grants/previous.htm (accessed October 2007).

Exemption of Marketing Application Fee

The Prescription Drug User Fee Act (PDUFA) enacted in 1992 authorized the FDA to levy three types of user fees—application, establishment, and product fees—on marketing applications for new drugs or certain biological products to expedite review.[27] Through the Food and Drug Administration Modernization Act of 1997 (FDAMA), Congress exempted sponsors of designated orphan drugs from the application fee for the orphan indication, but left in place the establishment and product fees to be waived on a case-by-case basis.[28] Subsequently, the Prescription Drug User Fee Amendments of 2007 allowed FDA to exempt sponsors of designated and approved orphan drugs from product and establishment fees, if their gross revenue did not exceed $50 million dollars in the preceding year. These fee exemptions represent significant cost-saving benefit for sponsors, since the PDUFA user fees are expected to increase substantially each year. In fiscal year 2008, for example, the application fee amounts to $1,178,000 for a standard marketing application requiring full review of clinical data, and $589,000 for an application not requiring review of clinical data or a supplemental application requiring review of clinical data.[29] Additionally, the product fee is $65,030 for each product, and the establishment fee is $392,700 for each establishment.

Written Recommendations for Investigations of Orphan Drugs

In addition to financial incentives, the Act also includes a regulatory incentive—written recommendations from the FDA for the preclinical and clinical investigations necessary for marketing approval of an orphan drug.[30] A sponsor may submit a request for such recommendations through OOPD.[31] Once the request is determined to meet the applicable regulatory requirements, OOPD will forward it to the FDA review division concerned for formal review and recommendations. While a drug need not be a designated orphan drug to qualify for such assistance, the sponsor must provide adequate information to show it is intended for a rare disease or condition in the United States. The request for written recommendations may be made at any stage of drug development. It may be denied, however, if the FDA deems that there is insufficient information about the drug, the disease, the overall investigational plan, or the scientific rationale for its use.

Since the FDA-wide implementation of the informal multidisciplinary pre-IND consultation program, the written recommendations provision has been

---

[27] Public Law No. 102–571 (1992).

[28] Subtitle A—Fees Relating to Drugs—of the Food and Drug Administration Modernization Act of 1997 (Public Law No. 105–115).

[29] See http://www.fda.gov/OHRMS/DOCKETS/98fr/07-5052.htm (accessed October 2007).

[30] See section 525 of the FDCA (21 USC Section 360aa), "Recommendations for Investigations of Drugs for Rare Diseases or Conditions."

[31] Code of Federal Regulations Title 21 316 Subpart B.

rarely invoked. Through the pre-IND program, the sponsor can obtain from the FDA written advice, supplemented by teleconferences or meetings as needed, on the preclinical and clinical drug development process.[32] Recently, the FDA and the European Medicines Agency (EMEA) have agreed to undertake a pilot program to provide parallel scientific advice to sponsors of breakthrough drugs, including orphan drugs.[33] This program aligns closely with the FDA pre-IND and end-of-phase 2 consultations. Interested sponsors may submit a "Request for Parallel Scientific Advice" to the FDA and EMEA describing why such advice would be beneficial to their drug development process. Because of different jurisdictional requirements and perspectives, sponsors should not expect to always receive similar recommendations from the two agencies.

THE FDA OFFICE OF ORPHAN PRODUCTS DEVELOPMENT

In May 1982, the FDA created the Office of Orphan Products Development in the Office of the Commissioner to address the public interest in the problems of inadequate orphan drugs.[34] At present, OOPD is administratively responsible for orphan-drug designations, the Orphan Product Grants Program, and humanitarian-use device designations. OOPD also serves in an advisory role to the FDA review divisions on issues related to orphan products. Infrequently but importantly, OOPD takes an active part in resolving orphan drug shortage problems. In addition, OOPD closely interacts with the medical research communities, the pharmaceutical industry, other government agencies, patient advocacy groups, and international regulatory authorities to promote the development of orphan products.

ORPHAN-DRUG DESIGNATION

According to the Orphan Drug Regulations, more than one sponsor may seek and obtain orphan designation of a previously unapproved drug for the treatment, prevention, or diagnosis of a rare disease or condition in the United States, or of a drug that is being investigated or already approved for a common disease when there is also a rare disease or condition for which it may be useful.[35] Each sponsor must independently submit its own request to OOPD. A sponsor may also request orphan designation of a drug that is the

---

[32] See http://www.fda.gov/cder/about/smallbiz/pre_IND_qa.htm (accessed October 2007).

[33] See http://www.fda.gov/oia/pilotprogram0904.html (accessed October 2007). This pilot program was initiated under the auspices of the confidentiality arrangement between the European Commission, the EMEA, and FDA in 2003 (http://www.fda.gov/oia/arrangements0904.html). The program provides a mechanism for FDA, EMEA, and sponsors to exchange their views on scientific issues during the development phase of new drugs.

[34] Haffner ME. Orphan products: origins, progress, and prospects. Annu Rev Pharmacol Toxicol 1991; 31:603–620.

[35] Code of Federal Regulations Title 21 316.20(a).

same as a previously approved drug for the same rare disease or condition. In such case, the sponsor must provide a plausible hypothesis that its drug may be clinically superior to the previously approved drug (see discussions under "Determination of Sameness of Two Orphan Drugs" and "Clinically Superior Orphan Drugs").

The orphan-drug designation request may be filed at any time during the drug development process, but prior to the submission of the marketing application of the drug for the orphan indication.[36] While the request should be made as early as possible to maximize the tax credit benefit, it should not be prematurely submitted without adequate nonclinical and/or clinical evidence to support the scientific rationale for the intended use of the drug.

Format and Content of an Orphan-Drug Designation Request

OOPD requires two paper copies of a signed and dated request for orphan-drug designation.[37] The request may also be submitted via electronic format through the use of physical media.[38] The following information must be provided:

- The name and address of the sponsor's primary contact person (or the U.S. resident agent, if the sponsor is not based in the United States), through whom all communications are made on the sponsor's behalf.
- The proposed designation for use.[39]
- The generic name and trade name, if any, of the drug.
- The name and address of the manufacturer of the drug, if it is not manufactured by the sponsor.
- A description of the disease or condition of interest.
- The reasons why the drug is needed.
- A description of the drug and the scientific rationale for its use to include all available data from nonclinical in vitro and/or in vivo experiments, and results of pertinent clinical investigations, if any, whether they are published or unpublished, positive, negative, or inconclusive.

---

[36] Code of Federal Regulations Title Section 316.23(a).

[37] Code of Federal Regulations Title Section 316.20.

[38] See "Draft Guidance for Industry: Providing Regulatory Submissions in Electronic Format for Orphan Drug and Humanitarian Use Device Designation Requests and Related Submissions" available at http://www.fda.gov/orphan/esub/esub.htm (accessed October 2007).

[39] The *designated use* of an orphan drug, i.e., treatment, prevention, or diagnosis of a rare disease or condition, should be distinguished from the *indication for use* of a drug, which is based on results of safety and effectiveness data from clinical studies of the drug. They may not always be the same. For example, a drug may be designated based on its plausible pharmacologic activity for the treatment of spinal muscular atrophy (SMA). The sponsor, however, may elect to investigate its therapeutic use in only type 1 SMA patients. Therefore, if approved, the indication for use of the drug would be limited to treatment of type 1 SMA. As elsewhere discussed, the orphan-drug marketing exclusivity would also be restricted to only this subset.

- Documentation with authoritative references to demonstrate that the targeted disease or condition does not exceed the numerical prevalence threshold of 200,000 persons at the time the request is submitted.
- Should the targeted disease or condition affect more than 200,000 persons in the United States, a report by an independent certified public accountant containing data on: (*i*) development, production, and distribution costs already incurred, or expected to incur, prior to and after the submission of the designation request, and during the first seven years of marketing of the drug and (*ii*) the projected revenues from sales during the first seven years of marketing for the orphan indication in the United States.
- A summary of the regulatory history of the drug in the United States and foreign countries to include the investigational status, marketing approval, and adverse regulatory action, if any.
- A statement whether the sponsor is the real party in interest of the development, production, and sales of the drug.

Recently, the FDA and the EMEA have adopted the Common EMEA/FDA Application Form for Orphan Medicinal Product Designation. This standardized application form is intended to lessen the burden of filing two separate, differently formatted requests when a sponsor desires to seek orphan designation of its drug in both jurisdictions.[40] The sponsor may also use this application form even if it intends to request orphan designation from only the FDA.

According to the Orphan Drug Regulations, only the generic name and trade name, if any, of the drug are required in the request.[41] In the absence of these names, a chemical name, an amino acid sequence, or a nucleotide sequence, should be given. If none of these are available (or applicable), the sponsor should provide a detailed description of how and from what the drug is prepared. A company code name is unacceptable for purposes of orphan-drug designation. It may be useful to provide the proposed/accepted international nonproprietary name, the anatomical therapeutic chemical code, proposed strength, pharmaceutical form, and route of administration of the drug, if available.

It bears noting that consistent with the intent of the Act, orphan status is granted to a potentially "promising" drug—one with a demonstrable medical plausibility for effectiveness—that merits the economic and regulatory incentives for development.[42] Since the orphan designation process usually takes place at an early stage in drug development—often with little or no available clinical experience with the drug—it is important that the sponsor present in

---

[40] 2 Federal Register 63,615 (2007). Available at: (http://www.fda.gov/OHRMS/DOCKETS/98fr/E7-21971.pdf) (accessed November 2007).

[41] Code of Federal Regulations Title 21 Section 316.20(b).

[42] See the preamble to the Orphan Drug Act (Public Law No. 97–414) and Code of Federal Regulations Title 21 Section 316.25(a)(2).

detail all relevant data on the drug's activity in appropriate in vitro and/or in vivo preclinical models of the proposed disease or condition for review. Results of comparative studies of the drug with others known to be active in these models are often informative and desirable. When available, clinical data from studies of the drug in the disease or condition of interest—even if preliminary—need to be included in the request. Clearly, results from controlled studies or a meta-analysis comparing the drug's efficacy data to those obtained with comparable, preferably approved, drug(s) are more useful than descriptive data from non-comparative studies.

To qualify for orphan designation, the disease or condition for which the drug is intended to treat must affect fewer than 200,000 persons in the United States.[43] If the disease or condition has an average duration of less than one year (excluding those with a chronic relapsing/remitting course), the FDA has generally considered the average annual number of affected persons as an acceptable estimate. For a vaccine, diagnostic drug, or preventive drug, the number of persons to whom the drug may be administered must be less than 200,000 per year.

In general, acceptable sources of prevalence typically include epidemiologic data from peer-review journals, authoritative textbooks, and monographs. Prevalence information may also be obtained, in some cases, from available datasets from government agencies such as the Centers for Disease Control and Prevention or the National Institutes of Health, well-maintained proprietary or nonproprietary health services databases, rare disease registries, national health surveys, or pharmaceutical databases.[44] When the disease or condition is less well-defined, when the estimated prevalence closely approximates the statutory numerical threshold, or when the reliability of available prevalence information is an issue, multiple data sources should be used to confirm the prevalence, if possible. When out-of-date information is used to establish the prevalence, the sponsor should provide an explanation why it is reasonable to do so, and make appropriate adjustment as necessary. If the overall prevalence is extrapolated from a subpopulation data, a justification on the validity of such extrapolation should be included. In the absence of adequate prevalence information of a disease or condition in the United States, it is reasonable to infer from foreign prevalence data, provided that they are free from epidemiologic or demographic bias. If all else fails, the sponsor should submit substantiated information from at least three independent experts in the field.

Regardless of what source information is used to derive prevalence, the sponsor should, to the extent possible, demonstrate that the data in use are not compromised by inherent selection, compilation, and reporting errors or bias. If

---

[43] Code of Federal Regulations Title Sections 316.20(b)(8)(i) and 316.21(a)(b).

[44] For cancer prevalence in the United States, the FDA has considered data from the Surveillance, Epidemiology, and End Results Program of the National Cancer Institute as a definitive source of information.

so, means to minimize them should be discussed. The sponsor should describe in full the methods and calculations used to derive the prevalence. All source ("raw") data, proprietary or nonproprietary, published or unpublished, and cited references should be submitted for verification purposes.

Where orphan designation is sought for multiple drugs intended for use as fixed-combination drugs in a single dosage form, or as a combination product, the sponsor should provide a rationale for the use of each drug, an explanation how each makes a contribution to the claimed effects, and why such concurrent use is necessary.[45] At present, where a combination product is comprised of a drug and a medical device, the drug may receive orphan designation if it is the constituent part responsible for the "primary mode of action."[46]

Granting, Revocation, and Amendment of Orphan-Drug Designation

Upon receipt of an orphan-drug designation request, OOPD reviews the information primarily to determine the following:

- Whether or not there is adequate evidence to believe the targeted disease or condition is rare in the United States at the time the request is submitted.
- If the drug is intended for a disease or condition affecting more than 200,000 persons in the United States, whether or not there exists an adequate justification that there is no reasonable expectation of cost recovery by sales of the drug for the orphan indication in the United States.[47]
- Whether or not there is sufficient scientific rationale to establish a medically plausible basis for expecting the drug to be effective for the intended use.[48]
- Whether or not there is a plausible hypothesis of clinical superiority, if the drug is the same drug as a previously approved orphan drug for the same use.

If the designation criteria are met, OOPD will grant the designation request and notify the sponsor in writing. If not, OOPD may, by its discretion, either refuse to grant the sponsor's request or place it in abeyance while asking for additional information and/or explanations. Failure on the sponsor's part to provide satisfactory

---

[45] See Code of Federal Regulations Title 21 Section 300.50 and Code of Federal Regulations Title 21 Section 3.2 for regulatory information on fixed-combination drugs and combination products, respectively.

[46] See Code of Federal Regulations Title 21 Section 3.2(m) for the definition of *primary mode of action* with respect to a combination product.

[47] Following the 1984 amendment of the Orphan Drug Act to allow orphan designation of drugs for diseases or condition affecting less than 200,000 persons in the United States, only three drugs have been designated on the cost recovery basis thus far: Subutex[R] and Suboxone[R] for opioid dependence and Evista[R] for reduction of breast cancer risk in postmenopausal women. Because of the lack of in-house expertise, it is likely that such designation requests may not be reviewed entirely by OOPD.

[48] The FDA's Orphan Drug Development Program. 4 US Reg Rep 1987; 1–6.

responses will result in a denial of the request. OOPD will publish the designation in a publically available list of designated orphan drugs.[49]

An orphan-drug designation may be revoked if the FDA subsequently finds that the request contained an untrue statement of material fact, omitted required material information, or if the drug was in fact not eligible for designation at the time the request was submitted.[50] A revocation of the orphan designation will also result in suspension or withdrawal of the sponsor's exclusive rights to market the drug, if such exclusivity is in effect, but not the marketing approval. To protect the sponsor's good-faith investment and to eliminate the unpredictability of investment risk eligibility for orphan drug status is determined in the basis of facts and circumstances as of the date the designation request is filed. An orphan designation cannot be revoked if the prevalence of the targeted disease or condition increases to more than 200,000 persons after the drug is designated.[51]

At any time prior to the marketing application approval of a designated orphan drug, the sponsor may apply for an amendment to the designated use if the proposed change is based on new and unexpected findings about the drug, unforeseen developments in the treatment or diagnosis of the disease or condition, or if the FDA recommends such change.[52] The amendment would be granted if the FDA finds the original request was made in good faith, and the change would not result in exceeding the prevalence or cost recovery thresholds upon which the drug was originally designated.

Determination of Sameness of Two Orphan Drugs

The primary incentive of the Act is the seven-year marketing exclusivity during which the FDA is barred from approving another same drug for the same orphan use. Therefore, the question of whether one drug is the same as another is crucial to the protection of this exclusivity. Since any undermining of this exclusivity would discourage development of orphan drugs, the Orphan Drug Regulations go at length to define what constitute the sameness of two orphan drugs.[53]

For small chemical molecules, two drugs intended for the same use would be considered the same if they contained an identical *active moiety*—the part of the drug other than the parts that make it a salt, an ester, or other noncovalent derivative (such as a complex, chelate, or clathrate)—that is responsible for the physiologic or pharmacologic action of the drug. This definition reflects the long-standing principle that any changes to the chemical structure of a drug's

---

[49] A periodically updated list of designated orphan drugs can be found at http://www.fda.gov/orphan/designat/list.htm (accessed October 2007).

[50] Code of Federal Regulations Title 21 Section 316.29(a).

[51] Code of Federal Regulations Title 21 Section 316.29(c).

[52] Code of Federal Regulations Title 21 Section 316.26.

[53] Code of Federal Regulations Title 21 Section 316.3(b)(13).

active moiety other than the formation of salt, ester derivative, or other non-covalent modifications would render the drug a new molecular entity.

For large molecules such as proteins, polysaccharides, or polynucleotides, a certain degree of heterogeneity is invariably common. Furthermore, it is possible to make minor structural modifications to these molecules without significantly affecting their pharmacological activity. Therefore, to ensure that inconsequential structural changes would not be sufficient to make a second drug a different drug to circumvent exclusivity, the Orphan Drug Regulations define the sameness of two large molecules intended for the same use on the basis of the *principal molecular structural features* as follows:

- Two protein drugs would be considered the same if their structural differences were because of minor changes in the amino acid sequence, posttranslational events, or infidelity of transcription or translation.[54] For example, changes to a protein, such as a single amino acid substitution at an unimportant site in the molecule, glycosylation, or PEGylation, would not render it a different protein.[55] A peptide that mimics the active site of a protein drug per se would not be considered a different drug.[56]
- With respect to monoclonal antibodies, the complementarity determining (hypervariable) regions of the heavy and light chain variable regions are viewed by the FDA as the principal molecular structural features. Hence, two monoclonal antibody drugs would be considered the same if the amino acid sequences of the complementarity determining regions were the same or if there were only minor amino acid differences between them.[57]
- Two polysaccharide drugs would be considered the same if their saccharide-repeating units were identical—even if the number of units were to vary—or if the structural differences were due to post-polymerization modifications.[58]
- Two polynucleotide drugs consisting of two or more distinct nucleotides would be considered the same if they possessed an identical sequence of

---

[54] Transcription refers to the process by which genetic information from a gene is copied into a messenger ribonucleic acid (mRNA). Translation refers to the process by which the mRNA is decoded to produce a specific protein according to the rules specified by the genetic code. Any further modifications to the protein after translation are referred to as post-translational. Examples of posttranslational modifications include the enzymatic attachment of sugar side groups to the amino acids called glycosylation, and the folding of the linear strand of amino acids into a complex three-dimensional shape called tertiary structure.

[55] Therapeutic protein molecules may be chemically conjugated to a strand of the polyethelene glycol (PEG) polymer, a process known as PEGylation, to help improve their safety and effectiveness.

[56] See FDA's response to comment 21 in the Supplementary Information of Orphan Drug Regulations, final rule (57 Federal Register 62,076) (1992).

[57] See "Guidance for Industry—Interpreting Sameness of Monoclonal Antibody Products under the Orphan Drug Regulations" available at: http://www.fda.gov/cber/gdlns/orphan.htm (accessed October 2007).

[58] A polysaccharide is a complex polymer made up of many carbohydrate (sugar)-repeating units. Examples of common polysaccharides include starch, cellulose, and glycogen. Any modifications to the polysaccharide after polymerization are referred to as "post-polymerization."

purine and pyrimidine bases (or their derivatives) bound to an identical sugar backbone.[59,60,61]

- Two closely related, complex, partly definable drugs, such as two live viral vaccines, would be considered to be the same.[62]

Obviously, the above regulatory definitions of sameness of two orphan drugs provide considerable protection to the innovator sponsor of an approved orphan drug against a second sponsor's attempt to defeat its marketing exclusivity by introducing insignificant chemical or molecular structural change to the drug. Nevertheless, if the second sponsor could show that such a chemical or structural modification, regardless how minor, would make its drug a clinically superior drug, then the follow-on drug could be considered a different drug and could enjoy full orphan-drug incentives for development as discussed below.

Clinically Superior Orphan Drugs

The orphan-drug marketing exclusivity ensures that the first sponsor to obtain the FDA approval of an orphan drug will be protected from competitors "free-riding" on its innovative efforts. Nevertheless, to ensure the exclusivity would not stifle the prompt availability of therapeutically or diagnostically superior follow-on drugs to patients in need, the Orphan Drug Regulations stipulate that a drug possessing the same active moiety or principle molecular structural features as that of a previously approved orphan drug will be considered a different drug, if it can be shown to be clinically superior.[63] Such a drug may receive orphan designation to enjoy the premarketing development incentives, provided the sponsor could present a plausible hypothesis that the drug may be proven clinically superior to the already approved drug. To receive marketing approval,

---

[59] A polynucleotide is a polymer comprised of repeating units called nucleotides. A nucleotide consists of three components: a base (adenine, guanine, cytosine, or thymine), a sugar, and a phosphate group. The sugars of sequential nucleotides are linked together via the phosphate groups and together they form the backbone of a polynucleotide. The unique sequence of the bases attached to the backbone determines the specificity of the polynucleotide.

[60] The definition of sameness of two polynucleotide drugs in the Orphan Drug Regulations was crafted in the early 1990s and did not anticipate new developments in therapeutic polynucleotides. As such, it may result in little or no exclusivity protection to new polynucleotide drugs such as antisense drugs. An antisense drug is made up of a short sequence of nucleotides (oligonucleotides). Under the current definition, while the mere addition or deletion of nucleotide(s) to an antisense drug may not significantly affect the activity of the drug, it will render it a different drug.

[61] The current Orphan Drug Regulations also do not include a definition of sameness of two gene transfer drugs (gene therapies) employing the same gene but with a different vector or transfer system.

[62] As another example, the FDA previously considered two animal-derived lung surfactants to be the same since their complex compositions were considered to be closely related and only partly definable.

[63] Code of Federal Regulations Title 21 Section 316.3(b)(13).

however, the sponsor must show clear evidence of clinical superiority. If approved, the drug will carry its own marketing exclusivity independent that of the first approved drug.

Clinical superiority is defined in the Orphan Drug Regulations as "a significant therapeutic advantage over and above that provided by the already approved orphan drug" in one or more of the following ways:[64]

- The drug must confer greater effectiveness as assessed by its effect on a clinically meaningful endpoint in adequate and well control clinical studies.[65,66] Generally, this would require the same level of evidence needed to support a comparative effectiveness claim for two different drugs, such as through direct comparative clinical studies.
- The drug must provide greater safety, for example, by eliminating an ingredient or contaminant associated with relatively frequent adverse effects, in a substantial portion of the target population. Such a demonstration may not always require direct comparative clinical studies.
- In rare cases, where neither greater effectiveness nor greater safety can be shown, a second drug may be considered clinically superior if it makes a major contribution to patient care.[67] While the regulations do not define what constitutes a "major contribution," they make clear that this third basis for clinical superiority is narrowly construed so that only truly important differences can result in such a finding. It does not intend to open the flood gates to allow approval of any drug that can confer a minor convenience over the previously approved drug; otherwise the marketing exclusivity would be worthless.

---

[64] Code of Federal Regulations Title 21 Section 316.3(b)(3). Although the current definition of clinical superiority presently refers only to the *therapeutic advantage*, if the drug is a diagnostic drug, it is safely assumed that the *diagnostic advantage* of the drug would be of interest.

[65] It is reasonable to assume that greater effectiveness may also be assessed by the drug's effect on a *surrogate endpoint* that is reasonably predictive of clinical benefit in adequate and well-controlled clinical studies, if the drug is to be approved on that basis. See Code of Federal Regulations Title 21 Sections 314.510 and 601.41 for explanations on the use of surrogate endpoints for purposes of accelerated approval of drugs for serious or life-threatening diseases.

[66] See Code of Federal Regulations Title 21 Section 314.126 for definition of an adequate and well-controlled clinical study.

[67] The drug Sandostatin® (octreotide acetate) was approved for treatment of severe diarrhea and flushing associated with carcinoid tumors, and profuse watery diarrhea due to vasoactive intestinal peptide-producing tumors. The drug would have to be injected up to four times a day (or 120 times a month) to control the symptoms. The FDA subsequently granted orphan designation and eventually approval with orphan-drug marketing exclusivity to Sandostatin® LAR®, a long-acting depot formulation of octreotide acetate on the basis of a major contribution to patient care, since the drug would need to be injected only once a month to achieve the same treatment effect as that of Sandostatin.

Designation of a Drug for Use in an "Orphan" Subset of a Common Disease

In general, a drug is designated as an orphan drug for the diagnosis, treatment, or prevention of a rare disease or condition. Nevertheless, a drug may also be designated for use in a rare subset of patients with a common disease or condition, if the sponsor can present a medically plausible explanation why the remaining persons with the same disease or condition are not appropriate candidates for use of the drug.[68] Such explanation is mandatory to avoid the so-called "salami slicing" of a common disease or condition into small artificial subsets simply to qualify a drug for orphan designation.

The plausible bases for restricting the use of a drug to a subset of patients include, but are not limited to, its toxicologic profile, pharmacologic property, mechanism of action, biopharmaceutic characteristics, or previous clinical experience. The following are some hypothetical examples of reasonable "medically plausible" subsets. If a drug is so toxic that its use would be clinically confined to patients' refractory or intolerant of other less toxic treatments, then these patients might constitute a medically plausible subset for purposes of orphan-drug designation. A group of patients with a receptor-positive tumor may be considered a medically plausible subset if the drug in question requires interaction with the receptor to confer its therapeutic or diagnostic effect. An inhalation drug shown to produce adequate local drug exposure in the lungs but subtherapeutic blood levels may well be expected to treat only the medically plausible subset of patients with the pulmonic manifestation of the disease.

As the field of pharmacogenomics advances, it may be possible to identify subsets of individuals who respond differently to certain drugs due to their genetic variability in drug-metabolizing enzymes, drug transporters or receptors.[69] Consequently, the use of these drugs may be selectively restricted to only the subset of patients known to be treatment responders based on their genetic make-up to optimize benefit and minimize harm. If such a subset meets the statutory prevalence threshold for a rare disease or condition, it is likely that the development of these drugs would qualify for orphan drug incentives.[70]

---

[68] See section II.B, paragraph 6 of notice of proposed rulemaking entitled "Orphan Drug Regulations" [56 Federal Register 3338 (1991)] and Code of Federal Regulations Title 21 Section 316.20(b)(6). Such subset is often referred to as a *medically plausible* subset. The regulatory term medically plausible subset is often misconstrued to denote a medically recognizable or a medically distinct cohort of patients.

[69] Sadée W, Dai Z. Pharmacogenetics/genomics and personalized medicine. Hum Mol Genet 2005; 14(spec no. 2):R207–R214.

[70] Maher PD, Haffner ME. Orphan drug designation and pharmacogenomics: options and opportunities. BioDrugs 2006; 20(2):71–79.

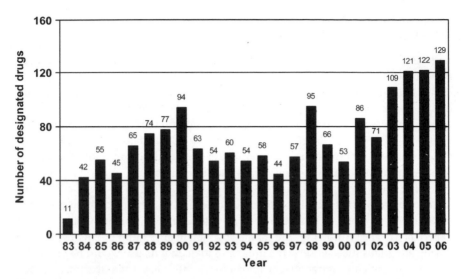

Figure 1   Annual number of orphan drugs designated by OOPD.

24 YEARS OF ORPHAN DRUG EXPERIENCE IN THE UNITED STATES

From the time the Act was passed in 1983 to June 2007, OOPD received 2477 orphan designation requests; of these, 1749 (71%) have been granted (Fig. 1).[71] Approximately 69% of designated drugs were chemical drugs, and 31% were biological products. During the same period, 316 orphan drugs, mostly developed by drug companies, have been approved for marketing. In contrast, a 1980 survey found only 47 orphan drugs that had ever been approved in the United States.[72,73] Of these, 34 were marketed by drug companies and 13 were made available through government agencies. Furthermore, only 10 of the 34 were developed solely by drug companies without the support of a government agency or a university. Collectively, the 316 approved orphan drugs benefit up to 12 million Americans suffering from over 180 different rare diseases or conditions. About 70% of approved orphan drugs were chemical drugs (approved under section 505(b) of the FDCA); and 30% were biologic products (approved under section 351 of the Public Health Service Act) (Fig. 2). More than half of the approved orphan drugs (167) targeted diseases or conditions affecting 30,000 persons or less in the United States. Approximately 25% of orphan drugs were approved for various types of rare cancer, 11% for disorders related to blood and the immune

---

[71] See http://www.fda.gov/orphan/designat/list.htm (accessed October 2007).

[72] Ashbury CH. The Orphan Drug Act. The first 7 years. JAMA 1991; 265(7):893–897.

[73] Subcommittee on Health and Environment of the Committee on Energy and Commerce, "Preliminary Report of the Survey on Drugs for Rare Diseases." Committee Print 97–BB, 97th Congress, 2nd Session (1982).

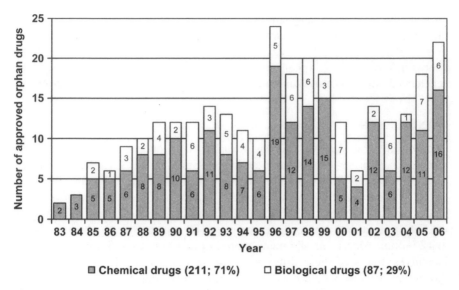

□ **Chemical drugs (211; 71%)**   □ **Biological drugs (87; 29%)**

Figure 2 Annual number of orphan drugs approved by the FDA.

system, 10% for endocrine disorders, 10% for metabolic disorders, and 8% for neurologic disorders. Less than 8% were approved for each of the other categories of rare diseases or conditions. Additionally, many orphan drugs have been made available early in their development through expanded access venues to patients who are not enrolled in the clinical trials, particularly those who cannot be satisfactorily treated by alternative drugs.[74]

Orphan drugs are subject to the same approval standards as nonorphan drugs.[75,76] The statutory requirements for demonstrating safety and effectiveness are not any less for orphan drugs than for any other drugs, that is, the evidence must be substantiated through adequate and well-controlled clinical investigations. Orphan drugs have enjoyed expedited development and regulatory approval. Between 1998 and mid-2007, 45% of drugs approved by the FDA

---

[74] The treatment use of an experimental drug—by way of a treatment protocol or a treatment IND—is governed under Code of Federal Regulations Title 21 Section 312.34. It is colloquially known as *compassionate use* and aims at making a promising experimental drug available to patients with a serious or immediately life-threatening disease who have no alternative treatment, and who may not be eligible to enroll in clinical trials with the drug. The FDA recently published a proposed rule titled "Expanded Access to Investigational Drugs for Treatment Use" to clarify existing regulations and to add other types of expanded access for treatment use of an investigational new drug (71 Federal Register 75,147) (2006).

[75] See the FDA's response to comment 74 in the Supplementary Information of Orphan Drug Regulations, final rule (57 Federal Register 62,076) (1992).

[76] Haffner ME. Adopting orphan drugs—two dozen years of treating rare diseases. N Engl J Med 2006; 354(5):445–447.

through the FDAMA-mandated fast track drug development program were orphan drugs.[77,78] Of the 149 drugs that underwent priority marketing application review since 1999, 44 (30%) were orphan drugs.[79] And since 2000, approximately 15% of orphan drugs were approved by the FDA through the accelerated approval provision compared with only 5% of nonorphan drugs.[80]

CONCLUSION

The Orphan Drug Act of 1983 has been hailed as one of the most successful pieces of healthcare legislation in the United States. It has since been emulated around the world: Singapore introduced orphan drug legislation in 1991, followed by Japan in 1993, Australia in 1997, and the European Union in 1999. Under the Act, more than 300 safe and effective drugs have been approved by the FDA to treat, prevent, or diagnose over 180 orphan diseases bringing hope to 12 million Americans and many more in other countries. Without the Act's incentives, many of these drugs would have never been developed, or their development likely would have been significantly delayed.

ACKNOWLEDGEMENTS

The author thanks E. Dickinson, Esq, T. Cote, MD, MPH, and M. Jones, for expert assistance.

---

[77] Section 112 of the Food and Drug Administration Modernization Act of 1997 (Public Law No. 105–115) amended the FDCA by adding new section 506 (21 USC Section 356) known as the *fast track products* provision. Under this provision, drugs intended to treat serious or life-threatening diseases or conditions and showing potential to address unmet medical needs are placed through a fast track drug development program that, among others, includes the following eligibilities: (1) six-month priority review time of the marketing application (versus 10-month standard review time); (2) rolling submission of completed portions of the marketing application as they become available; and (3) accelerated approval based on the drug effect on a less than well-established surrogate endpoint but reasonably predictive of clinical benefit, or a clinical endpoint other than survival or irreversible morbidity through adequate and well-controlled clinical studies (see Code of Federal Regulations Title 21 Section 314.510).

[78] See http://www.fda.gov/cder/rdmt/internetftap.htm (accessed October 2007).

[79] See http://www.fda.gov/cder/rdmt/default.htm (accessed October 2007).

[80] See http://www.fda.gov/cder/rdmt/accappr.htm (accessed October 2007).

7

CMC Sections of Regulatory Filings and CMC Regulatory Compliance During Investigational and Postapproval Stages

Prabu Nambiar

Vertex Pharmaceuticals, Inc., Cambridge, Massachusetts, U.S.A.

Steven R. Koepke

SRK Consulting, LLC, Walkersville, Maryland, U.S.A.

INTRODUCTION

The chemistry, manufacturing, and controls (CMC) section of a regulatory filing [investigational new drug (IND), IND amendments, IND annual reports, new drug application (NDA) or biologics license application (BLA), postapproval CMC supplements, NDA annual reports] contains detailed information pertaining to the characteristics, manufacturing, and quality aspects of the drug substance and drug product. Under the International Conference on Harmonization (ICH) common technical document (CTD) format,[1] the CMC section is referred to as the quality section and the structure is outlined in the ICH CTD guidance.[2] This chapter first discusses the details of the quality section of a CTD, followed by how CMC changes are managed during the IND development phases and postapproval stages. As this book addresses the Food and Drug Administration

---

[1] ICH M4: organization of the CTD. Available at: http://www.fda.gov/cder/guidance/4539O.PDF.

[2] ICH M4Q: the CTD–Quality. Available at: http://www.fda.gov/cder/guidance/4539Q.PDF.

(FDA) regulatory affairs, the focus of the discussions is primarily based on the U.S. FDA expectations and requirements.

PHARMACEUTICAL QUALITY

The quality section, which is the module 3 in a CTD (ICH M4Q), describes how the drug substance and the drug product are manufactured and how the consistency of their quality will be assured from batch to batch. The contents of these quality sections will evolve with time and experience in both quantity and detail of information. The quality section of a marketing application (CTD/NDA) describes the CMC processes for commercial product, and therefore these sections of a marketing application are very detailed. However, for an IND application, while the same basic information is required, it may be supplied in much less detail because of the preliminary stage of development. The CMC information filed in an IND or NDA/CTD is reviewed by the agency to ensure that the drug substance and drug product meet the "quality standards" and do not pose any significant safety risk or compromise efficacy during the intended use in the targeted patient population.

Although in each phase of the investigation sufficient information should be submitted to assure the proper identification, quality, purity, and strength of the investigational drug, the amount of information needed to make that assurance will vary with the phase of the investigation, the proposed duration of the investigation, the dosage form, and the amount of information otherwise available. For example, although stability data are required in all phases of the IND to demonstrate that the new drug substance and drug product are within acceptable chemical and physical limits for the planned duration of the proposed clinical investigations, if very short-term tests are proposed, the supporting stability data can be correspondingly very limited. It is expected that with the progression of a product through the phases of the IND, additional information will be provided. The process of updating/amending the CMC information for an IND through the development phases is outlined in later sections of this chapter. The final application should contain the information necessary to ensure the identity, strength, quality, and purity of the product. The information to be provided in the quality module (module 3) of a marketing application should include the following information about the drug substance and drug product.

Drug Substance

General Information (Nomenclature/Structure/Physicochemical Properties)

Nomenclature. All appropriate names or designations for the drug substance should be provided along with any codes, abbreviations, or nicknames used in the application to identify the drug substance. Any "official" names (USAN, INN, BAN, CAS, etc.) that have not yet been finalized should be identified as proposed.

Structure. This first section contains only summary information relating to structure and other characteristics. More detailed information concerning proof of structure is to be provided in the characterization section. Information that is expected to be provided here includes

1. one or more drawings to show the overall chemical structure of the drug substance, including stereochemistry,
2. molecular formula, and
3. molecular weight.

For a naturally derived protein drug substance, the information should include

1. the number of amino acid residues,
2. the amino acid sequence indicating glycosylation sites or any other post-translational modifications, and
3. a general description of the molecule (e.g., shape, disulfide bonds, subunit composition).

General properties. A list of the general physicochemical properties of the drug substance should be provided. Relevant properties are those physical, chemical, biological, and microbiological attributes relating to the identity, strength, quality, purity, and/or potency of the drug substance and, as appropriate, drug product. The information should include, as appropriate, the following:

1. A general description of the drug substance (e.g., appearance, color, physical state)
2. Melting or boiling points
3. Optical rotation
4. Solubility profile (aqueous and nonaqueous, as applicable)
5. Solution pH
6. Partition coefficients
7. Dissociation constants
8. Identification of the physical form
9. Biological activities

For a naturally derived protein drug substance, additional information should be included, such as:

1. Isoelectric point
2. Extinction coefficient
3. Any unique spectral characteristics

Manufacture

This section is divided into several subsections that as a whole describe the manufacturing process and its controls on both process and materials.

Manufacturer(s). The name, address, and manufacturing responsibility should be provided for each firm (including contract manufacturers and testing laboratories) and each site (i.e., facility) that will be involved in the manufacturing or testing of the drug substance.

Method of manufacture. This section should include a schematic flow diagram that gives the steps of the manufacturing process and shows where each material enters the process. The entire manufacturing process from the starting materials to the final drug substance released for testing should be depicted. This schematic flow diagram should be accompanied by a narrative description of the manufacturing process that represents the sequence of manufacturing steps undertaken and should include the scale of production. The narrative provided should include more details than that provided in the flow diagram. The description should identify all process controls along with any associated numeric ranges, limits, or acceptance criteria. Any process controls that are considered critical process controls should be highlighted. All critical operating parameters, environmental controls, process tests and all tests performed on intermediates, postsynthesis materials, and unfinished drug substance should be listed along with their associated numeric ranges, limits, or acceptance criteria. The noncritical controls should be listed separately from the critical tests to distinguish them from the critical tests that constitute the specification for the intermediate, postsynthesis material, or unfinished drug substance.

Materials from biological origin should include additional detailed information on isolation procedures, preparation procedures, and procedures to maintain traceability of biological materials. A discussion regarding the risk of adventitious agents and a statement that any bovine-derived materials originate in bovine spongiform encephalopathy (BSE)-free countries should also be provided. For materials that may have biological origin, specific tests and acceptance criteria to control microbial contamination should also be included in the specification. A discussion assessing the risk with respect to potential contamination with adventitious agents should be provided when appropriate.

If the drug substance is to be sterile, validation information relating to any sterilization process (e.g., drug substance, packaging components) should be submitted.

The application should also contain a process development section in the drug product section in which a description and history of the manufacturing process for the drug substance throughout the various development phases should be provided, and this will be described later.

Characterization (Structure Elucidation)

Data and analysis to support the determination of the structure of the drug substance should be provided. The chemical structure of the drug substance should be confirmed using physical and chemical techniques such as elemental analysis, mass spectrometry (MS), nuclear magnetic resonance (NMR) spectroscopy, ultraviolet (UV) spectroscopy, infrared (IR) spectroscopy, X-ray crystallography, and any other relevant tests (e.g., functional group analysis, derivatization, complex formation). For naturally derived proteins, the primary, secondary, tertiary and, if applicable, quaternary structures should be confirmed using appropriate techniques such as amino acid compositional analysis, full amino acid sequencing, peptide mapping, and mass spectrometry. Additional tests (e.g., isoform analysis, carbohydrate composition or sequence) may be warranted for glycoproteins.

Information on drug substance impurities should also be provided as part of characterization. A discussion of the actual and potential impurities most likely to arise during manufacture, purification, and storage of the drug substance should be provided. Impurities of all kinds (e.g., organic, inorganic, residual solvents) should be included in the discussion. For drug substances of biological origin and semisynthetic drug substances, the description of impurities should include, if appropriate, those related to the natural origin of the material [e.g., pesticide residues, heavy metals due to the concentration of metals by certain plant species, and related substances whose concentrations vary with changes in harvesting conditions (species, location, season, organ)].

Control of Drug Substance (Specifications)

The proposed specifications for the drug substance used to produce the drug product should be provided. A specification is defined as a list of tests, references to analytical procedures, and appropriate acceptance criteria, which are numerical limits, ranges, or other criteria for the tests described. Guidance on setting specifications is outlined in guidance ICH Q6A; for biotechnology products, the guidance is outlined in ICH Q6B.[3] The specification establishes criteria to which each batch of drug substance should conform to be considered acceptable for its intended use. *Conformance to specification* means that the drug substance, when tested according to the listed analytical procedures, will meet the listed acceptance criteria. The specification sheet should list all tests to which each batch of a drug substance will conform and the associated acceptance criteria and should also include a reference to the analytical procedures that will be used to perform each test. The acceptance criteria are the associated numerical limits, ranges, or other criteria for the tests described (for further guidance, see ICH Q6A). To support the proposed specifications, a description of relevant batches manufactured and the results of these batch analyses should be

---

[3] ICH Q6A specifications: test procedures and acceptance criteria for new drug substances and new drug products: chemical substances. Available at: http://www.fda.gov/OHRMS/DOCKETS/98fr/122900d.pdf.
ICH Q6B specifications: test procedures and acceptance criteria for biotechnological/biological products. Available at: http://www.fda.gov/cder/guidance/Q6Bfnl.PDF.

provided. Batch analysis, which is a collation of analytical data for all the tests included in the specifications, should be provided for all drug substance batches used for (*i*) nonclinical studies, (*ii*) drug product clinical efficacy and safety, bioavailability, and bioequivalence, and (*iii*) primary stability studies. Batch analysis data should also be provided for any other batches that are being used to establish or justify specifications and/or evaluate consistency in manufacturing. It is recognized that analytical methods may change during the course of development and the batch analysis reports should include information concerning the analytical method utilized. The information submitted on each of the batches should include a description of the batch. The description should include the following:

1. Batch identity (i.e., batch number) and size
2. Date of manufacture
3. Site of manufacture
4. Manufacturing process, where applicable
5. Use of batch (e.g., clinical, stability)

The agency will utilize all available information to evaluate the submitted application. A written justification for the proposed drug substance specifications based on the relevant development data, information on impurities, standards in an official compendium, batch analyses data, stability studies, toxicology data, and any other relevant data should be submitted along with the proposed specifications. Specification for impurities should include organic and inorganic impurities and residual solvents. Guidance on impurities in new drug substance and residual solvents are outlined in ICH Q3A and Q3C, respectively.[4]

Reference Standards or Materials

Information on any reference standards or reference materials used for testing of the drug substance (active pharmaceutical ingredient) should be provided. These should include any postulated or actual impurity or related substance reference standards. If the reference standard is obtained from an official source, this should be stated. When the reference standard is not from an official source, it should be fully characterized by the applicant.

Container Closure System

A description of the container closure system for the drug substance should be provided, including the identity of materials of construction of each primary packaging component and its specifications. The same type of information

---

[4] ICH Q3A impurities in new drug substances. Available at: http://www.fda.gov/cder/guidance/4164fnl.pdf.
ICH Q3C residual solvents. Available at: http://www.fda.gov/cder/guidance/Q3Cfnl.pdf.

should be provided for any functional secondary packaging components. Only a brief description should be provided for any secondary packaging components that do not provide additional protection. The suitability of the container closure system should be discussed with respect to protection from moisture and light, compatibility of the materials of construction with the drug substance, including the potential for sorption to container, and leaching.

Stability

A summary of all relevant stability studies conducted, protocols used, and the results of the studies should be provided. ICH guidance on stability studies is outlined in ICH Q1A, Q1B, Q1C, Q1D, and Q1E; guidance for biotechnology products is outlined in ICH Q5C.[5] (Note: The ICH Q1F guidance discussing stability studies for hot or humid zones has been withdrawn as of June 2006.) The discussion should include, for example, (*i*) a summary of stability batches tested, storage conditions used, attributes tested, shelf life acceptance criteria, test schedule, amount of data available, and analysis of data (including a summary of any statistical analyses performed) and (*ii*) conclusions regarding the label storage conditions and retest or expiration dating period. A postapproval stability protocol and stability commitment should be provided for monitoring the drug substance over the course of the application lifetime.

Drug Product

Description and Composition of the Drug Product

This section should include a brief description of the dosage form, the container closure system, and a statement of composition of the drug product. The composition statement describes the qualitative and quantitative formulation of the drug product as intended for use. The composition statement must contain a list of all components used in the manufacture of the drug product regardless of whether or not they appear in the finished drug product. The composition statement should include: (*i*) quality of the material used (i.e., United States Pharmacopeia (USP), American Chemical Society (ACS), technical, etc.),

---

[5] ICH Q1A(R2) stability testing of new drug substances and products. Available at: http://www.fda.gov/cder/guidance/5635fnl.pdf.

ICH Q1B photostability testing of new drug substances and products. Available at: http://www.fda.gov/cder/guidance/1318fnl.pdf.

ICH Q1C stability testing for new dosage forms. Available at: http://www.fda.gov/cder/guidance/1319fnl.pdf.

ICH Q1D bracketing and matrixing designs for stability testing of new drug substances and products. Available at: http://www.fda.gov/cder/guidance/4985fnl.PDF.

ICH Q1E evaluation of stability data. Available at: http://www.fda.gov/cder/guidance/5531fnl.pdf.

ICH Q5C stability testing of biotechnological/biological products. Available at: http://www.fda.gov/cder/guidance/ichq5c.pdf.

(*ii*) the function of the component, (*iii*) the amount of the component on a per unit basis, (*iv*) the total weight, volume, or other appropriate measure of the unit on a lot basis, and (*v*) any additional explanatory information.

Pharmaceutical Development

The pharmaceutical development section should contain information on the development studies conducted to establish that the dosage form, formulation, manufacturing process, container closure system, microbiological attributes, and usage instructions are appropriate for the purpose specified in the application. The studies included in this section are in addition to those routine control tests conducted on a lot-by-lot basis according to specifications (e.g., release testing, stability testing). A brief description of each of the components of this section follows (see also the draft guidance ICH Q8).[6]

Components of the drug product

Drug substance.   Any key physicochemical characteristics (e.g., water content, solubility, particle size distribution, polymorphic form, solvation or hydration state, pH, dissociation constant [pKa]) of the drug substance that can influence the performance or manufacturability of the drug product should be discussed. This includes the compatibility of the drug substance with the excipients used in the drug product. For combination drug products, the compatibility of the two (or more) drug substances with each other should also be discussed.

Excipients.   The choice of excipients, their concentration, and the characteristics that may influence the drug product performance or manufacturability should be discussed in context to the respective role of each excipient. Any excipient ranges present in the batch formula should be justified with data in this section. The use of any functional excipients (e.g., antioxidants, penetration enhancers) to perform throughout the intended drug product shelf life should also be demonstrated. The use of any novel excipients (those that are used in the United States for the first time in a human drug product or by a new route of administration) should be discussed and justified. It should be noted that the manufacturing, chemistry, and controls information for any novel excipient should be provided in the same level of detail as that provided for a new drug substance. This information would be expected to be included in an appendix.

Drug product

Formulation development.   A brief summary describing the development of the drug product taking into consideration the proposed route of administration and usage should be provided. For modified release drug products, a detailed

---

[6] ICH Q8 Q8(R1) pharmaceutical development. Available at: http://www.fda.gov/cder/guidance/8084dft.pdf.

description of the release mechanism (e.g., erodible matrix system, barrier erosion, diffusion) should be included. Any parameters relevant to the performance or manufacturability (e.g., powder flow characteristics) of the drug product should be addressed. Physicochemical and biological properties such as pH, osmolarity, dissolution, redispersion, reconstitution, particle size distribution, aggregation, polymorphism, rheological properties, biological activity or potency, and/or immunological activity can be relevant.

Overages. An overage is a fixed amount of the drug substance in the dosage form that is added in excess of the label claim. Any overages included in the formulation should be justified. It should be noted that normally overages in drug products can only be justified by manufacturing process losses or inability to dispense the total amount of product.

Manufacturing process development. The selection and optimization of the manufacturing process, in particular critical aspects of the process, should be explained. It is important that in this section the differences between the manufacturing processes used to produce lots for the clinical safety and efficacy, bioavailability, bioequivalence, or primary stability batches and the process be identified. Information on the manufacturing process differences between the production of the clinical batches that support efficacy or bioequivalence and primary stability batches and the procedures and equipment proposed for production batches should be provided. The information should be presented in a way that facilitates comparison of the processes and the corresponding batch analyses information (e.g., tables). Differences in equipment (e.g., different design, operating principle, size), manufacturing site, and batch size should be delineated for each submitted batch.

Container closure system. Container closure system refers to the sum of packaging components that together contain and protect the dosage form. A brief description of the container closure systems and the container closure system used for storage and transportation of drug products should be provided. The suitability of the container closure systems should be discussed and taken into consideration, the choice of materials, protection from moisture and light, compatibility of the materials of construction with the dosage form (including sorption to container and leaching), safety of materials of construction, and performance (such as reproducibility of the dose delivery from the device when presented as part of the drug product). Any additional relevant information to support the appropriateness of the container closure system or its use should be provided as warranted.

Microbiological attributes. For sterile products in particular, the microbiological attributes of the drug product, drug substance, and excipients should be discussed.

Compatibility. The compatibility of the drug product with any diluents (e.g., constitution, dilution of concentrates, admixing) or dosage devices specified in the drug product labeling and the compatibility of the drug product with likely coadministered drug products should be addressed to provide appropriate and supportive information for the labeling. The information should be used to identify in the labeling of diluents and other drug products that are compatible with the drug product as well as those that are found to be incompatible. Compatibility studies should assess, for example, precipitation, sorption onto injection vessels or devices, leachables from containers and administration sets, and stability. The design and extent of the compatibility studies depend on the type of drug product and its anticipated usage.

Manufacture (Manufacturer(s)/Method of Manufacture)

Manufacturer. The name, address, and manufacturing responsibility should be provided for each firm (including contract manufacturers, packagers, and testing laboratories) and each site (i.e., facility) that will be involved in the manufacturing, packaging, or testing of the drug product. Each site should be identified by the street address, city, state, and the drug establishment registration number.

Method of manufacture. A batch formula should be provided that includes a list of all components used in the manufacturing process, their amounts on a per batch basis, including overages, a reference to their quality standards, and any explanatory notes. Batch formulas should be provided for the intended validation batch sizes of each formulation.

A description of the manufacturing process and process controls should be provided, including a flow diagram of the manufacturing process. The submitted flow diagram should include the following:

- The entire manufacturing process giving the steps of the process and showing where materials enter the process. The diagram should identify each of the critical steps and any manufacturing step where, once the step is completed, the material might be held for a period of time before the next processing step is performed.
- The identity of the material being processed in each step.
- The identification of any critical process controls and the points at which they are conducted.
- The type of equipment used in each step of the process.

A manufacturing process description, including packaging stages, which represents the sequence of steps undertaken and the scale of production, should be provided. This description should provide more detail than that provided in the flow diagram. In lieu of the manufacturing process description, a master batch record containing all pertinent information may be provided. Steps in the manufacturing process should have the appropriate process controls identified and associated numeric values submitted.

All critical process controls and their associated numeric ranges, limits, or acceptance criteria should be identified and justified. Any research studies or information that supports the justification should be included. For sterile products, validation information relating to the adequacy and efficacy of any sterilization process should be submitted. When applicable, validation information should be provided for processes used to control adventitious agents.

Control of Excipients (Specifications)

Compendial—nonnovel excipients. When a compendial excipient is tested according to the monograph standard, no additional testing need be submitted unless pertinent to the quality of the final product.

Noncompendial—nonnovel excipients. Information for each individual excipient should be submitted. Generally, additional CMC information for the excipient will be required and should be provided with reference to a drug master file (DMF) (if applicable).

Novel excipients. Full CMC information on novel excipients should be included in an appendix or referenced to a DMF (if applicable).

Excipients of human or animal origin. Any excipient of human or animal origin should be identified and a specification submitted, regardless of whether or not the excipient appears in the finished drug product (e.g., processing agent).

The analytical procedures used for testing the excipients should be provided.

Control of Drug Product (Specifications)

The proposed specifications for the drug product should be provided. The specifications establish criteria to which each batch of drug product should conform to be considered acceptable for its intended use. *Conformance to specification* means that the drug product, when tested according to the listed analytical procedures, will meet the listed acceptance criteria. A specification is one part of the strategy to control drug product quality. They are proposed and justified by the manufacturer and approved by the agency. Specifications are established to confirm the quality of drug products rather than to establish full characterization and should focus on those characteristics found to be useful in ensuring product quality as it relates to safety and efficacy. ICH Q6A provides guidance for proposing acceptance criteria, which should be established for all new drug substances and new drug products, i.e., *universal* acceptance criteria, and for those that are considered specific to individual drug substances and/or dosage forms.

- Description—a qualitative statement about the state (e.g. solid, liquid) and color of the new drug substance.
- Identification—an identifying test should be specific for the new drug substance, e.g., IR spectroscopy or two orthogonal chromatographic procedures.
- Assay—a specific, stability-indicating procedure should be included to determine the content of the new drug substance.
- Impurities—organic and inorganic impurities and residual solvents are included in this category. For further information on impurities in new drug product, refer to ICH Q3B[7] (also refer to ICH Q3A and ICH Q3C).

In addition to the universal specifications for drug substance and drug product, it is expected that additional specifications specific to both the drug substance and drug product will be necessary to control the quality of the product. These additional specifications will be dependent on the properties of the drug substance, type of dosage form, the route of administration, and the patient population.

- Dissolution—a measure of the rate of release of the drug substance from the drug product.
- Uniformity of dosage units—this term includes both the mass of the dosage form and the content of the active substance in the dosage form; a pharmacopeial procedure should be used.
- Water content—a test for water should be included where appropriate.
- Sterility—all parenteral products should have a test procedure and acceptance criterion for evaluation of sterility.
- Extractables/leachables—generally, where development and stability data show evidence that extractables from the container or closure systems are consistently below levels that are demonstrated to be acceptable and safe, elimination of this test can normally be accepted. Extractables would also be expected from implants.

For complex products such as drug-device combinations (e.g., metered dose inhalers), additional specifications related to the performance of the device should be included. Information should be provided for all analytical procedures listed in the specification. Analytical validation information for all analytical procedures used in the specifications, including experimental data, should be

---

[7] ICH Q3B impurities in new drug products. Available at: http://www.fda.gov/cder/guidance/7385fnl .pdf.

provided. Validation of an analytical procedure is the process of demonstrating that analytical procedures are suitable for their intended use.

Batch analysis, which is a collation of analytical data for all tests included in the specifications, should be provided for all batches used for clinical efficacy and safety, bioavailability, bioequivalence, and primary stability studies. Batch analysis data should also be provided for any other batches that are being used to establish or justify specifications and/or evaluate consistency in manufacturing. It is recognized that analytical methods may change during the course of development and the batch analysis reports should include information concerning the analytical method utilized. The information submitted on each of the batches should include a description of the batch. The description should include the following:

- Batch identity (i.e., batch number), strength, and size
- Date of manufacture
- Site of manufacture
- Manufacturing process, where applicable
- Container closure system
- Use of batch (e.g., bioavailablility, stability)
- Batch number of the drug substance used in the drug product
- Batch number of any novel excipients that are not compendial

All expected drug product impurities should be listed in this section of the application, whether or not the impurities are included in the drug product specification. Drug substance process impurities that could carry over to the drug product should be listed here even if they are not degradants and are normally controlled during drug substance testing. It is expected that a cross-reference will be provided for the qualified level of an impurity.

Degradation products. Degradation products of the active ingredient can arise during drug product manufacture or as reaction products of the active ingredient with an excipient and/or immediate container closure system. Attempts should be made to identify all degradation products found at significant levels in the drug product (ICH Q3B).

Residual solvents. The level of residual solvents in a drug product should be controlled in the specifications. Because these are known compounds, the identity and presence of residual solvents in the finished drug product can usually be confirmed by using routine analytical techniques.

Miscellaneous drug product impurities. Any miscellaneous drug product impurity is an impurity other than (*i*) a degradation product, (*ii*) a residual solvent, or (*iii*) an extraneous contaminant that is more appropriately addressed as a good manufacturing practice (GMP) issue (e.g., metal shavings). Miscellaneous drug product impurities include, for example, container closure system leachables, excipient degradants, heavy metals, aluminum, and ethylene oxide residuals.

Justification of Specification(s)

Justification for the proposed drug product specifications should be provided. The justification should be based on relevant development data, batch analyses, characterization and qualification of impurities, stability studies, and any other relevant data. Data from the clinical efficacy and safety, bioavailability, bioequivalence, and primary stability batches and, when available and relevant, development and process validation batches should be considered in justifying the specification. If multiple manufacturing sites are planned, data from these sites should be provided to help establish the relevant tests and acceptance criteria. This is particularly true when there is limited initial experience with the manufacture of the drug product at any particular site. Proposed acceptance criteria can include a reasonable allowance for analytical and manufacturing variability.

Reference Standards or Materials

Information on the reference standard or reference materials used in testing the drug product should be provided. The information on the reference standards for drug substance and drug substance impurities will be provided in the drug substance section and need not be replicated here. A list of available reference standards should be provided in this section for any impurities that are unique to the drug product. The reference standards could be for impurities from drug substance and excipient interactions, impurities formed during drug product manufacturing, or an excipient impurity or leachable from the container closure system that is included in the drug product specification.

Container Closure System

A description of the container closure system for the drug product should be provided, including the identity of materials of construction of each primary packaging component and its specification. This information should include the composition, specifications, and architectural drawings of all primary packaging materials. The same type of information should be provided for functional secondary packaging components as is provided for primary packaging components. For nonfunctional secondary packaging components (e.g., those that neither provide additional protection nor serve to deliver the product), only a brief description should be provided.

Stability

The types of studies conducted, the protocols used in these studies, and results of the studies should be summarized. This summary should include (*i*) a summary of stability batches tested, storage conditions used, product attributes tested, shelf life acceptance criteria, test schedule, amount of data available, and analysis of data (including a summary of statistical analyses, if performed), (*ii*) conclusions regarding the labeled storage conditions and the proposed shelf life, and (*iii*) conclusions regarding in-use storage conditions and shelf life, if applicable. Detailed results from these stability studies undertaken on primary stability batches should be included.

It is important that the analytical procedures used to generate the data in each of the stability studies be identified. A summary of any changes in the analytical procedures should be provided if the analytical procedure was changed over the course of generating the stability data. The summary should identify when an analytical procedure changed, the differences between the analytical procedures, and the impact of the differences with respect to the data being reported. A postapproval stability protocol and stability commitment should be provided for monitoring the drug product over the course of the application lifetime.

Constitution or dilution studies performed as part of formal stability studies to confirm product quality through shelf life should also be reported in this section of the application. This is in addition to the data submitted in the compatibility section of the drug product. The design and any results from drug product stress testing and thermal cycling studies should be provided here. The information should be used, as appropriate, to support the validation of analytical procedures.

Additional Information for Biotechnology Products

Viral adventitious agents and transmissible spongiform encephalopathy agents. All developmental or approved products manufactured or processed in the same areas as the applicant's products should be identified when there is potential for cross-contamination with transmissible spongiform encephalopathy (TSE) agents. For nonoral, nontopical products, this information should also be provided when there is potential for cross-contamination with viral adventitious agents. Information should be included on the design features of the facility and procedures to prevent cross-contamination of areas and equipment.

For protein products. A diagram should be provided illustrating the manufacturing flow, including movement of raw materials, personnel, waste, and intermediates in and out of the manufacturing areas. Information should be presented with respect to adjacent areas or rooms that may be of concern for maintaining integrity of the product. Information on all development or approved products manufactured or manipulated in the same areas as the applicant's product should be included. A summary description of the product-contact equipment and its use (dedicated or multiuse) should be provided. Information on preparation, cleaning, sterilization, and storage of specified equipment and materials should be included, as appropriate. Information should be included on procedures (e.g., cleaning and production scheduling) and design features of the facility (e.g., classifications) to prevent contamination or cross-contamination of areas and equipment where operations for the preparation of cell banks and product manufacturing are performed.

CMC REGULATORY COMPLIANCE

After review and approval/acceptance of the CMC information by the agency, the CMC processes and procedures described in the IND/CTD/NDA become a binding commitment. Thus, all future batches of that particular drug substance and drug product will be manufactured by the processes and procedures described in the regulatory filing(s) so that they meet the quality criteria described in the application. Continuing to maintain this commitment is referred to as CMC Regulatory Compliance. The details of how the CMC procedures are followed by a firm in a compliant manner are governed by the firm's operating procedures defined under GMP. The QC/QA departments perform the compliance verification by QC release testing, batch record review, and product release. The agency may also verify the CMC Regulatory Compliance during the GMP inspections. For any reason, if the sponsor has to deviate from a filed or approved process or procedure, the resulting product cannot be used in the clinic or put in commerce until the sponsor has taken the necessary regulatory steps as outlined below. In accordance with GMP, formal change-control procedures are followed to implement the changes in a systematic manner.

MANAGING CMC CHANGES AND MAINTAINING CMC REGULATORY COMPLIANCE

Changes to established CMC processes and procedures are routinely needed because of any one or many of the reasons in this nonexhaustive list:

1. Continuous improvement
   a. Quality
   b. Efficiency
   c. Cost
2. Adaptation of new science and technology
3. Adapting to new scientific/clinical findings
4. Adapting to supplier/vendor situations
5. Changing clinical/market needs
6. Complying with regulatory changes
7. Complying with compendial changes
8. Transfer of products/facilities to new owners
9. Expansion into new markets

Changes are more frequent during IND stages but also continue to happen after approval of the NDA. It is important that a sponsor/firm assess the nature of the change(s) and ensure that the change(s) has no significant impact on the quality/safety profile of the drug substance or drug product. Depending on the nature of the change and its potential impact on the quality of the product, the sponsor will have to file the information to the agency and get their acceptance or approval prior to implementation of the change and thus maintain CMC Regulatory Compliance. For a drug at the IND stage, significant CMC changes and new CMC information are communicated to the FDA via IND information amendments [21 Code of Federal Regulations (CFR) 312.31(a)(1)]; a summary of significant changes are also summarized in IND Annual Reports [21 CFR 312.31(a)(1)]. It should be noted that close attention should be paid to those attributes of a drug product that are requested in the "Pharmaceutical Development" section. These are the components of an application that have the greatest potential to adversely affect the identity, strength, quality, and purity of the product. For an approved product, CMC changes are submitted in multiple ways, depending on the nature of the change (21 CFR 314.70). A prior approval supplement (PAS) or a changes being effected (CBE) supplement should be filed for major and moderate changes respectively; minor changes are reported in NDA annual reports. Only after following the appropriate regulatory process can the product resulting from the change be used in the clinic or commercial purpose. Under the GMP system of a company, a well-defined change-control process is used to make sure that all clinical and/or commercial supplies are CMC regulatory compliant.

Managing Changes During IND Stages

Generally, an IND for a new chemical entity or a new biological entity is filed with CMC processes that are not optimized. This is primarily because of time and cost constraints to develop a thoroughly optimized process. In addition, the cost of goods is not a critical factor at this stage in development. Given the industry competition, uncertainties about the viability of the drug, and uncertainties about the final dose/dosage form at the initial stages, companies file an IND with minimal CMC processes, making sure that the quality of the product does not affect the safety of the study patients. The regulations emphasize a graded nature of CMC information needed as the drug development progresses under an IND. 21 CFR 312.23(a)(7)(i) requires that an IND for each phase of investigation include *sufficient* CMC information to ensure the proper identity, strength, quality, purity, or potency of the drug substance and drug product.[8] Note that the regulations say "sufficient" information, as appropriate to the phase of investigation.

The phase 1 CMC regulatory review focuses on ensuring the identity, strength, quality, purity, and potency of the investigational new drugs as they relate to safety. The safety of the clinical supplies are generally assured by

---

[8] INDs for phase 1 studies of drugs and biotech products (Nov. 1995). Available at: http://www.fda.gov/cder/guidance/phase1.pdf.

making sure that their quality is equal or better than the supplies used for IND-enabling toxicology studies. In addition, attention should also be paid to make sure that the following safety risk factors are absent.

1. Product made with unknown or impure components.
2. Product possessing structures of known or likely toxicity.
3. Product not stable through clinical study duration.
4. Impurity profile indicates health hazard.
5. Strength or impurity profile insufficiently defined.
6. Poorly characterized master or working cell bank.
7. Lack of sterility assurance for injectables.

Because of the fairly rudimentary nature of CMC development at the IND stage, the CMC processes for the drug substance and drug product change routinely, as the drug progresses through the clinical phases of development. Some of the common/potential drug substance and drug product CMC changes are outlined in Table 1. Any of these changes, independently or in combination, has the potential to affect the identity, strength, quality, purity, or potency of the investigational drug as they relate to safety of the drug. Therefore, the FDA expects the sponsor to carefully assess the nature of the change(s) to determine if it can affect the safety of the product directly or indirectly.

Change assessment for the drug substance involves comparison of the quality by analyzing the before and after batches for purity, impurity profile, residual solvents, solid-state properties, and stability. For drug products, change assessment depends on the nature of the dosage form; usually studies include analyzing the before and after batches for dissolution/disintegration (for solid oral dosages), impurity profile, dose uniformity, pH/particulates/reconstitution time/sterility (for injectables), preservative effectiveness, functionality testing (for drug-device combination products, such as metered dose inhalers), leachables/extractables, and stability. The following factors should be kept in context, as the change assessment is carried out for the drug substance and product:

1. Clinical development stage of the drug (technical and scientific understanding of the drug substance/product and the manufacturing processes continue to increase as the development continues; commensurately, the level of complexity of change assessment will also continue to increase).
2. Where in the process is change being made? A change in the earlier step in multistep drug substance synthesis process is likely to have a lesser impact on the final drug substance and hence the drug product than a change in the final step of the synthesis.
3. Availability of sensitive analytical methods to detect the changes pre- and postchange. Having the appropriate and highly sensitive method will allow the change assessment with higher level of confidence; e.g., monitoring low levels of a highly toxic impurity.

Table 1 Common/Potential Drug Substance and Drug Product CMC Changes

Drug Substance	
CMC Parameter	Potential Change
Physicochemical/Solid state form	Salt form
	Crystal morphology
	Particle size
Manufacture	Site
	Scale
	Equipment
Process	Synthetic route
	Reagents/Solvents
	Conditions (temperature/volume)
	Starting materials/Vendor
Packaging	Container-Closure System
Specifications	Analytical tests
	Test methods
	Acceptance limits
Stability	Retest date
Drug Product	
CMC Parameter	Potential Change
Dosage	Dosage form
	Strength
	Components/Composition
Manufacture	Site
	Scale
	Equipment
Process	Unit operations
	Conditions (temperature/volume)
	Excipients/Vendors
Packaging	Container-Closure system
Specifications	Analytical tests
	Test methods
	Acceptance limits
Stability	Shelf life

Abbreviation: CMC, chemistry, manufacturing, and controls.

4. Which quality criteria are affected by the change? For example, the significance of a slight increase in the levels of a highly toxic impurity is very high compared with a slight decrease in the purity of the drug substance.

An ideal case would be that the new CMC process continues to produce drug substance and/or drug product of comparable quality with no impact on safety. Changes with a significant potential to affect the safety of the product are communicated to the FDA by IND information amendments. Comparability data demonstrating the absence of adverse impact on the quality and safety are usually included in the submission. In the event that the drug substance and/or drug product from the new process do not meet the comparability criteria, sponsors should perform appropriate qualification and/or bridging studies to support the safety and bioavailability of the material to be used in the clinical trials.

As the investigational drug reaches phase 2 and then moves on to phase 3, the agency expects more detailed CMC information to be submitted via IND amendments. Details about the level of CMC information required for phase 2 and phase 3 are outlined in the FDA guidance.[9]

By the end of phase 2 studies, it is more assured that the drug is likely to become a commercial product and the likely dosage form(s), dosage strength(s), and container-closure system are more clearly defined. As a result, the CMC processes start to get "locked-in" during the phase 3 stage. Usually, the anticipated CMC changes between phase 2 supplies and those to be used in phase 3 are discussed with the FDA during the end-of-phase 2 (EOP2) meeting.[10] Planned comparability or bridging studies are also discussed at this meeting to get a buy-in from the agency on the scientific approaches to demonstrate equivalency of the pre- and postchange products.

The phase 3 clinical supplies and the CMC processes to manufacture them are expected to be representative of the commercial product and processes. These supplies are also used for ICH stability studies to define the retest date for the drug substance and the expiry date for the drug product. By this time, the commercial manufacturing operations also start to gear up and technology transfer activities are carried out gradually. Ideally, no major changes are expected after this stage except for unforeseen circumstances. Certain kinds of major changes in CMC processes at phase 3 stage could necessitate clinical studies to demonstrate equivalency (e.g., bioequivalency studies for modified release dosage) and also initiate new ICH stability studies. Such events could potentially cause significant delays to the completion of phase 3 clinical studies and hence the NDA filing and approval timeline. Therefore, advanced and careful planning is recommended before finalization and initiation of phase 3 studies and subsequent major CMC changes. In the event that such a major CMC change is unavoidable, a follow-up meeting or a teleconference with the agency is recommended to have a mutual agreement on the path forward. It should be noted that CMC changes made in the later stages of development, particularly in phase 3 clinical studies, may have to be treated similarly to postapproval changes to an NDA for demonstration of comparability.

---

[9] INDs for phase 2 and phase 3 studies: chemistry, manufacturing, and controls information (May 2003). See http://www.fda.gov/cder/guidance/3619fnl.pdf.

[10] IND meetings for human drugs and biologics: chemistry, manufacturing, and controls information. Available at: http://www.fda.gov/cder/guidance/3683fnl.pdf.

Finally, by the completion of phase 3 studies, sponsors meet with the FDA at a pre-NDA meeting to discuss the format and content of the submission. In addition, sponsors might also provide an outline on how they intend to present in the NDA the details of resolving outstanding CMC issues discussed during the EOP2 meeting. Full details of product development information, commercial processes, and quality criteria are included in the NDA/CTD (in accordance with the ICH M4Q guidance), which get reviewed and approved by the FDA.

Biotechnology-derived products are especially sensitive to what may be perceived to be small changes in the drug substance–manufacturing process. Much of the regulation and required data requirements are based on actual experience obtained in the review by the agency on these classes of products. The following changes to a product, production process, quality controls, equipment, or facilities have been found to have caused detrimental effects on products even where validation or other studies have been performed and would require regulatory review prior to implementation because of the potential effect on identity, strength, quality, and purity of the resultant product.

- Process changes including, but not limited to,
  - extension of culture growth time, leading to significant increase in number of cell doublings beyond validated parameters.
  - new or revised recovery procedures.
  - new or revised purification process, including a change in a column.
  - a change in the chemistry or formulation of solutions used in processing.
  - a change in the sequence of processing steps or addition, deletion, or substitution of a process step.
  - reprocessing of a product without a previously approved reprocessing protocol.
- Scale-up requiring a larger fermentor, bioreactor, and/or purification equipment (applies to production up to the final purified bulk).
- New lot of, new source for, or different in-house reference standard or reference panel (panel member), resulting in modification of reference specifications or an alternative test method.
- Change of the site(s) at which manufacturing, other than testing, is performed, addition of a new location, or contracting of a manufacturing step in the approved application, to be performed at a separate facility.
- Conversion of production and related area from single to multiple product manufacturing area.
- Changes in the location (room, building, etc.) of steps in the production process, which could affect contamination or cross-contamination precautions.

Dependent on the product and its use, these drug substance– (and drug product) manufacturing changes may require in vivo studies to demonstrate the absence of adverse effects such as immunogenicity. The FDA guidance issued in

1996 and ICH guidance Q5E provide additional details of demonstration of comparability of biotechnological products resulting from changes in their manufacturing process.[11,12] In complex or not so obvious cases, it is prudent for the sponsor to discuss the comparability protocol with the FDA prior to execution to avoid any gaps in regulatory expectations.

Managing Changes During Postapproval Stages

CMC processes and procedures approved in an NDA/BLA are bound to change postapproval for any one or combination of the reasons outlined in section "CMC Regulatory Compliance" of this chapter. The common/potential drug substance and drug product changes outlined in the previous section are applicable to the postapproval stages as well.

Any of the mentioned changes, independently or in combination, has the potential to adversely affect the identity, strength, quality, purity, or potency of the drug as they may relate to the safety or effectiveness of the drug. The holder of an approved application under section 505 of the Food, Drug and Cosmetic Act must assess the effects of the change before distributing a drug product made with a manufacturing change [§ 314.70(a)(2)]. The NDA holder must establish if the change is a major, moderate, or a minor one on the basis of its potential to have an adverse effect on the identity, strength, quality, purity, or potency of a drug product as these factors may relate to the safety or effectiveness of the drug product.

As outlined in 314.70(b), 314.70(c), 314.70(d), and the FDA guidance on changes to an approved NDA,[13] a major change is a change that has a *substantial* potential, a moderate change is a change that has a *moderate* potential, and a minor change is a change that has a *minimal* potential to have an adverse effect on the identity, strength, quality, purity, or potency of a drug product, as these factors may relate to its safety or effectiveness. A major change requires the submission of a PAS and subsequent review and approval by the FDA prior to distribution of the drug product made using the change. A moderate change requires the submission of a CBE supplement; a CBE could be classified as CBE-30, whereby the NDA holder has to wait 30 days from the date of submission for the distribution of the drug product made using the change. If the FDA informs the applicant within 30 days of receipt of the supplement that information is missing, distribution must be delayed until the supplement has been amended to provide the missing information. Alternatively, a CBE could be classified as CBE-0, whereby for certain moderate changes, the product

---

[11] Demonstration of comparability of human biological products, including therapeutic biotechnology-derived products. Available at: http://www.fda.gov/cder/guidance/compare.htm.

[12] ICH Q5E comparability of biotechnological/biological products subject to changes in their manufacturing process. Available at: http://www.fda.gov/cder/guidance/6677fnl.pdf.

[13] Changes to an approved NDA or ANDA (April 2004). Available at: http://www.fda.gov/cder/guidance/3516fnl.pdf.

Table 2 Postapproval CMC Changes and the Reporting Categories

Type of change	Extent of potential adverse effect on product quality[a]	Reporting category
Major	Substantial	PAS
Moderate	Moderate	CBE (CBE-0 or CBE-30)
Minor	Minimal	AR

[a]Product quality = identity, strength, quality, purity or potency.
Abbreviations: CMC, chemistry, manufacturing, and controls; PAS, prior approval supplement; CBE, changes being effected; AR, annual report.

distribution can occur when the FDA receives the supplement. Minor changes are described in the NDA annual report.

The type of postapproval CMC change and the reporting category are summarized in Table 2. An assessment of the effects of a change on the identity, strength, quality, purity, and potency of the drug product should include a determination that the drug substance intermediates, drug substance, in-process materials, and/or drug product affected by the change conform to the approved specifications. Change assessment is typically done by comparing the analytical test results of several pre- and postchange batches of the intermediate/drug substance or drug product, as appropriate and determining if the test results are equivalent and the pre and postchange products are comparable. In addition, the FDA recommends that the NDA holder perform additional testing (chemical, physical, microbiological, biological, bioavailability, and/or stability profiles), when appropriate, to make more precise change assessment and demonstrate comparability. The FDA's scale-up and postapproval changes (SUPAC) guidance also provide very valuable information to sponsors regarding the change assessments.[14]

Details of reporting categories for the following major CMC parameter changes are outlined in the changes to an approved NDA or ANDA guidance.

- Components and composition
- Manufacturing sites
- Manufacturing process

---

[14] SUPAC IR: immediate release solid oral dosage forms. Available at: http://www.fda.gov/cder/guidance/cmc5.pdf.
SUPAC MR: modified release solid oral dosage forms. Available at: http://www.fda.gov/cder/guidance/1214fnl.pdf.
SUPAC IR/MR manufacturing equipment addendum. Available at: http://www.fda.gov/cder/guidance/1721fnl.pdf.
SUPAC SS: nonsterile semisolid dosage forms. Available at: http://www.fda.gov/cder/guidance/1722dft.pdf.
SUPAC SS: in vitro release testing and in vivo bioequivalence documentation. Available at: http://www.fda.gov/cder/guidance/1447fnl.pdf.

- Specifications
- Container closure system
- Labeling
- Miscellaneous changes
- Multiple related changes

These reporting categories are consistent with the SUPAC guidance; any difference in recommended reporting categories in previously published guidances is superseded by the changes to an approved NDA or ANDA guidance. It should be noted that reporting category of the change does not in any way change the nature of requirements or amount of data required to justify the proposed change. The required studies must be performed, and the resulting data supplied to the FDA. The reporting category simply changes the timing and method of providing that information to the FDA for their review. In complex or not so obvious cases, it is prudent for the sponsor to discuss postapproval change assessment and filing strategy with the FDA prior to execution to avoid any gaps in regulatory expectations.

If an assessment indicates that a change has adversely affected the quality of the drug product, the FDA recommends that the change be submitted in a PAS regardless of the recommended reporting category for the change.

As mentioned in the previous section "Managing Changes during IND Stages," biotechnology-derived products are especially sensitive to what may be perceived to be small changes in the drug substance–manufacturing process. Dependent on the product and its use, these drug substance–(and drug product) manufacturing changes may require in vivo studies to demonstrate the absence of adverse effects such as immunogenicity. The FDA guidance issued in 1996 and ICH guidance Q5E provide additional details of demonstration of comparability of biotechnological products resulting from changes in their manufacturing process. In complex or not so obvious cases, it is prudent for the sponsor to discuss comparability protocol, postapproval change assessment, and filing strategy with the FDA prior to execution to avoid any gaps in regulatory expectations.

RECENT DEVELOPMENTS AT THE FDA AND THE IMPACT OF cGMP FOR THE 21ST CENTURY INITIATIVE ON POSTAPPROVAL CMC CHANGE MANAGEMENT

The FDA introduced the pharmaceutical current good manufacturing practices (cGMPs) for the 21st century initiative in, August 2002, (cGMP initiative; http://www.fda.gov/cder/gmp/index.htm) to enhance and modernize the regulation of pharmaceutical manufacturing and product quality and to encourage companies to innovate and adopt state of the science and technology in pharmaceutical manufacturing. A final report on "Pharmaceutical cGMPs for the 21st Century—A Risk-Based Approach" was published in

September 2004.[15] According to this report, the FDA's existing practice of drug regulation may have contributed to pharmaceutical companys' reluctance to adapt state-of-the art technologies in their manufacturing processes and equipment.

One of the goals of the cGMP Initiative is to create a regulatory paradigm that will encourage pharmaceutical manufacturers to use modern quality management systems, and risk management approaches to facilitate their decision making and implementation of manufacturing processes to reliably produce pharmaceuticals of high quality. Under this new paradigm, pharmaceutical manufacturers are ultimately responsible for ensuring the quality of their products subject to the FDA regulatory oversight. This is expected to offer significant regulatory relief in terms of postapproval change in management practice for the industries. Accordingly, the FDA has been working to revise 21 CFR 314.70 to support this new paradigm[16] and issuing new guidance to promote the risk-based approach to cGMP. One of the regulatory tools that the FDA is focusing on for the postapproval CMC change management is the "Comparability Protocol," and draft guidance were issued on this topic in 2003.[17]

A comparability protocol is a well-defined, detailed, written plan for assessing the effect of specific CMC changes on the identity, strength, quality, purity, and potency of a specific drug product, as these factors relate to the safety and effectiveness of the drug substance or drug product. A comparability protocol describes the changes that are covered under the protocol and specifies the tests and studies that will be performed, including the analytical procedures that will be used, and acceptance criteria that will be achieved to demonstrate that specified CMC changes do not adversely affect the product. This is an optional submission for companies and can be submitted as part of the original NDA/CTD or as a separate PAS. Upon approval of the comparability protocol, a sponsor can implement the change under a reduced-reporting category, as agreed in the comparability protocol submission/acceptance. Therefore, prudent use of comparability protocols is expected to reduce postapproval CMC regulatory burden to a great extent.

CONCLUSION

CMC Information for the drug substance and drug product of an investigational and commercial drug is provided in the quality module of a dossier submitted in CTD format. It is inevitable that the information will continue to change because

---

[15] Pharmaceutical cGMPs for the 21st Century—A Risk-Based Approach Final Report—Fall 2004. Available at: http://www.fda.gov/cder/gmp/gmp2004/GMP_finalreport2004.htm.

[16] Federal register/vol. 72, no. 3 / Friday, January 5, 2007/Notices. Available at: http://a257.g .akamaitech.net/7/257/2422/01jan20071800/edocket.access.gpo.gov/2007/pdf/E6-22588.pdf.

[17] Comparability protocols—chemistry, manufacturing, and controls information (DRAFT). Available at: http://www.fda.gov/cder/gmp/5427dft.pdf.
Comparability protocols protein drug products and biological products—chemistry, manufacturing, and controls information (DRAFT). Available at: http://www.fda.gov/cber/gdlns/protcmc.pdf.

of various improvements and necessities throughout development and post-approval. It is the sponsor's responsibility to perform adequate assessment of the changes to demonstrate that the changes have adverse affect on the identity, strength, quality, purity, or potency of the drug as they may relate to the safety or effectiveness of the drug. Communicating the changes and the change assessments to the FDA by appropriate regulatory process is critical for maintaining CMC regulatory conformance and complying with the Food, Drug, and Cosmetic Act. Constant communication and coordinated team work among the research and development (R&D), manufacturing, quality (QA/QC), toxicology, clinical, commercial, and regulatory team members of the project is extremely important to proactively plan for the changes and implement them in a timely manner to avoid any interruptions in product supply and potential delays in drug development and marketing, as well as maintaining regulatory compliance.

8

Overview of the GxPs for the Regulatory Professional

Bob Buckley and Robert Blanks

Idenix Pharmaceuticals, Inc., Cambridge, Massachusetts, U.S.A.

INTRODUCTION TO THE GxPs

GxP (Good—Practices) is an acronym commonly used in the drug, device, or biologic industry to describe a collection of regulations, guidance, and industry standards employed in several aspects of drug development and commercialization, including manufacturing, nonclinical research, and clinical research. The big three GxPs, for which we will attempt to provide a high-level and practical overview in this chapter, include good laboratory practice (GLPs), good manufacturing practice (GMPs), and good clinical practice (GCPs).

The GxPs singular purpose is to ensure that medication available to the public is both safe and effective. Unfortunately, the previous statement has not always held true and the evolution of the GxPs is grossly, but fairly, generalized, as a series of reactions to scientific misconduct, medical tragedies and human rights violations, and the resulting media attention each received. These events have directly, if not immediately, resulted in a number of ethical doctrines and regulations, while many more have evolved over time. Not surprisingly, the concepts described in all three GxPs are similar. These concepts include the need for independent oversight, written procedures, change control, and good documentation practices.

GxP requirements in the United States are administered by the Food and Drug Administration (FDA) through a series of regulations and guidances whose definitions are described below. In general, the regulations and guidances do not specify how a company meets the requirements defined in these documents but allow each company to determine their own path to compliance. However, there are expectations within the industry that have become the accepted norm or commonly practiced procedure in achieving compliance often referred to generically as "industry standards."

Regulation	enforceable instruction that is codified and is meant to provide the minimum standard that must be met to comply with the law.
Guidance	or guidance document is a recommended approach to comply with regulations for a given process. An FDA guidance document typically represents the agency's current thinking on a topic; however, alternative approaches may be taken to comply with regulations. Guidances are not enforceable by FDA, but if an alternative approach is taken, it should be discussed with the Agency.
Industry standards	a generic term used to describe the accepted norms and commonly practiced procedures to achieve a given task within the industry.

In this chapter, we will briefly review the origins of the GxPs to provide a brief historical basis for today's standards, and we will focus on what we feel are a few of the "key" regulations, and guidelines that one should be familiar with as a Regulatory Affairs professional; however, the reader must be cautioned that this is merely the tip of the iceberg. We will also attempt to provide practical tips and examples of how to implement GxP in the real world and supply the reader with a list of valuable Web sites to expand their GxP knowledge (exposing more of the iceberg) and to keep handy as a GxP reference guide.

INTRODUCTION TO GOOD LABORATORY PRACTICES

GLPs are the regulations and guidance that govern the nonclinical laboratory studies that support investigational new drug applications (INDs)/investigational device exemptions (IDEs) and ultimately marketing applications. Nonclinical studies, per FDA definition, includes in vivo and in vitro experiments in which test articles (including drugs, devices, and biologics) are studied prospectively in test systems under laboratory conditions to determine their safety.[1] The results from these nonhuman experiments provide predictive evidence that the dose selected to move into human trials should be safe, and GLPs are intended to provide assurance that the data are credible. GLPs define the quality processes and working environment under which studies are planned, performed, monitored, recorded, archived, and reported.[2] It is important to note that GLP is not synonymous with good science, as GLPs provide the procedural controls, not the detail to design scientifically sound studies. A study conducted according to GLPs gives the sponsor the ability (in theory anyway) to submit data to a number of regulatory authorities worldwide, as the data were derived in accordance with globally recognized standards.

Some scientists with limited experience working in an FDA-regulated environment oftentimes will claim that they "use" GLPs and may become rather offended when you challenge them to the contrary. While they may use good laboratory techniques, the fact that the GLPs is confined to nonclinical studies is not always well understood, and the phraseology associated with GLPs is commonly confused.

You will recognize some common themes within this overview of GLPs, which we will also discuss in the GMP and GCP overviews in this chapter, the importance of independent oversight, written procedures, change control, and good documentation practices. To have an understanding of the GLPs today, it is important to recognize some of the reasons why they became necessary and where they evolved from.

History of the GLPs

As with GMPs and GCPs, the origination of GLPs is rooted in a series of missteps by industry. In the 1970s, suspicion arose as to the validity of nonclinical safety data submitted in a couple of new drug applications (NDAs) by a major pharmaceutical company, Searle (Omaha, Nebraska, U.S.). Further inspections of several nonclinical studies and test facilities, of both Searle and other companies, indicated the lack of oversight during nonclinical studies. There was evidence of inadequate control of these studies, including replacing dead animals with new ones without the proper documentation, deleting necropsy observations because the pathologist received no specimens of lesions, or substituting hematology results from a control group not associated with the study. Congress held a series of hearings (Kennedy Hearings, 1975) to address these issues. Subsequently, the FDA promulgated a series of proposed GLP regulations in 1976, which were finalized in 1978 under

---

[1] Code of Federal Regulations Title 21 Section 58.3(d).

[2] Organisation for Economic Cooperation and Development Principles on Good Laboratory Practice, ENV/MC/CHEM(98)17, 1997.

21 Code of Federal Regulations (CFR) 58[3] and came into effect in 1979. In the preamble to the final rule, the FDA stated that the GLP regulations "is based on the investigatory findings by the agency that some studies in support of the safety of regulated products have not been conducted in accord with acceptable practice, and that accordingly data from such studies have not always been of quality and integrity to assure product safety."[4]

The Environmental Protection Agency (EPA) soon followed with their own proposed GLP regulations, equivalent to the FDA's, in 1979 and 1980 because of similar problems with the integrity of submitted nonclinical safety data for chemicals. In fact, one of the same testing facilities (IBT) that the FDA had found having inadequate controls was responsible for a majority of the nonclinical safety studies submitted in support of new pesticides. These regulations were finalized in 1983 (40 CFR 160[5] and 40 CFR 792[6]). In 1981, the Organisation for Economic Cooperation and Development (OECD) published their version of the GLPs[7] to promote the mutual acceptance of nonclinical safety data for chemicals and, thereby, eliminate a nontariff trade barrier for the import or export of chemicals.

The FDA revised the GLP regulations in 1987[8] to allow for greater flexibility in the operation of nonclinical laboratories while still protecting the public safety. Most of these changes were to clarify the wordings of the original GLP regulations that test facilities were interpreting too strictly. Other changes included altering the definition of control article to exclude feed and water given control animals, allowing the quality assurance unit (QAU) to determine the phase of the study to inspect instead of having to inspect all phases, and eliminating the need to put proposed starting dates and completion dates in the protocol.

GLPs Today

U.S. GLP Regulations

The U.S. regulations that cover the GLPs of interest for this textbook (drugs/devices/biologics) are within Title 21 of the U.S. CFR. Title 21 of the CFR applies to products regulated by FDA, and 21 CFR Part 58 is titled *Good Laboratory Practice for Nonclinical Laboratory Studies*. FDA GLP regulations apply to safety studies of food and color additives, animal food additives, human and animal drugs, medical devices for human use, biologic products, and electronic products.[9] The generic term "good laboratory practice" also applies to regulations governed by the U.S.

---

[3] 43 Federal Register, 59986, December 22, 1978.

[4] 43 Federal Register, 59986, December 22, 1978.

[5] 48 Federal Register 53946, November 29, 1983.

[6] 48 Federal Register 53946, November 29, 1983.

[7] "Decision Concerning the Mutual Acceptance of Data in the Assessment of Chemicals," 1981 [C(81) 30 (Final)].

[8] 52 Federal Register 33768, September 4, 1987.

[9] Code of Federal Regulations Title 21 Section 58.1(a).

EPA, regulating studies conducted on pesticide products,[10] and studies relating to health effects, environmental effects, and chemical fate testing;[11] however, we will not be discussing EPA GLPs here (Table 1).

GLPs are applicable to those nonclinical studies that are intended to support INDs/IDEs and marketing applications. Nonclinical studies conducted by sponsors in preparing for their IND/IDE-supporting studies (such as a dose range finding study) do not need to be GLP compliant, and these exploratory studies will be less expensive to run non-GLP. Once the exploratory studies have yielded enough data to provide a solid scientific hypothesis, the regulatory pathway (nonclinical studies required) to advance the product into human clinical trails via an IND/IDE are described in general terms in the following guidance documents:

- International Conference on Harmonization (ICH) M3, Nonclinical Safety Studies for the Conduct of Human Clinical Trials for Pharmaceuticals. Available at: http://www.fda.gov/cder/guidance/1855fnl.pdf.
- ICH S6a, Preclinical Safety Evaluation of Biotechnology-Derived Pharmaceuticals. Available at: http://www.fda.gov/cder/guidance/1859fnl.pdf.
- ICH S7a, Safety Pharmacology Studies for Human Pharmaceuticals ICH S7a. Available at: http://www.fda.gov/cder/guidance/4461fnl.htm.
- FDA Guidance for Industry, Estimating the Maximum Safe Starting Dose in Initial Clinical Trials for Therapeutics in Healthy Volunteers. Available at: http://www.fda.gov/cder/guidance/5541fnl.pdf.

GLP Guidance Documents

Guidance documents related to GLPs are issued by FDA and ICH, two organizations discussed in almost every chapter of this textbook but also by the OECD. The OECD was originally an organization established in post–World War II Europe to help reconstruct the economic stability of the region; however, today it's an international organization (including the United States), which issues guidance documents on a number of very broad topics including economic, environmental, and social issues. While the OECD guidance documents are viewed as guidance in the United States, the OECD Principles of Good Laboratory Practice have been adopted as legislation by some European Community member states and is enforceable in these countries. The OECD has issued 15 guidance documents titled *The Series on Principles of Good Laboratory Practice and Compliance Monitoring*.

---

[10] Code of Federal Regulations Title 21 Section 160.
[11] Code of Federal Regulations Title 21 Section 792.

Table 1 Complete List of 21 CFR 58 GLP Requirements

Subpart A general provisions
- 58.1 Scope
- 58.3 Definitions
- 58.10 Applicability to studies performed under grants and contracts
- 58.15 Inspection of a testing facility

Subpart B organization and personnel
- 58.29 Personnel
- 58.31 Testing facility management
- 58.33 Study director
- 58.35 Quality assurance unit

Subpart C facilities
- 58.41 General
- 58.43 Animal care facilities
- 58.45 Animal supply facilities
- 58.47 Facilities for handling test and control articles
- 58.49 Laboratory operations areas
- 58.51 Specimen and data storage facilities

Subpart D equipment
- 58.61 Equipment design
- 58.63 Maintenance and calibration of equipment

Subpart E testing facility operation
- 58.81 Standard operating procedures
- 58.83 Reagents and solutions
- 58.90 Animal care

Subpart F test and control articles
- 58.105 Test and control article characterization
- 58.107 Test and control article handling
- 58.113 Mixture of articles with carriers

Subpart G protocol for and conduct of a nonclinical laboratory study
- 58.120 Protocol
- 58.130 Conduct of a nonclinical laboratory study

Subpart H – I (Reserved)

Subpart J records and reports
- 58.185 Reporting of nonclinical laboratory study results
- 58.190 Storage and retrieval of records and data
- 58.195 Retention of records

Subpart K disqualification of testing facilities
- 58.200 Purpose
- 58.202 Grounds for disqualification
- 58.204 Notice of and opportunity for hearing on proposed disqualification
- 58.206 Final order on disqualification
- 58.210 Actions upon disqualification
- 58.213 Public disclosure of information regarding disqualification
- 58.215 Alternative or additional actions to disqualification
- 58.217 Suspension or termination of a testing facility by a sponsor
- 58.219 Reinstatement of a disqualified testing facility

No. 1, OECD Principles of Good Laboratory Practice (as revised in 1997)
No. 2, Revised Guides for Compliance Monitoring Procedures for Good Laboratory Practice (1995)
No. 3, Revised Guidance for the Conduct of Laboratory Inspections and Study Audits (1995)
No. 4, Quality Assurance and GLP (as revised in 1999)
No. 5, Compliance of Laboratory Suppliers with GLP Principles (as revised in 1999)
No. 6, The Application of the GLP Principles to Field Studies (as revised in 1999)
No. 7, The Application of the GLP Principles to Short-Term Studies (as revised in 1999)
No. 8, The Role and Responsibilities of the Study Director in GLP Studies (as revised in 1999)
No. 9, Guidance for the Preparation of GLP Inspection Reports (1995)
No. 10, The Application of the Principles of GLP to Computerised Systems (1995)
No. 11, The Role and Responsibilities of the Sponsor in the Application of the principles of GLP (1998)
No. 12, Requesting and Carrying Out Inspections and Study Audits in Another Country (2000)
No. 13, The Application of the OECD Principles of GLP to the Organisation and Management of Multi-Site Studies (2002)
No. 14, The Application of the Principles of GLP to In Vitro Studies (2004)
No. 15, Establishment and Control of Archives that Operate in Compliance with the Principles of GLP (2007)[12]

For those who are interested in learning more about the difference in GLP regulations, a comparison chart of FDA, EPA, and OECD GLPs is posted on the FDA Web sites at: http://www.fda.gov/ora/compliance_ref/bimo/comparison_chart/.

One key OECD guidance document is the "The Application of the OECD Principles of GLP to the Organisation and Management of Multi-Site Studies."[13] This document defines the management of a GLP study that is conducted at more than one site, a trend that has been growing for the last decade. A simplistic example of a multisite GLP study would be a study where one laboratory may analytically confirm the uniformity, concentration, and stability of the test article and dose the animals with the test article, but send the animal serum samples to a separate laboratory to conduct the bioanalytical analyses. Though the work conducted for this

---

[12] See: http://www.oecd.org/document/63/0,3343,en_2649_34381_2346175_1_1_1_1,00.html.

[13] The Application of the OECD Principles of GLP to the Organisation and Management of Multi-Site Studies, ENV/JM/MONO(2002)9, 2002.

type of study set up may take place in separate laboratories within a single company (either geographically remote or organizationally distinct locations) or at two (or more) separate companies, the study is viewed as a single study. Since a multisite study is a single study, communication becomes critically important.

The GLP concepts within 21 CFR 58 Subparts A to K and the OECD guidance documents mirror some of the common themes repeated throughout this GxP chapter, i.e., the need for independent oversight, written procedures, change control, and good documentation practices. Subparts A to K are shown in full in Table 1, and the full list of OECD guidance documents are listed above. Instead of regurgitating the contents of the regulations and guidance, we will summarize some of the key highlights from them both.

Organization and Personnel

Both the FDA and the OECD delineate the requirement for nonclinical laboratory facility management to create several key personnel roles to conduct a GLP study, mainly the role of the study director, principal investigator, and the QAU, all of which are defined below:[14,15]

Study director	The individual responsible for the overall conduct of the nonclinical laboratory study.
Principal investigator	The individual who, for a multisite study, acts on behalf of the study director and has defined responsibility for delegated phases of the study. The study director's responsibility for the overall conduct of the study cannot be delegated to the principal investigator(s); this includes approval of the study plan and its amendments, approval of the final report, and ensuring that all applicable Principles of Good Laboratory Practices are followed.[16]
QA program/QAU	A QA program is a defined system, and the QAU is the personnel who are independent of the study conduct that execute the program, which is designed to assure test facility management of compliance with the Principles of Good Laboratory Practices.

---

[14] Code of Federal Regulations Title 21 Section 58.3.

[15] OECD Principles on Good Laboratory Practice, ENV/MC/CHEM(98)17, 1997, Section 2, Definitions of Terms.

[16] It should be noted that the term "Principal Investigator" does not appear in 21 CFR 58 but is an OECD term that has been adopted as multisite studies are now commonplace.

As with GMPs, the GLPs require that management ensure that there is adequate staffing, equipment, and facilities to conduct the nonclinical experiments in compliance with GLPs in addition to an adequate training program to ensure personnel are properly trained to perform their duties.

One key management function is the formal appointment of the study director and investigators. The study director is responsible for the scientific conduct of the study, including planning, documentation, and approval of its protocols and reports. They must coordinate with the QAU and management to ensure GLP compliance. The study director is responsible for the scientific and regulatory assessment of a project and must have the appropriate experience and knowledge of GLP principles and regulations to allow them to successfully perform their task. The management's decision to replace a study director must be documented.[17] Within a multisite study, the study director faces an additional challenge of being responsible for all study activities; some of these may be conducted by other companies. The study director should ensure that all test sites used in a multisite study are acceptable. To do this, the study director may visit the different facilities, but in practice this is more the exception than the rule, and is not required. Most often what is required is that each test site names a principal investigator whom the study director will communicate with directly. Direct communication is critical and must be allowed by the sponsor,[18] though the sponsor would be best served to be copied on all communications between all sites in a multisite study.

The role of QAU is critical in establishing and maintaining GLP compliance. The QAU, as defined by GLPs, must be independent of the study conducted, which is a common element of a quality organization across the GxPs. Some of the key responsibilities of the QAU are to

- Maintain a master schedule of all GLP studies conducted at the test facility
- Maintain copies of protocols
- Conduct inspections of studies at intervals adequate to assure integrity of the study
- Submit written reports to management and study directors
- Assess and document deviations from protocols and standard operating procedures (SOPs)

---

[17] Pharmaceutical Technology Europe Magazine, Applying Good Laboratory Practice Regulations, 6/1/03 by Hana Danan. Available at: http://www.ptemag.com/pharmtecheurope/article/articleDetail .jsp?id=60144&pageID=1&sk=&date=.

[18] The Application of the OECD Principles of GLP to the Organisation and Management of Multi-Site Studies, ENV/JM/MONO(2002)9, 2002.

- Review final study reports for data accuracy and sign a statement specifying dates of inspection and when findings were reported to management and study director
- Maintain a SOP/policy detailing the roles and responsibilities of the QAU

In the case of a multisite study, there should be a distinction between the lead QAU and test site QAU. The lead QAU is the one that oversees the study director. A test site QAU is the unit that provides the quality oversight of the additional facilities where principal investigators are conducting certain phases of the study. The lead QAU maintains all QAU responsibilities except for the oversight and inspection of the activities carried out by the principal investigator(s). Test site QAU(s) provide a statement relating the GLP compliance of the principal investigator's activities to the lead QAU prior to the completion of the study report.

Facilities and Equipment

Both the facilities and equipment used in a GLP study must be appropriately designed. For a facility, this means the building must be of adequate size and design to quarantine incoming and/or sick animals, segregate different studies and animal species, and provide appropriate workflow and work areas for all the different functional areas conducting a GLP study. Environmental controls, to prevent infestation and contamination, must be employed. Test/control article storage must also be adequate to preserve the identity, strength, purity, and stability of the test/control articles and mixtures. Equipment, or analytical instrumentation, used in a GLP study must be appropriately qualified, inspected, cleaned, maintained, calibrated, and standardized, all of which must be accompanied by supportive documentation. The design, setup, and maintenance of both GLP facilities and equipment must be adequate to minimize the risk of test/control article, test system, or sample mix-ups and/or cross-contamination. These same principles apply to facilities and equipment in a GMP environment.

Testing Facility Operations

One key aspect under the Subpart E heading of the FDA GLPs and the OECD guidelines is the requirement that SOPs shall be established for, but not limited to, the following topics (Table 2):[19,20]

---

[19] Code of Federal Regulations Title 21 Section 58.81(b).

[20] OECD Principles on Good Laboratory Practice, ENV/MC/CHEM(98)17, 1997, Section 7, Standard Operating Procedures.

Table 2 FDA and OECD Required SOP Topics/Categories

FDA	OECD
Animal room preparation	Test and reference items
Animal care	Apparatus, materials, and reagents
Receipt, identification, storage, handling, mixing, and method of sampling of the test and control articles	Record keeping, reporting, storage, and retrieval
Test system observations	Test system (where appropriate)
Laboratory tests	Quality assurance procedures
Handling of animals found moribund or dead during study	
Necropsy of animals or postmortem examination of animals	
Collection and identification of specimens	
Histopathology	
Data handling, storage, and retrieval	
Maintenance and calibration of equipment	
Transfer, proper placement, and identification of animals	

It should be noted that the table above is a listing of required SOP topics and not SOP titles. While this is only a small list, these topics will encompass a great number of procedures. It is commonplace for contract nonclinical laboratories to maintain hundreds of SOPs; such is the life of the QAU. In conducting a GLP study under such a large number of SOPs, deviations from the SOPs may occur. In such circumstances, per GLPs, the study director, and the principal investigator in the case of multisite studies, should acknowledge these deviations in the raw data.

Other notable requirements of Subpart E are the labeling requirements for reagent/solutions and animal care requirements. The animal care requirements, generally speaking, highlight the need for isolation of newly received animals from outside sources until their health status is determined, identification and segregation of animals, keeping the animal cages and area cleaned, and providing the animals with noncontaminated feed and water.[21]

Test and Control Article

The drug, device, or biologic under development during nonclinical evaluation is generically referred to as a test article. All test articles used in GLP studies must have a documented "chain of custody," i.e., records of receipt,

---

[21] Code of Federal Regulations Title 21 Section 58.90.

use, and return, including dates and amounts of material.[22] Methods of synthesis or manufacturing of the test article must be documented.[23] However, test articles during this stage of development do not need to be made under GMPs (an overview of GMPs will be provided in the next section). Test articles are required to be "characterized," meaning that the identity, strength, purity, and composition are determined and documented. The stability of the test article as well as the test article in the mixture given to animals needs to be determined either prior to study initiation of the study or concomitantly with the ongoing study, and a retention sample of the test and control articles must be kept for all studies lasting more than four weeks.[24] Characterization and stability may be conducted by the nonclinical laboratory itself or the study sponsor in accordance with GLPs. Test article characterization is essential to ensure that the drug, device, or biologic being advanced through nonclinical development is representative of what will be used in the "first in man" study. Failure to do so will result in inadequate toxicology coverage for human clinical trials and potentially necessitate the need to repeat nonclinical safety studies.

Protocols, Records, and Reports

Each GLP study is to be conducted according to an approved, written protocol (or study plan as referenced in the OECD). The FDA and the OECD required contents of GLP protocols are listed in 21 CFR 58.120 and OECD Principles of GLP Section 8, respectively. The FDA requires that the protocols be signed by the study director and the sponsor. The OECD requires the study director's approval signature on all GLP protocols and the sponsor and test facility management's approval where required by national regulation. Alternatively, deviations from or amendments to a GLP protocol requires only the study director's approval signature per both FDA and OECD,[25,26] although sponsor review and approval of significant deviations and amendments is often the recommended practice.

All original test facility records and documentation that are the result of original observations and activities in a study are considered the raw data. This includes both manual (laboratory notebooks, worksheets, etc.) and automated data (chromatograms, telemetry data, balance printouts, etc.). Where raw data is acquired through automated computer systems for the generation, measurement, or assessment of data intended for regulatory

---

[22] Code of Federal Regulations Title 21 Section 58.107(d).

[23] Code of Federal Regulations Title 21 Section 58.105(a).

[24] Code of Federal Regulations Title 21 Section 58.105(d).

[25] Code of Federal Regulations Title 21 Section 58.120(b).

[26] OECD Principles on Good Laboratory Practice, ENV/MC/CHEM(98)17, 1997, Section 8.1, Study Plan.

submission, 21 CFR 11 applies, and these systems must be validated to assure the integrity and quality of the raw data. Additional guidance on the application of GLP to computerized systems is available from OECD.[27]

As with the study protocols, the contents of study reports per FDA and OECD requirements are listed in 21 CFR 58.185 and OECD Principles of GLP Section 9, respectively. FDA and OECD regulations require that the study director sign the final report. The QAU must prepare and sign a statement indicating when the QAU inspections of the study took place and the inspection findings were reported to facility management, the study director, and to principal investigators (in the case of multisite studies).

It is important to remind Regulatory Affairs professionals that study reports do not necessarily have to be final or audited reports to submit the tabulated, integrated summarized data to the FDA for initiation of the IND. If, however, the integrated summary is based on unaudited reports, sponsors should submit an update to their integrated summary within 120 days of FDA's receipt of the integrated summary. If the audit of the individual reports did not result in a change to the integrated summary data, an update still must be submitted stating no changes.[28,29]

Compliance with GLPs

The FDA's inspection program for nonclinical laboratories is their Bioresearch Monitoring Program, often referred to as BIMO. The Bioresearch Monitoring Program was established in 1977 by a task force with representation from the drug, biologic, device, radiologic product, veterinary drug, and food branches of the FDA. This task force established an inspection program for nonclinical (animal) laboratories as well as clinical investigators, research sponsors, contract research organizations (CROs), bioequivalence laboratories, and Institutional Review Boards (IRBs).

FDA uses Compliance Program Guidance Manuals (CPGMs) as procedures for its field personnel to conduct these inspections. The purpose of each CPGM is to assure the quality and integrity of safety data submitted to FDA, with the ultimate goal of protecting human research subjects. The FDA has issued the following CPGMs enforced by the Bioresearch Monitoring Program,

---

[27] The Application of the Principles of GLP to Computerised Systems, OCDE/GD(95)115, 1995.

[28] FDA Guidance for Industry. Content and Format of Investigational New Drug Applications (INDs) for Phase I Studies of Drugs, Including Well-Characterized, Therapeutic, Biotechnology-derived Products. November 1995.

[29] FDA Guidance for Industry. Q & A Content and Format of Investigational New Drug Applications (INDs) for Phase I Studies of Drugs, Including Well-Characterized, Therapeutic, Biotechnology-derived Products. October 2000.

Table 3 CPGM and the Regulations They Enforce

CPGM	FDA Regulation BIMO Enforces
CPGM for good laboratory practice for nonclinical laboratories	Part 58—good laboratory practice for nonclinical laboratory studies
CPGM for clinical investigators	Part 50—protection of human subjects
CPGM for sponsors, monitors, and contract research organizations	Part 312—IND Part 812—IDE Part 511—new animal drugs for investigational use
CPGM for IRBs	Part 56—IRBs
CPGM for in vivo bioequivalence compliance program	Part 320—bioavailability and bioequivalence requirements Parts 50, 56, and 312 also enforced by this CPGM

Abbreviations: CPGM, Compliance Program Guidance Manual; FDA, Food and Drug Administration; IND, investigational new drug application; IDE, investigational device exemptions; IRB, Institutional Review Board.

and they are available on the Web at: (http://www.fda.gov/oc/gcp/compliance.html) (Table 3).

The objective of BIMO inspections of nonclinical laboratories is

- To verify the quality and integrity of data submitted in a research or marketing application.
- To inspect (approximately every 2 years) nonclinical laboratories conducting safety studies that are intended to support applications for research or marketing of regulated products.
- To audit safety studies and determine the degree of compliance with GLP regulations.[30]

FDA's Bioresearch Monitoring Program inspects commercial nonclinical laboratories without prior notification in most cases. There are two classifications of inspections: surveillance inspections and directed inspections.

---

[30] Compliance Program Guidance Manual. Bioresearch Monitoring: Good Laboratory Practice (Nonclinical laboratories). February 21, 2001. Available at: http://www.fda.gov/ora/compliance_ref/bimo/7348_808/48-808.pdf.

Surveillance inspections:	are periodic, routine determinations of a laboratory's compliance with GLP regulations. These inspections include a facility inspection and audits of ongoing and/or recently completed studies.
Directed inspections:	are assigned to achieve a specific purpose, such as
	verifying the reliability, integrity, and compliance of critical safety studies being reviewed in support of pending applications.
	investigating issues involving potentially unreliable safety data and/or violative conditions brought to the FDA's attention.
	reinspecting laboratories previously classified OAI (usually within 6 months after the firm responds to a warning letter).
	verifying the results from third party audits or sponsor audits submitted to the FDA for consideration in determining whether to accept or reject questionable or suspect studies.[31]

Both the biennial surveillance inspection program and any directed inspections of nonclinical laboratories are data-driven processes and are often conducted by a team of BIMO investigators, depending on the nature of the facility being inspected or the reason ("for cause") for the directed inspection. FDA field personnel conducting facility audits are referred to as investigators. We also use the term investigator in multisite GLP activities and the conduct of GCP studies at clinical trial sites, so the terminology sometimes can be confusing. The FDA investigators will interview key personnel who typically will include a QAU representative, the study director(s) for those studies being reviewed, and potentially facility management representatives, the archivist, and technicians within the laboratories and/or animal care facilities. Tours of the facility will be taken to determine the conditions, layout, and workflow of the employees, test systems, test/control articles, and in-process samples. SOPs will be reviewed and raw data will be reviewed to confirm that the laboratory is in compliance with its own SOPs, and that the SOPs adequately ensure compliance with GLPs. The inspection will typically include the evaluation of at least one

---

[31] Compliance Program Guidance Manual. Bioresearch Monitoring: Good Laboratory Practice (Nonclinical laboratories). February 21, 2001. Part II, Section C, Types of Inspections.

completed GLP study. The audit of the completed study will include a comparison of the protocol and amendments, raw data, other records, and specimens against the final report to ensure that the protocol requirements were met and that the final report accurately reflects the conduct and findings of the GLP study. A typical audit may last three to four business days, but can vary greatly.

As with all FDA GxP inspections, the inspectional and administrative follow-up procedures are similar across the GxPs, and an explanation of the FDA process is included in section "GMP Inspections and Consequences" of this chapter.

INTRODUCTION TO CURRENT GOOD MANUFACTURING PRACTICES

Current good manufacturing practices (cGMPs) are the regulations that govern the manufacture of human and veterinary drugs, biologics, and medical devices to endure the identity, strength purity, and quality of the finished product. The cGMP are based on the fundamental principles of quality assurance: (*i*) quality safety and effectives must be designed and built into the product, (*ii*) quality cannot be inspected or tested into the product, and (*iii*) each step of the manufacturing process must be controlled to maximize the likelihood that the product will be acceptable.[32] Sponsors, even if part or all of the manufacturing activities are outsourced, are responsible for ensuring that their products comply with cGMPs throughout the product development lifecycle from development to commercialization. The FDA enforces these regulations primarily through inspections, and failure to comply will result in various regulatory actions.

History of the cGMPs

It is important for the Regulatory Affairs professional to understand that the evolution of cGMP regulations have emerged mostly as a result of missteps by medical product manufacturers.

The regulatory basis for cGMPs is the Food, Drug and Cosmetic Act (FD&C) first published in 1938 after a public health crisis involving Elixir Sulfanilamide. This sulfa drug was dissolved in diethylene glycol, an analogue of antifreeze, and as a result over a hundred people died, many of them children. Subsequently, the Act was quickly passed by Congress and required that all drugs be labeled with directions for safe use and mandated the preapproval of all new drugs. The initial use of the term, "good manufacturing practices," is recorded in the Act, as it sets tolerances for poisonous substances that cannot be avoided by the observance of GMP. The law also formally authorized facility inspections and gave the FDA authority to enforce compliance with the Act.

However, the general use of the term "current good manufacturing practice" did not become prevalent until the Kefauver–Harris Amendments to the FD&C in

---

[32] Juran, Quality Control Handbook. 4th ed. McGraw-Hill, 1988.

1962. Under these amendments, a drug is adulterated if: "The methods used in, or the facilities or controls used for, its manufacture, processing, packaging, or holding do not conform to or are not operated or administered in conformity with cGMP to assure that such drug meets the requirements of this Act as to safety and has the identity and strength, and meets the quality and purity characteristics, which it purports or is represented to possess."[33] The amendments require that all drugs be shown to be safe and effective before being marketed and gave the FDA greater oversight of clinical trials and access to manufacturers' production records. The amendments were precipitated by a health crisis that occurred outside the United States, involving Thalidomide. Thalidomide, a sedative, was given to thousands of pregnant European women and resulted in over 8000 children with birth defects. The FDA refused to approve the drug in the United States despite pressure from the applicant. It should be noted that the FDA reviewer in charge received the highest governmental civilian award, the Civilian Medal of Honor, for *not* approving the Thalidomide application.

Modern day drug cGMP regulations are a result of a regulatory revisions published in 1978.[34] Additional amendments were proposed in 1996,[35] but have since been withdrawn by the agency in anticipation of a more comprehensive cGMP initiative (see Pharmaceutical cGMPs for the 21st Century-A Risk-Based Approach, FDA Sept. 2004). The cGMP regulations as they apply to drugs and biologics can be found in the CFR Title 21 parts 210 and 211 (21 CFR 210 and 211).

The cGMP regulations for medical devices were promulgated in 1978 as a result of the Medical Device Amendments to the FD&C in 1976.[36] The Medical Device Amendments were adopted in response to another health crisis caused by the Dalkon Shield intrauterine device. The Dalkon shield caused numerous injuries to women and resulted in one of the largest class action lawsuits ever against the manufacturer. The subsequent passage of the Medical Device Amendments requires different levels of FDA premarketing oversight, depending on the classification of the device. In the ensuing years after 1978, the FDA interpretation of the cGMPs evolved to more closely resemble the medical device requirements set by the International Organization of Standardization (ISO). In 1996, FDA published a final rule revising the cGMP requirements for medical devices incorporating them into a quality system regulation (QSR).[37] The regulations are codified in 21 CFR 820.

Although not discussed in detail in this chapter, additional cGMPs regulations exist to cover more unique medical products. These include the cGMPs for blood and blood products that can be found in the 21 CFR 606 and cGMPs

---

[33] United States Code Title 21 Section 351(a)(2)(B) (FDCA § 501 (a) (2) (b)).

[34] 43 Federal Register 45,104, (September 29, 1978).

[35] 61 Federal Register 20,104, May 3, 1996.

[36] United States Code Title 21 Section 351(a)(2)(B) (FDCA § 515 (a) (2) (b)).

[37] 61 Federal Register 52,448, October 7, 1996.

for positron emission tomography (PET) Drugs Products 21 CFR 212 (proposed), which has yet to be codified into law.

cGMPs Today

In recent regulatory publications by the FDA and ICH, the CGMPs are converging toward a single set of regulations for all medical products that are applicable throughout the ICH community. Concepts found in medical device cGMPs, as well as international standards (e.g., ISO, EU GMPS, PIC/S), are being integrated into drug cGMPs. There is a greater emphasis on understanding process performance, use of modern analytical techniques, and continual process improvement. cGMPs are being applied as appropriate throughout the product lifecycle from pharmaceutical development to product discontinuation. Management responsibilities are being identified to assure compliance to cGMP regulations. The hope for this evolution in cGMPs is for sponsors to have greater regulatory latitude and subsequently reduce the number of regulatory changes submitted to the health authorities while continuing to manufacture products that are consistently safe and effective.

A major initiative by the FDA in August 2002 titled "Pharmaceutical cGMPs for the 21st Century-A Risk-Based Approach" launched a series of guidelines and to promote a more modern, comprehensive approach to cGMPs for drug products. The initiative's five major objectives are:

- Encourage the early adoption of new technologic advances by the pharmaceutical industry.
- Facilitate industry application of modern quality management techniques, including implementation of quality systems approaches, to all aspects of pharmaceutical production and quality assurance.
- Encourage implementation of risk-based approach that focuses both industry and Agency on critical areas.
- Ensure that regulatory review, compliance, and inspection policies are based on state-of-the-art pharmaceutical science.
- Enhance the consistency and coordination of FDA's drug quality regulatory programs, in part, by further integrating enhanced quality systems approached into the Agency's business process and regulatory policies concerning review and inspection activities.[38]

---

[38] Pharmaceutical CGMPS for the 21st Century-A Risk-Based Approach Final Report September 2002.

Two major guidelines published by the FDA to address the needs descri-bed in the Pharmaceutical cGMPs for the 21st century report were "PAT—A Framework for Innovative Pharmaceutical Development, Manufacturing and Quality Assurance" and "Quality Systems Approach to Pharmaceutical cGMP Regulations." The FDA's guidance "Quality Systems Approach to Pharmaceu-tical cGMP Regulations" outlines concepts where process analytical technology (PAT) can be used to increase manufacturing efficiency while still working within the framework of cGMPs. This guideline emphasizes the need for the sponsor to build in or design a quality process on the basis of the desired attributes of the product, a concept originally found in the medical device cGMPs. In addition to quality by design, the guideline emphasizes the need for extensive process development and understanding. Process understanding requires the identification of critical sources of variability, the ability to manage variability, and the knowledge that the management of variability will result in a quality product. Using the knowledge obtained during process development and analytical tools during the processing allows for more regulatory flexibility in defining the parameters that produce a quality product. The FDA guidance "Quality Systems Approach to Pharmaceutical cGMP Regulations" provides a systematic approach to meeting 210 and 211 CFR while incorporating more modern, universally recognized concepts of quality. The quality system approach, another concept originally found in the medical device cGMPs, identifies four critical elements associated with a successful quality program; senior management support, sufficient resources, manufacturing operations partnership, and continual self-evaluation. The guidance also describes the FDA's six systems approach to inspections, dividing manufacturing into five systems: production, facilities and equipment, laboratory controls, materials, and packaging and labeling. The sixth system, quality, encompasses the other five.

Concurrent with the recent cGMP publications by the FDA, there has been the publication of several ICH cGMP applicable guidelines, "Q8 Pharmaceutical Development," "Q9 Quality Risk Management," and "Q10 Pharmaceutical Quality System." These guidelines espouse the same concepts put forth by the FDA in "Pharmaceutical cGMPs for the 21st Century" such as quality by design, risk management, and quality systems. The ICH guideline "Q8 Pharmaceutical Devel-opment" promotes the idea of prospectively designing quality on the basis of the product's indication, method of administration, and physiologic properties. The concept of product lifecycle management and improvement is introduced with a focus on the early development of a drug product. "Q9 Quality Risk Management" integrates risk management, a common notion that is found throughout the medical device regulations, into pharmaceutical development and provides the tools to achieve the goals of ICH "Q8 Pharmaceutical Development." Risk identification, analysis, and evaluation allow manufacturers to manage variability in their pro-cesses with greater regulatory flexibility. "Q10 Quality Systems" is the international equivalent of the FDA's guidance "Quality Systems Approach to Pharmaceutical cGMP Regulations" and provides a modern, quality framework for meeting cGMPs, as appropriate, throughout the different stages of product development from inception to discontinuation. On the basis of ISO standards, this guideline's requirements for a successful quality system include management support plus continual process and quality system improvement.

The basic premise for cGMPs is that "quality should be built into the product, and testing alone cannot be relied on to ensure product quality."[39] Through quality, one can achieve the desired identity, strength, purity, and other quality characteristics of the final product and, therefore, be assured that the final product meets the required levels of safety and effectiveness. In general, the cGMPs require

- The establishment of a quality system and an independent group to oversee the quality system.
- A system for monitoring process performance and product quality to ensure a state of control is maintained.
- The documentation of process performance and product quality through written records.
- A change management system to assure that all changes are properly evaluated and documented.
- A corrective action and preventative action system to address items that may affect process performance and product quality.

GMP Regulations and Guidance

The specific cGMP regulations for drugs and medical devices, as summarized in Table 1, address all areas that impact process performance and product quality; personnel, components, procedures, equipment, and facilities. Personnel must be qualified and trained to perform their function. Materials used in the process must meet specified quality attributes and controlled in a manner to prevent mix-ups. Procedures must be established and followed for the manufacture, testing, cleaning, and validation activities associated with the product. Equipment must be properly identified, cleaned, and maintained to prevent cross-contamination. Facilities must be suitable for their intended purpose with proper lighting, air handling, plumbing, and sanitation. Although design controls, which require that the desired product performance characteristics are established prior to production, are found only in the medical device cGMPs, this concept is now being promulgated for pharmaceutical cGMPs in the FDA's guidance "Quality Systems Approach to Pharmaceutical cGMP Regulations" and ICH's guidance "Q10 Quality Systems" (Table 4).

---

[39] Food and Drug Administration Quality Systems Approach to Pharmaceutical CGMP Regulations.

Table 4 Subparts of 21 CFR 211, 21 CFR 600, and 21 CFR 820

	Subpart topic		
Subpart	21 CFR 211	21 CFR 600	21 CFR 820
A	General provisions	General provisions	General provisions
B	Organization and personnel	Establishment standards	Quality system requirements
C	Buildings and facilities	Establishment inspection	Design controls
D	Equipment	Reporting of adverse events	Document controls
E	Control of components and drug product containers and closures		Purchasing controls
F	Production and process control		Identification and traceability
G	Packaging and labeling control		Production and process controls
H	Holding and distribution		Acceptance activities
I	Laboratory controls		Nonconforming product
J	Records and reports		Corrective and preventive action
K	Returned and salvaged drug products		Labeling and packaging control

The cGMP expectations for active pharmaceutical ingredients (APIs) are equivalent to those outlined in the drug product cGMP regulations (21 CFR 210 and 211). ICH's guidance for Industry "Q7A Good Manufacturing Practice Guidance for Active Pharmaceutical Ingredients" further clarifies the application of cGMPs to APIs (both chemical and biologic) and intermediates. This guidance recognizes the differences between API and drug product production and, most importantly, defines the point at which API production should be under cGMP control.

Other guidelines exist that apply cGMPs to a specific area or topic (e.g., "Sterile Drug Products Produced by Aseptic Processing—Good Manufacturing Practice" or "Application of the Device Good Manufacturing Practice (GMP) Regulation to the Manufacture of Sterile Devices") and still others will continue to be published by the FDA and ICH.

cGMPs apply throughout the product's lifecycle, but the stringency of cGMPs increases from initial clinical trials to commercialization. Early-stage development products are given greater flexibility in their approach to cGMP compliance than commercial products because process knowledge is limited at this stage. Therefore, the level of controls needed to achieve investigational product quality differs from that of a commercial product. For example, pharmaceutical GMPs require that the production process be validated, which is impractical for an investigational product where sometimes only one or two batches have been manufactured. This concept is expressed in several FDA guidelines, including the " INDS-Approaches to Complying with cGMP During Phase 1" (since withdrawn, but still representative of the agency's thinking), "1991 Guideline on the Preparation of Investigational New Drug Products (Human and Animal)," "Content and Format of investigational new drug applications (INDs) for Phase 1 Studies of Drugs, Including Well –Characterized Therapeutic, Biotechnology Product," and "INDs for Phase 2 and Phase 3 Studies Chemistry, Manufacturing, and Controls Information." The ICH guidance "Q7A Good Manufacturing Practice Guidance for Active Pharmaceutical Ingredients" contains a specific section regarding the application of cGMPs to investigational APIs. On a cautionary note, reasoned judgment should apply in establishing the level of cGMPs for investigational products as the Agency can put on clinical hold or terminate an IND if there is "evidence of inadequate quality control procedures that would compromise the safety of an investigational product."[40]

Given the number of companies today that outsource the manufacture, packaging, and labeling activities for their medical products, how GMPs apply to these companies deserves special mention. The ICH guidance for Industry "Q10 Quality Systems" specifically states that the pharmaceutical quality system extends to the oversight and review of outsourced activities, and this idea is reiterated in the FDA guidance for Industry "Quality Systems Approach to Pharmaceutical cGMP Regulations." Statutory pharmaceutical cGMP requirements, under 21 CFR 211, require that the quality control unit "accepts/rejects products manufactured, packed or held under contract by another company."[41] Therefore, even companies that do not manufacture their own products must have an appropriate quality system. Oversight is established through written agreements, called quality agreements, which define quality roles and responsibilities between the contract giver and contract acceptor. In addition, quality agreements describe change management expectations, audit activities, and communication mechanisms.

Compliance with cGMPs

FDA and other regulatory authorities assure compliance with cGMPs through their routine and preapproval inspection program. In general, routine inspections are scheduled to occur biennially, while preapproval inspections occur prior to

---

[40] Food and Drug Administration Guidance for Industry "INDS-Approaches to Complying with CGMP during Phase 1," p. 4.

[41] Code of Federal Regulations Title 21 Part 211.22 (a).

the approval of an NDA or PMA. In reality, due to limited FDA resources, inspections may not happen in these timeframes and is more dependent on the compliance history of the firm. It is important to note that the FDA may inspect a firm at anytime.

There are several FDA internal inspection-related documents available, all of which contain various compliance programs and instructions for agency personnel to follow during inspections. These documents include the FDA CPGM[42] and the FDA Inspection Reference.[43] Both the CPGM and Inspection Reference provide important information regarding the agency's expectations during the inspections of different systems and/or product types. Some examples are:

- Drug Manufacturing Inspections
- Sterile Drug Process Inspections
- Guide to Inspection of Computer Systems in Drug Processing
- High Purity Water Systems
- Inspection of Medical Device Manufacturers
- Medical Device Premarket Approval and Postmarket Inspections
- Inspection of Biologic Drug Products

The biennial inspection program strictly audits the firm for compliance with GMPs, while an FDA preapproval inspection also includes ensuring that the information, especially the Chemistry, Manufacture and Control (CMC) information, submitted in the regulatory application is in agreement with the company's data on site (e.g., stability, manufacturing processes, and test methods). Any inaccuracies found can be considered a cGMP violation and can lead to the approval of the application being withheld.

GMP Inspections and Consequences

An inspection is initiated by the FDA's presentation on site of the FDA Form 482 (Notice of Inspection) and, if there are observations of noncompliance with cGMPs upon completion of the inspection, concluded with the presentation of FDA Form 483 (Inspectional Observations). From the 483 observations, an Establishment Inspection Report (EIR) is generated by the FDA for internal review and classification. The inspection is classified No Action Indicated (NAI), no substantive GMP noncompliance, Voluntary Action Indicated (VAI), substantive cGMP noncompliance but no further regulatory action required, and

---

[42] See: www.fda.gov/ora/cpgm/default.htm.

[43] See: www.fda.gov/ora/inspect_ref/default.htm.

Official Action Indicated (OAI), meaning further administrative and/or judicial regulatory actions are required.[44]

The consequences of noncompliance are multifold. Administrative actions include the issuance of a warning letter that states that the company is in violation of laws or regulations (i.e., specific 21 CFR 211, 21 CFR 600, or 21 CFR 820 violations) and failure to correct such violations may result in further FDA action without warning. The company has 15 days to respond to the letter. Other administration actions include application action (e.g., withdraw approval of IND, IDE, NDA, BLA, or PMA) and FDA-initiated product recalls. The FDA Application Integrity Policy (AIP)[45] and Compliance Policy Guide (CPG) 7150.09, "Fraud, Untrue Statements of Material Facts, Bribery, and Illegal Gratuities" allows for the agency to defer substantive review of applications if there is evidence of fraudulent data and requires the company to undergo a series of corrective actions to reestablish the integrity of the data.[46] If warranted, the violations may be referred to the FDA Office of Criminal Investigations for potential judicial actions, including, injunction, seizure, and prosecution. A felony conviction on FDA-related charges results in debarment.

A firm must respond to any inspectional observations in a thorough and timely manner, either by outlining the corrective action to be taken and timing of these corrective actions or disputing the findings with supportive data. Adequately addressing an FDA inspector's concern during an inspection can prevent an observation from being noted on the 483 Form. Adequately addressing any observations on the 483 Form can prevent the issuance of a warning letter or, if a warning letter is issued, prevent further administrative or judicial action. Even for a finding of VAI, a firm should respond to the observations as the FDA can issue an untitled letter or regulatory meeting to notify the firm that the findings are expected to be corrected. It is important to keep the Agency informed of the firm's progress in instituting the corrective actions, especially if there are numerous serious observations that require a long-term corrective action plan or if the timing or corrective action plan itself changes. The FDA will conduct a follow-up inspection to ensure that all of the items in the warning letter have been addressed appropriately.

The failure to respond to the substantive 483 observations can be a costly mistake and the responsibility ultimately falls upon the head of the company. In the landmark decision, United States versus Park, the president of a 36,000-employee company was found responsible for storing food in a warehouse under unsanitary condition. The court found that "persons responsible for exercising supervisory authority have a duty not only to seek out and remedy violation but to prevent them, thus imposing upon that person a duty to take affirmative action."[47]

---

[44] Office of Regulatory Affairs Field Management Directive No. 86.

[45] FR FDA 09/10/91 Notice 56 Fr 46191 - Fraud, Untrue Statements Of Material Facts, Bribery, And Illegal Gratuities; Final Policy.

[46] See: www.fda.gov/ora/compliance_ref/frn/fraud_ill_grat.html.

[47] 421 U.S. 658 (1975).

   The FDA latest enforcement tool to ensure cGMP compliance is the policy
of disgorgement, a sanction based on the premise that the firm is not entitled to
profits gained by illegal means, which allows the FDA to impose huge fines. In
2001, Schering Plough paid a $500 million dollar fine as part of a consent decree
for cGMP violations in their New Jersey and Puerto Rico manufacturing facilities.
In addition to the fine, the approval of Clarinex® was delayed for about a year and
ultimately the President and Chief Operating Officer resigned.[48]

cGMP References

There are multiple cGMP references available to the Regulatory Affairs professional. By accessing the information available in the regulations, Federal Register,
guidelines, and policies, the Regulatory Professional can keep abreast of the
Agency's thoughts in this area. The Federal Register is the daily official publication of the U.S. government and where all proposed and final federal rulemaking
(including the FDA regulations) can be accessed by the public. FDA-related
Federal Register items can be accessed at www.accessdata.fda.gov/scripts/oc/
ohrms/index.cfm or one can subscribe via email to a daily list of the Federal
Register table of contents at http://listserv.access.gpo.gov. Many other useful
email subscriptions are available from the FDA and can be accessed at https://
service.govdelivery.com/service/user.html?code=USFDA, including updates on
the latest regulatory guidelines. Another important site is electronic Freedom of
Information (FOI) room that contains useful information on cGMPs, including
recent warning letters and 483 Observations. This information is available for
drugs, biologics, and devices and for the Office of Regulatory Affairs (ORA). The
FDA's ORA (www.fda.gov/ora/about/default.htm) contains valuable information
on compliance and inspectional activities. Additional references to access information regarding cGMPs available on the Internet are listed in the reference
section of this chapter. This listing of Internet resources also contains a few useful
international GMP references because of the harmonization cGMPs and the global
nature of most companies today.

INTRODUCTION TO GOOD CLINICAL PRACTICES

The regulations, guidance, and industry standards that make up the GCPs are
intended to provide assurance that the safety and well-being of human subjects
participating in research has been protected *and* that the research yields quality
scientific data. A trial conducted in full adherence to GCPs gives the sponsor the
ability (in theory anyway) to submit data to a number of regulatory authorities
worldwide as the data was derived in accordance with a globally recognized
standard, if not in compliance with each and every local regulation.

   It is commonly accepted that the GCPs are far less descriptive than both
the GLPs and GMPs, resulting in significant "gray area" open for interpretation.

---

[48] Food & Drug Letter, June 7, 2002.

While a sponsor enjoys the benefit of choosing their best practice for GCP compliance, ad hoc interpretation without supporting written procedures can breed inconsistency and inefficiency. You will recognize some common themes within this overview of GCPs, which are also discussed in the GLP and GMP overviews in this chapter, the importance of independent oversight, written procedures, change control, and good documentation practices. To have an understanding of the GCPs today, it is important to recognize some of the reasons why they became necessary and where they evolved from.

History of the GCPs

The human subject has always been and, at least for the time being, is still the gold standard for human physiology experimentation. Today in the industry we use the more palatable words "investigation," "research," or "trial" when describing experimentation in man; however, the evolution of the GCPs and our collective awareness to human subject rights and protection is surprisingly a relatively recent development.

Certainly, a regulator or historian would argue that the following selection of events leading to the creation of the GCPs is an oversimplification. Guilty as charged. But for the purposes of this chapter, which is intended to be more practical than theoretical, we chose to highlight just a couple of post–World War II events which laid the foundation for the GCPs.

1947	The Nuremberg Code is written following the Nuremberg Trials, in which Nazi doctors were tried (and some sentenced to death) for the bizarre human experimentation they conducted in the name of science during World War II. The first of the 10 principles of the Code states that "the voluntary consent of the human subject is absolutely essential"; however, the Code falls short, in that it is interpreted to apply only to nontherapeutic human research, and is not applied uniformly for all human research subjects.
1962	U.S. Congress passes the Kefauver–Harris Amendments to the FD&C. In addition to requiring the FDA to evaluate new drugs for efficacy, the amendments establish the requirement for obtaining the informed consent of human research subjects.
1964	The World Medical Association meets in Helsinki, Finland, and adopts a document setting forth the ethical principles for medical research involving human subjects. The Declaration of Helsinki, as it came to be known, makes some of the principles set

| | forth in the Nuremberg Code applicable to clinical (therapeutic) research, and thus applicable to drug development studies. The Declaration of Helsinki has been amended several times since its inception, most recently clarified with a release in Tokyo, 2004.[49] |

1966   The New England Journal of Medicine publishes a landmark article by Dr. Henry K. Beecher titled "Ethics and Clinical Research." In his article, Dr. Beecher describes 22 research studies published in major medical journals, which he believed were examples of "unethical or questionably ethical studies."

1972   The *New York Times* publishes an expose on the Tuskeegee syphilis study conducted by the U.S. Public Health Service. The study began in 1932, documenting the natural progression of syphilis in African-American sharecroppers in Macon County, Alabama. When these men enrolled into the study there was no effective treatment for the disease; however, a decade into the study, penicillin was shown to be a safe and effective treatment for syphilis. The men in the study went decades without receiving penicillin for their syphilis though they were led to believe they were receiving treatment. The study continued in this fashion until the *Times* article exposed their mistreatment.

1974   The National Commission for the Protection of Human Subjects of Biomedical and Behavioral Research is formed with the primary goal to establish the basic ethical principles and policies to conduct human subject research in the United States. The *Times'* uncovering of the Tuskegee study and Dr. Beecher's article six years earlier are often cited as precursors for the Commission's formation.

1979   The National Commission for the Protection of Human Subjects of Biomedical and Behavioral Research publishes the Belmont Report, identifying three basic ethical principles of human subject research: respect for persons, beneficence, and justice. Very simply stated:

---

[49] The Declaration of Helsinki is included in the U.S. Federal Regulations 21CFR 312.120(c)(4) as a minimum standard for FDA's acceptance of clinical trial data gathered from foreign studies not conducted under an IND.

Respect for persons = Acknowledge the subject's
autonomy and protect those
subjects whose autonomy is
diminished

Beneficence = Minimize potential harm to the
subject and maximize their
potential benefit

Justice = Distribute the benefits and
burdens of research fairly.
Avoid exploiting a subject
population who would not
benefit from the research for
the sake of convenience.

1980   Federal regulations governing the Protection of Human
Subjects (21 CFR 50) are published in the Federal
Register

The Protection of Human Subjects regulations changed the way clinical research was conducted in the United States during the 1980s, and paved the way for additional regulations governing human subject research in the 1980s and 1990s.

GCPs Today

U.S. GCP Regulations

The U.S. regulations that cover the GCPs are contained within Titles 21 and 45 of the U.S. CFR. Unlike GLP and GMP, there is no part of the U.S. CFR titled "Good Clinical Practice"; so you can stop looking.

Title 21 of the CFR applies to products regulated by FDA. The CFR regulations under Title 21 that apply equally across drug, device, and biologic trials are cited in Table 5.

The CFR regulations under Title 21 that apply to a specific type of product (drug, biologic, or device) research regulated by the FDA are cited in Table 6.

Title 45 of the CFR applies to Public Welfare. The CFR regulations under Title 45 apply to research conducted by the Department of Health and Human Services (HHS) or conducted or funded in whole or in part by any of the governmental agencies that have adopted these standards, and are contained in 45 CFR Subtitle A – Department of HHS; Part 46 Protection of Human Subjects, which is similar to those FDA regulations governing Protection of Human Subjects and IRBs at 21 CFR Parts 50 and 56, respectively.

Table 5 Title 21 Parts/Subparts that Apply to Drugs, Devices, and Biologic Clinical Trials

Title/part	21 CFR 11	21 CFR 50	21 CFR 54	21 CFR 56
	Electronic records; electronic signatures	Protection of human subjects	Financial disclosure by clinical investigators	IND
Applies to	Drug/device/ biologic	Drug/device/ biologic	Drug/device/ biologic	Drug/device/ biologic
Subpart		Subpart topic		
A	General provisions	General provisions		General provisions
B	Electronic records	Informed consent of human subjects		Organization and personnel
C	Electronic signatures	Reserved		IRB functions and operations
D		Additional safeguards for children in clinical investigations		Records and reports
E				Administrative actions for noncompliance

Abbreviations: IND, Investigational new drug application; IRB, Institutional Review Board.

45 CFR Part 46 is often called the "Common Rule," referring to its common adoption by 17 U.S. governmental agencies. It should be noted, however, when research involving products regulated by the FDA is funded, supported, or conducted by FDA and/or HHS, both the HHS and the FDA regulations apply.[50] There are several differences between the FDA regulations and the HHS regulations for the protection of human subjects. A chart comparing the differences in these regulations is posted on the FDA Web site at http://www.fda.gov/oc/gcp/comparison.html. Another regulation related to GCPs and regulated by HHS is the Privacy Rule under 45 CFR Part 160 and 164, often referred to as HIPAA, an acronym for the Health Insurance Portability & Accountability Act of 1996. HIPAA was enacted to provide efficiencies in the transfer of health-related electronic data and to provide protection for the confidentiality and security of health data identifiable to an individual patient, "protected health information." HIPAA is not regulated by FDA, and as such,

---

[50] See: http://www.fda.gov/oc/ohrt/irbs/faqs.html.

Table 6 Title 21 Parts/Subparts that Apply to a Specific Type of Product, Either Drugs, Devices, or Biologic Clinical Trials

Title/part	21 CFR 312	21 CFR 314	21 CFR 601	21 CFR 803	21 CFR 812	21 CFR 814
	IND	Applications for FDA approval to market a new drug	Licensing	Medical device reporting	IDE	Premarket Approval of Medical Devices
Applies to:	Drug/biologic	Drug	Biologic	Device	Device	Device
Subpart			Subpart topic			
A	General provisions	General provisions	General provisions	General provisions	General provisions	General
B	IND	Applications	Establishment licensing	Generally applicable requirements for individual adverse event reports	Application and administrative action	Premarket Approval Application (PMA)
C	Administrative actions	Abbreviated applications	Product licensing	User-friendly reporting requirements	Responsibilities of sponsors	FDA Action on a PMA
D	Responsibilities of sponsors and investigators	FDA action on applications and abbreviated applications	Diagnostic radio-pharmaceuticals	Importer reporting requirements	IRB review and approval	Administrative Review RESERVED

E	Drugs intended to treat life-threatening and severely debilitating illnesses	Hearing procedures for new drugs	Accelerated approval of biologic products for serious or life-threatening illnesses	Manufacturer reporting requirements	Responsibilities of investigators	Postapproval Requirements
F	Miscellaneous	RESERVED	Confidentiality of information		Records and reports	RESERVED
G	Drugs for investigational use in laboratory research animals or in vitro tests	Miscellaneous provisions				RESERVED
H		Accelerated approval of new drugs for serious or life-threatening illnesses				Humanitarian Use Devices
I		Approval of new drugs when human efficacy studies are not ethical or feasible				

Abbreviations: IND, investigational new drug application; IDE, investigational device exemptions; IRB, Institutional Review Board.

will not be discussed in depth here; however, it is important to note that the investigator, as the health care provider, is considered a "covered entity" under HIPAA, but the sponsor is not. Although sponsors are not regulated under HIPAA, it is good business practice for sponsors to ensure that investigator-informed consent forms (ICF) comply with HIPAA requirements as per 45 CFR 164.508 and the language allows the sponsor future access to the study data obtained under that consent. For further information regarding HIPAA and its impact on clinical research, visit the HHS Web site dedicated to the topic at http://privacyruleandresearch.nih.gov/.

As noted previously, the regulations governing GCPs are not overly detailed and in many cases are open for broad interpretation. However, this is where guidance documents (aptly titled, don't you think?) can provide useful guidance.

GCP Guidance Documents

There are a number of guidance documents related to GCPs, and a listing of FDA and ICH guidance documents can be accessed via the FDA Web site (http://www.fda.gov/opacom/morechoices/industry/guidedc.htm). The most comprehensive "how-to" GCP guidance document was created by the ICH in 1996 (ICH E6). This guidance was subsequently published by the FDA in the Federal Register on May 7, 1997 and is applicable to drug and biologic trials, but not applicable to device trials; though we would say that the principles of GCPs listed in the document also apply to device trials, and device trial sponsors would be well served to make use of many of the recommendations included in ICH E6. The ICH E6 guideline "is intended to define 'Good Clinical Practice' and to provide a unified standard for designing, conducting, recording, and reporting trials that involve the participation of human subjects."[51] As with all guidance documents published by FDA, the ICH E6 guideline represents FDA's "current thinking" onGCP.

The principles of ICH E6 are paraphrased below:

- Clinical trials should be conducted ethically, consistent with the Declaration of Helsinki (which we already discussed in this section) and applicable regulatory requirements.
- Rights, safety, and well-being of subjects are paramount.
- Benefits of study must outweigh risks.
- Study to adhere to protocol that has been reviewed and approved by an ethics committee (EC) (IRB).
- Study must be scientifically sound.

[51] 62 FR 25692 (5/7/97) International Conference on Harmonisation; Good Clinical Practice: Consolidated Guideline; Availability.

- Investigator(s) must be qualified.
- Informed consent must be obtained freely.
- Records must be maintained to allow for accurate reporting, interpretation, and verification.
- Confidentiality of records must be assured to respect the privacy and confidentiality of study subjects.
- Clinical trial supplies must meet GMPs.
- Systems and procedures should be implemented to assure the quality of the trial.

The ICH E6 guideline defines the responsibilities of IRBs, investigators, and sponsors, all of which we will discuss in this section as well. ICH E6 also defines the minimum information that should be included in a clinical protocol, an investigator's brochure (IB), and includes a list of required "essential" documents to be maintained during a clinical trial. A copy of the ICH E6 GCP guideline is a must for every regulatory, quality, or clinical professional conducting clinical trials on regulated investigational drugs, devices, or biologics. This document can be found online at http://www.fda.gov/cder/guidance/959fnl.pdf.

Who is a sponsor and how do they meet their obligations?

The sponsor of a clinical trial may be an individual, a drug/device/biologic company, or a CRO that has been paid to take on specific (or all) the obligations of the sponsor. The primary responsibility of a study sponsor is to ensure that trials are being conducted and quality data are generated, documented, and recorded in compliance with the IRB-approved study protocol, GCPs, and applicable regulatory requirements. As part of the IND description in chapter 2, we've discussed the process for submitting a protocol that is ethically and scientifically sound. We know that these protocol attributes are vetted by the IRB that has reviewed and approved the protocol in addition to the ICF, so we will begin discussing the practical application of GCPs with a review of IRB responsibilities.

IRB Responsibilities

The IRB [or research ethics board (REB)/EC/independent ethics committee (IEC)] is regulated by FDA under 21 CFR 56, IRBs for drug, device, and biologic trials. ICH guidance on investigator responsibilities is included in ICH E6 GCP Section 3. An IRB's primary responsibility is to provide independent oversight of a clinical trial to safeguard the rights, safety, and well-being of human subjects. IRBs generally are categorized as "local" IRBs, which are institutionally based entities responsible for the rights, safety, and well-being of research subjects at their own institution (e.g., hospital), or "central" IRBs, which are "for-profit" IRBs that hold the same responsibilities for patient safety.

The central IRB is not affiliated with, or may not even be in close geographic proximity to, the research.

The membership requirements of IRBs are defined in FDA regulation 21 CFR 56.107 and also in the ICH E6 guideline Section 3.2.1. IRBs are responsible for the initial and continuing review and approval of protocols and amendments, ICFs, recruitment advertising, IBs, available safety information, subject payments, and any other written information to be given to the subject. By regulation and guidance, IRBs must maintain written procedures to ensure that these responsibilities are met and must maintain adequate documentation of their review and approval activities. Review and approval of the research and related documents must be carried out during a convened meeting of the IRB in which a quorum is present, with the exception of those research activities allowed an "expedited review." An expedited review is a review of research conducted by an IRB chairperson, or by a single member or members of the IRB designated by the chairperson, whereby he/she can approve research (expedited review cannot disapprove research) that meets certain criteria listed in the federal register,[52] or approve of a minor change to previously approved research during the existing previously authorized approval period, one year or less, without a full quorum IRB meeting. The list of research activities allowed expedited review in the federal register can best be summarized as those not requiring an IND/IDE or those that involve no greater than minimal risk, with the most invasive procedure being twice weekly finger-stick blood draws. Expedited reviews are regulated by FDA and HHS regulation in 21 CFR 56.110 and 45 CFR 46.110, respectively.

The minimum standard for continuing review of research by an IRB requires annual reapproval; however, IRBs commonly require more frequent updates regarding the trial in the form of periodic written progress reports from the investigator. IRBs, generally speaking, are also becoming more proactive in conducting periodic investigator site inspections.

In theory, the obligation to obtain IRB approval sits with the investigator rather than the sponsor; however, in practice, and especially when a central IRB is involved, the sponsor may communicate directly with the IRB. Sponsors may submit protocols, ICFs, recruitment advertising, and any other documents required by the IRB for approval (IB, additional information given to study subjects, etc.) on behalf of all investigator sites using the central IRB. The role that the sponsor plays in communicating with central IRBs is changing, and FDA issued a guidance in March 2006 titled "Using a Centralized IRB Review Process in Multicenter Clinical Trials" (http://www.fda.gov/cder/guidance/OC2005201fnl.pdf). Sponsor communication directly with IRBs can be very beneficial to clearly understand if a review must be conducted by the full board

---

[52] Federal Register: November 9, 1998 (Volume 63, Number 216) Protection of Human Subjects: Categories of Research That May Be Reviewed by the Institutional Review Board (IRB) Through an Expedited Review Procedure. Available at: http://www.fda.gov/oc/ohrt/irbs/expeditedreview.html.

or via expedited review, as this may impact clinical trial timelines. A couple of regulatory exceptions to the standard investigator-IRB reporting obligation is with devices where it is a sponsor's responsibility to evaluate adverse device effects and report the results directly to the IRB[53] and when an informed consent waiver has been invoked under 21 CFR 50.24.[54]

The FDA-issued Information Sheet, Sponsor-Investigator-IRB Relationship (http://www.fda.gov/oc/ohrt/irbs/toc4.html), is a good resource for further understanding the interrelationship and interaction of these entities. This guidance also applies to devices as well as drugs and biologics.

Investigator Responsibilities

An investigator's responsibilities are regulated by the FDA under 21 CFR 312 60–69 for drug and biologic trials and under 21 CFR 812, Subpart E for device trials. ICH guidance on investigator responsibilities is included in ICH E6 GCP Section 4. For studies conducted under a U.S. IND/IDE, the sponsor submits either a Form FDA 1572 for drug and biologic trials or an investigator agreement for device trials, which is signed by the principal investigator. Sponsors should ensure that the investigator understands that they are committing to compliance via a signed document, in essence, a contract. While the specific responsibilities for investigators are similar, but not identical for drugs/biologics trials and device trials, the investigator commitments discussed below are paraphrased from Section 9 of the FDA Form 1572; however, the FDA has stated that "the general responsibilities are essentially the same."[55]

At the time of signing the Form 1572, the investigator has committed in writing to do the following:

Conduct the study in accordance with the protocol. The investigator is to follow the protocol as written, unless justified, to protect the safety, rights, or well-being of the subject. Nonemergency changes to the protocol may be made via a protocol amendment with prior sponsor and IRB approval. Minor logistical or administrative changes in the protocol [change of monitor(s), change of telephone number(s)] may not require a protocol amendment,[56] and may be documented through the use of an erratum or errata page. ICH E6 (Section 4.5.3) states that "the investigator, or person designated by the investigator, should document and explain any deviation from the approved protocol." The limitation here is that neither ICH nor FDA provides a definition of a protocol deviation. Sponsors use terms such as "deviation" and "violation," sometimes interchangeably, and some classify them as critical, major, or minor. There is no standardization in this terminology from sponsor to sponsor, so it is critical that

---

[53] Code of Federal Regulations Title 21 Section 812.150(b)(1).

[54] See: http://www.fda.gov/oc/ohrt/irbs/faqs.html.

[55] See: http://www.fda.gov/OHRMS/DOCKETS/98fr/07d-0173-gdl0001.pdf.

[56] International Conference on Harmonization E6 4.5.2.

the investigator receives clear direction from the sponsor on terminology of protocol deviations, violations, their classification (if any), and a means to document them to comply with ICH E6. FDA's device regulations are more descriptive than the drug or biologic regulations with regards to deviations from the protocol and the reporting requirements.[57]

Also of note, the protocol is expected to be followed as written. For example, if the protocol calls for a physician to conduct a physical exam, but state law allows nurse practitioners to conduct physical exams, the protocol must be followed.[58] Another example may be if sponsors indicate in their protocols that they are being conducted in accordance with ICH GCP, then ICH GCP must be followed.

Personally conduct or supervise the study. The investigator is wholly responsible for the care of study subjects and the conduct of the trial within his or her institution. Study tasks and investigator responsibilities may be delegated to appropriately qualified (and licensed in some cases) individuals, but the investigator is responsible for their supervision. ICH E6 requires documentation of these delegated tasks, and in May 2007, the FDA published a draft guidance titled "Protecting the Rights, Safety, and Welfare of Study Subjects – Supervisory Responsibilities of Investigators," which clarifies the FDA's expectations regarding an investigator's responsibilities (http://www.fda.gov/OHRMS/DOCKETS/98fr/07d-0173-gdl0001.pdf).

Inform patients and obtain their consent, ensuring IRB requirements are met. Informed consent is the process by which subjects are consented to participate in the study. IRBs review and approve the ICF to verify that the document contains all required elements. 21 CFR 50.25 describes the eight required elements of informed consent and another six additional elements to be included, if appropriate. ICH E6 has its own list of elements of informed consent in Section 4.8.10. A checklist of required elements of informed consent is included as an appendix at the end of this chapter. Obtaining informed consent from a study subject or their legally authorized representative is more than securing a signature on a document; it is a multistep process. An investigator must provide the subject with information regarding the study, the potential risks and benefits (as well as letting them know that there may be no benefit at all), the subject's role in the study, the opportunity for Q&A, and time to think about their decision and consult with family members or friends. Finally, the investigator must provide the subject with a copy of the consent form once it is signed and personally dated by the subject or their legally authorized representative. The process of obtaining consent should be appropriately documented so that it is clear that the subject was recruited and enrolled appropriately and that "informed consent was obtained prior to participation in the

---

[57] Code of Federal Regulations Title 21 Section 812.150(a)(4).

[58] Food and Drug Administration Draft Guidance Document "Protecting the Rights, Safety, and Welfare of Study Subjects—Supervisory Responsibilities of Investigators" May 2007.

study."[59] The point at which the study actually begins is sometimes a gray area. The FDA recognized this and issued an information sheet on the topic titled "Screening Tests Prior to Study Enrollment." This information sheet states that "consent must be obtained prior to initiation of any clinical procedures that are performed solely for the purpose of determining eligibility for research, including withdrawal from medication (wash-out). Procedures that are to be performed as part of the practice of medicine and which would be done whether or not study entry was contemplated, such as for diagnosis or treatment of a disease or medical condition, may be performed and the results subsequently used for determining study eligibility without first obtaining consent."[60]

There are exceptions from the requirement to obtain informed consent from a research subject before receiving an investigational product. These exceptions from informed consent are detailed in 21 CFR 50.23 and 50.24 and 45 CFR 46.116. There are also additional requirements that may require the assent of children in pediatric studies. 21 CFR 50.55 is entitled, requirements for permission by parents or guardians and for assent by children.

Report all adverse experiences. FDA regulations require an investigator to promptly report to the sponsor any drug or biologic adverse experience (AE) that may reasonably be regarded as caused by, or probably caused by, the drug. If the AE is alarming, the investigator shall report the AE immediately. A good source for definitions of AEs and serious adverse experiences (SAEs) and related terms for drugs and biologics is the ICH-E2A Guideline, "Clinical Safety Data Management: Definitions and Standards for Expedited Reporting," March 1995. The following are the definitions of an AE and SAE taken from the ICH guidance document:[61]

---

1. An adverse event (or adverse experience) can therefore be any unfavorable and unintended sign (e.g., including an abnormal laboratory finding), symptom, or disease temporally associated with the use of a medicinal product, whether or not considered related to the medicinal product.
2. An SAE or reaction is any untoward medical occurrence that at any dose
   - results in death,
   - is life-threatening,

     (NOTE: The term "life-threatening" in the definition of "serious" refers to an event in which the patient was at risk of death

---

[59] Code of Federal Regulations Title 21 Section 312.62(b).

[60] See: http://www.fda.gov/oc/ohrt/irbs/toc4.html#screening.

[61] International Conference on Harmonization E2A Guideline, "Clinical Safety Data Management: Definitions and Standards for Expedited Reporting," March 1995.

at the time of the event; it does not refer to an event which hypothetically might have caused death if it were more severe)

- requires inpatient hospitalization or prolongation of existing hospitalization,
- results in persistent or significant disability/incapacity, or
- is a congenital anomaly/birth defect of a medicinal product, whether or not considered related to the medicinal product.

The FDA regulations require an investigator to report unanticipated adverse device effects to the sponsor and to the IRB as soon as possible but no later than 10 working days after the investigator learns of the event.[62]

The FDA definition of an unanticipated adverse device effect is:

3. Any SAE on health or safety or any life-threatening problem or death caused by, or associated with, a device, if that effect, problem, or death was not previously identified in nature, severity, or degree of incidence in the investigational plan or application (including a supplementary plan or application), or any other unanticipated serious problem associated with a device that relates to the rights, safety, or welfare of subjects.[63]

Read and understand the IB. An IB is a compilation of the clinical and nonclinical data on the investigational product(s) that is relevant to the study of the investigational product(s) in human subjects.[64] The investigator must understand the relevant data to adequately oversee the investigation and adequately protect the safety and well-being of the subjects he/she enrolls in the trial.

Ensure all associates involved are informed of obligations. It is typically expected that an investigator will delegate tasks and investigator obligations to a study team. The study team may consist of nurses, physicians, pharmacists, nonlicensed individuals, etc. Section 6 of Form FDA 1572 is where sub-investigators are listed. Subinvestigators listed on the 1572 should be limited to those individuals who play a critical role in the treatment and/or evaluation of the study subjects in the study. The investigator is responsible for ensuring that all

---

[62] Code of Federal Regulations Title 21 Section 812.15(1).

[63] Code of Federal Regulations Title 21 Section 812.3(s).

[64] International Conference on Harmonization E6 1.36.

members of the study team are appropriately trained. The FDA's draft guidance, Protecting the Rights, Safety, and Welfare of Study Subjects—Supervisory Responsibilities of Investigators, indicates that the investigator should ensure that the study team is familiar with the protocol, understands the details of the investigational product, understands and are competent to perform tasks they've been delegated, are aware of their regulatory obligations, are informed of any pertinent changes and are retrained during the conduct of the trial (if necessary). While this draft document does not mention that the training must be documented, the old FDA adage could be applied in this case, "if it isn't written, it didn't happen."

Maintain adequate and accurate records (device/drug use records, subject case histories, record retention) and make available for inspection. The fundamental elements of data quality are that documentation be attributable, legible, contemporaneous, original, and accurate. This is often referred to as the ALCOA principle.[65]

The FDA defines an adequate and accurate case history to include the case report form (CRF) and supporting data including, e.g., ICFs, medical records, including physicians' and nurses' progress notes. 21 CFR 312.62(b) also notes that the case history for each subject shall document that informed consent was obtained prior to study participation. This is important to note for those studies whereby the date consented and date that the subject undergoes study-related procedures is the same. Unless times of consent are on the ICF and in the investigator's progress notes to verify the subject consented prior to participation, the case history file must contain documentation that the subject's consent was obtained prior to undergoing any study-related procedures.

Document retention periods must be satisfied by the investigator. The FDA requires retention for two years following the date of marketing application approval or two years after the investigation is discontinued and the FDA notified. ICH E6 is similar, though slightly different; however, it is important to note that different countries require different retention periods for certain documentation. Sponsors typically specify a period of time for document retention in their clinical trial agreement/contract with the investigator.

The FDA regulations speak to the investigator's obligation to allow FDA access to the study records, while ICH E6 indicates that the investigator is to allow record access to the monitor, auditor, IRB, and regulatory authority on request.[66,67]

---

[65] See: http://www.fda.gov/OHRMS/DOCKETS/98fr/04d-0440-gdl0002.pdf.

[66] Code of Federal Regulations Title 21 Section 312.68.

[67] International Conference on Harmonization E6 4.9.7.

Ensure an IRB that complies with 21 CFR Part 56 reviews and approves research, any changes to the research, and any unanticipated problems. The investigator is responsible for ensuring that an appropriately constituted IRB oversees the research, and that he/she enables the IRB to comply with its requirements by providing the IRB with all required reports and documents for review in compliance with regulations and the IRB's written procedures.

Comply with all other requirements. This all encompassing phrase could be interpreted as meaning compliance with all applicable state and local regulations or written procedures.

Measuring an investigator's compliance often does not include their adherence to SOPs, as investigators are not required by the FDA regulations to have SOPs. Many investigators still do not have SOPs in place, a notable exception being commercial clinical research entities—doctors who have gone into the business of conducting clinical trials instead of carrying a patient load. There have been recent FDA guidances published, both final and draft, that may be changing the expectations for SOPs at investigator sites. In May 2007, FDA published the final guidance document, "Computerized Systems Used in Clinical Investigations." This guidance document provides a list of "suggested" SOPs that need to be in place when using computerized systems to create, modify, maintain, or transmit electronic records, including when collecting source data at clinical trial sites. Also in May 2007, FDA published a draft guidance titled "Protecting the Rights, Safety, and Welfare of Study Subjects – Supervisory Responsibilities of Investigators." This draft guidance makes several references to an investigator's responsibility to have procedures for the overall supervision and oversight of the trial. While this draft document does not specifically say "written" procedures, the old adage "if it isn't written, it didn't happen" applies. The Supervisory Responsibilities of Investigators guidance, as noted previously, also clarifies and more explicitly explains the FDA's expectations of investigators with regards to appropriate delegation of tasks and training of study staff as well as highlighting the fact that the investigator is wholly responsible and accountable for the conduct of the study and for protection of the rights, safety, and welfare of study subjects. Time will tell, but this guidance may become a useful tool for the sponsor when establishing quality expectations with an investigator and his/her study staff.

Sponsor Responsibilities and Oversight of Clinical Trials

A sponsor's responsibilities are regulated by the FDA under 21 CFR 312.50–59 for drug and biologic trials and under 21 CFR 812, Subpart C for device trails. ICH guidance on sponsor responsibilities is included in ICH E6 GCP Section 5.

Although it appears that 13 out of a list of 13 principles of ICH GCP,[68] the very first obligation of a sponsor listed in the document is to implement quality

---

[68] International Conference on Harmonization E6 2.13.

systems and SOPs to ensure that trials are conducted and data are generated, documented, and reported in compliance with the protocol, GCP, and other applicable regulatory requirements.[69] The FDA device regulations require written monitoring procedures as part of the investigational plan.[70] The FDA drug and biologic regulations do not specifically require that sponsors have written procedures; however, guidance documents, which reflect the FDA's current thinking, do require SOPs. Additionally, implementing written SOPs is industry standard, definitely expected, and just good business practice. The number and type of SOPs a sponsor institutes may vary widely depending on how many activities are outsourced versus conducted in house. Below is a suggested list of SOPs to achieve GCP compliance.

- Investigator Site Selection
- Regulatory Document Collection, Review, and Submission
- Financial Disclosure
- Investigator Site Initiation
- Investigational Product Distribution and Tracking
- Clinical Monitoring of Investigator Site
- Investigator Site Close-out
- AE Reporting
- Quality Assurance Audits
- Required Documents for Study Master File and Document Retention
- Vendor (CRO) Qualification and Oversight
- Protocol Deviations
- Amending a Protocol
- FDA Inspection at Sponsor facility

To conduct the clinical trial, the study sponsor must ensure that investigators are qualified by education and experience and are trained on the conduct of the protocol. It is often a misconception in the popular press that investigators are qualified by the FDA, when in fact this is a sponsor responsibility, mandated by regulation. Sponsors typically collect curriculum vitaes and applicable licenses from investigators to check to see if they are qualified by training and experience, that the research is related to their field of practice, and that they are appropriately licensed to conduct those procedures required by the protocol.

Although actions on the part of the sponsor regarding 21 CFR 54 "Financial Disclosure By Clinical Investigators" is not required until filing a

---

[69] International Conference on Harmonization E6 5.1.1.

[70] Code of Federal Regulations Title 21 Section 812.25(e).

marketing application, the process of collection financial disclosure information from investigators begins at the time of study start-up for covered clinical trials [i.e., those that the applicant or the FDA relies on to establish that the product is effective (including studies that show equivalence to an effective product) or any study in which a single investigator makes a significant contribution to the demonstration of safety[71]]. Sponsors are required to disclose to the FDA any proprietary or equity interests held by the investigators, as this could potentially bias the study results by submitting a Form FDA 3455. If no financial interests and arrangements that fall under the 21 CFR 54 definitions exist, then the sponsor must certify the absence of these potential biases to the agency by submitting a Form FDA 3454. Since the marketing application may be submitted a number of years after completion of the study, this information is typically collected at the beginning of the study by having each investigator directly involved in the research complete and sign a questionnaire. Most sponsors have an SOP covering financial disclosure (see above). In addition to the regulation, the FDA has published a guidance document on the topic, Financial Disclosure by Clinical Investigators.[72]

To gain assurance that the study is being conducted according to set standards, the sponsor must monitor the progress of human research on an ongoing basis. Monitoring is defined in ICH E6 as the act of overseeing the progress of a clinical trial and of ensuring that it is conducted, recorded, and reported in accordance with the protocol, SOPs, GCPs, and the applicable regulatory requirements. The monitoring of a clinical trial may employ varying levels of oversight (e.g., frequency of study visits, depth, and detail of document review) depending on the size, duration, and complexity of the clinical trial design, plus the safety risk to study subjects. The most common method of clinical trial monitoring is through on-site visits made to the clinical trial site before the study begins and on a periodic basis until the study has been completed. Sponsors also use audits as another means to ensure compliance to GCPs.

The FDA originally issued a guideline for the monitoring of clinical investigations in 1988. In this document, FDA references a "pre-investigation" visit, which in practice is often carried out as a two-step process commonly referred to as investigator qualification (or site selection) and initiation.

An investigator qualification assessment may be conducted during an on-site visit to the investigator's site or by phone. From the agency's perspective, the purpose of the qualification assessment is to obtain information to assess the investigator's appropriateness to conduct the clinical trial, i.e., experienced staff, adequate facilities, time, and resources to assure patient safety. The sponsor will

---

[71] FDA's Guidance "Financial Disclosure for Clinical Investigators." Available at: http://www.fda. gov/oc/guidance/financialdis.html.

[72] FDA's Guidance "Financial Disclosure for Clinical Investigators." Available at: http://www.fda. gov/oc/guidance/financialdis.html.

also want to ensure that the investigator has access to appropriate subjects for recruitment as well as gauging the investigator's interest in conducting the trial.

The initiation covers more protocol-specific and GCP training. The initiation is typically conducted in one of two ways: an investigator's meeting, where all investigators participating in the study are trained on the protocol and GCPs by the sponsor or an on-site initiation visit where the CRA (or team of sponsor representatives) visits the clinical trial site and trains the investigator and his/her staff on the protocol and GCPs. Documentation of the investigator's training on the protocol, through attendance at an investigator's meeting or an on-site initiation visit should be maintained in the investigator site's study files as well as the sponsor's files before the site's enrollment of study subjects.[73]

Once a trial has begun, it is the sponsor's responsibility to monitor the conduct of the study at the investigator's site. Monitoring frequency is dependent on the size of the study, complexity of the protocol, safety risk to the study subjects, and the sponsor's philosophy on GCP compliance. A CRA will periodically visit an investigator's site during the active phase of the study when subjects are being seen and patient data is being collected. Visit frequency is study dependent and may vary greatly. Periodic (or interim) monitoring, as outlined in the FDA Monitoring Guideline, is required to assure that

---

- the investigator site's facilities continue to be acceptable for study purposes
- the investigator is following the study protocol/investigational plan
- any changes to the protocol have been reported to the sponsor and approved by the IRB
- the investigator is maintaining accurate, complete, and current records for each study subject
- the investigation is making accurate, complete, and timely reports to the sponsor and IRB
- the investigator is carrying out the activities he/she agreed to and has not delegated responsibilities to other previously unspecified staff

---

During an interim monitoring visit, the CRA is responsible for ensuring that all required documentation is maintained on site, that the protocol is being followed, the investigational product is accounted for, and that the rights, safety, and well-being of the study subjects are being protected. By conducting personnel interviews reviewing supporting documentation verifying source data during interim monitoring visits, the CRA can assure compliance with the protocol and GCPs.

---

[73] International Conference on Harmonization E6 8.2.20.

The ICH GCP Guideline Section 8, Essential Documents for the Conduct of a Clinical Trial, provides a quick and easy reference for required documents that need to be maintained at the study site. CRAs can use Section 8 of the ICH GCP guideline as a reference, or a study-specific checklist to ensure that the site is maintaining all required documents. To ensure that the investigator is following the study protocol, the CRA should review study subject medical records, study charts, and all appropriate documentation to ensure the subjects were being treated as dictated by the approved protocol.

The CRA should review investigational product dispensing/accountability logs and conduct a physical count of all investigational products on site to ensure that the investigator is appropriately dispensing and accounting for all investigational products. All investigational products must be stored in a manner that limits its distribution to those qualified and delegated by the investigator to do so. There must be adequate documentation to verify the chain of custody, i.e., shipping records that account for every unit of investigational product received and is maintained at appropriate storage conditions plus an accurate inventory accounting for all investigational product received, dispensed, recollected from study subjects, and returned to the sponsor or destroyed.

The CRA should ensure that the rights, safety, and well-being of study subjects were protected by the investigator and his/her staff. This is done initially through review of the ICF before study start-up to ensure that it contains all the required elements, and on an ongoing basis via a review of patient records to ensure they were appropriately consented before study participation, and that they are receiving quality care.

The FDA Monitoring Guideline discusses the sponsor's responsibility to "compare a representative number of subject records and other supporting documents with the investigator's reports.... " To fulfill this obligation, CRAs verify the accuracy of study data entered by the investigator's staff into the CRF against source documentation, which is commonly referred to as source document/data verification (SDV). Source documentation is the term used to describe where a study subject's information is first recorded. In some cases, the CRF may be considered source data; however, per ICH E6, the identification of any data to be recorded directly on the CRF and considered source documentation should be prospectively defined in the protocol.[74] As with monitoring visit frequency, study sponsors conduct SDV using different formulas to determine a representative sample. Some sponsors may choose to conduct 100% source data verification. Others may choose a plan whereby key safety and efficacy data, or a percentage of data, are only verified.

SDV provides assurance that the data recorded in the subject's records is completely and accurately transcribed to the CRFs. The CRF data eventually becomes the basis for marketing authorization submissions to FDA and other

---

[74] International Conference on Harmonization E6 Section 6.4.9.

regulatory authorities. SDV is described in the FDA's monitoring guideline as a means to provide assurance that:[75]

---

1. Information recorded in the investigator's reports is complete, accurate, and legible.
2. There are no omissions of specific data; such as concomitant medications or AEs.
3. Any missed study visits are noted in the reports.
4. Subjects who were dropped from or failed to complete the study are noted in the report with the reason adequately explained.
5. Informed consent was executed and adequately documented in accordance with federal regulations.

Another key item to look for during SDV is to ensure the presence of an appropriate "audit trail." An audit trail is required in both paper and electronic documentation systems in GCPs. An "audit trail" is a documentation that allows the reconstruction of the course of events. This allows someone reviewing the documentation to determine what data was changed, the original entry that was changed, why it was changed, by whom and when it was changed, and in cases where the need for the correction is not readily obvious, a brief explanation of why the change was necessary. The requirement for such documentation is referenced in ICH E6 Sections 4.9.3 and 5.18.4(n).

The description of a computerized system used in a clinical trial to create, modify, maintain, archive, retrieve, or transmit clinical data required to be maintained, or submitted to the FDA, can apply to many different types of computer applications used by IRBs, investigators, and sponsors. Sponsors have been dependent on computerized systems to store and manipulate study data for years; however, investigators were somewhat behind the times from a technology standpoint, but that is now rapidly changing. Although investigators have progressed with computerized record keeping, the application of 21 CFR 11 regulations may not be clear to all. The FDA's guidance for its field investigators states that "records in electronic form that are that created, modified, maintained, archived, retrieved, or transmitted under any records requirement set forth in agency regulations must comply with 21 CFR 11."[76] Guidance issued subsequently on the topic indicates that while this is true, the Agency intends to

---

[75] See: http://www.fda.gov/ora/compliance_ref/bimo/clinguid.html.

[76] Compliance Program Guidance Manual for FDA Staff, Bioresearch Monitoring: Clinical Investigators, October 1997. Available at: http://www.fda.gov/ora/compliance_ref/bimo/7348_811/default.htm.

interpret the scope of 21 CFR 11 narrowly and will exercise enforcement discretion with regard to some of the Part 11 requirements.[77]

All three entities, the IRB, investigator, and sponsor, bear the obligation to oversee, conduct, and monitor a clinical trial involving human subjects in compliance with GCP. The sponsor is additionally obligated by regulation to obtain the investigator's compliance. If the sponsor is unable to obtain compliance from the investigator, the sponsor is required to terminate the investigator's participation in the study as per 21 CFR 312.56 (b) and 21 CFR 812.46(a), for drugs, biologics, and devices, respectively. Additionally, the drug regulations require the sponsor to notify the FDA of the investigator's termination for noncompliance. However, the device regulations are silent on this topic.

Other key sponsor responsibilities covered by the GCPs are safety monitoring and clinical data management. The Pharmaceutical Research and Manufacturers of America (PhRMA) defines ongoing safety monitoring as a process whereby "all safety issues are tracked and monitored in order to understand the safety profile of the product under study. Significant new safety information will be shared promptly with the clinical investigators and any Data and Safety Monitoring Board or Committee (DSMB),[78] and reported to regulatory authorities in accordance with applicable law."[79] An investigator's responsibilities for safety reporting were briefly discussed in the previous section, and a sponsor's obligations for reporting safety data to regulatory authorities are discussed in the chapters covering INDs and medical device regulations. Further information regarding a sponsor's obligations for reporting of drug and biologic safety data can be found in ICH-E2A Guideline, "Clinical Safety Data Management: Definitions and Standards for Expedited Reporting," March 1995. For devices, additional detail can be found in the guidance for "Medical Device Reporting for Manufacturers," March 1997.[80]

"The discipline of Clinical Data Management includes paper and electronic case report form (CRF) design, clinical trials database design and programming, data acquisition and entry into the clinical trials database, data review, validation, coding and database finalization. Independent of how individual companies perform these tasks within their company, each company is obligated to ensure that the individuals performing these tasks follow Good

---

[77] FDA Guidance for Industry, Computerized Systems Used in Clinical Investigations, May 2007. Available at: http://www.fda.gov/OHRMS/DOCKETS/98fr/04d-0440-gdl0002.pdf.

[78] An independent data-monitoring committee that may be established by the sponsor to assess at intervals the progress of a clinical trial, the safety data, and the critical efficacy endpoints and to recommend to the sponsor whether to continue, modify, or stop a trial. Guidance on when a DSMB is needed is issued by the FDA, Establishment and Operation of Clinical Trial Data Monitoring Committees. Available at: http://www.fda.gov/cber/gdlns/clintrialdmc.pdf.

[79] PhRMA "Principles on Conduct of Clinical Trials and Communication of Clinical Trial Results" Revised June 2004. Available at: http://www.phrma.org/files/Clinical%20Trials.pdf.

[80] See: http://www.fda.gov/cdrh/manual/mdrman.html.

Clinical Practices."[81] The records and reports received and manipulated by the clinical data management function are regulated by FDA and addressed in ICH E6 guidance, and the electronic systems employed to handle the data are also governed by regulations and guidance. However, few guidances have been issued from FDA or ICH to provide these groups with direction with regard to clinical data management processes. The Society for Clinical Data Management, a professional organization not affiliated with a regulatory body, has issued a document titled "Good Clinical Data Management Practices," which is commercially available to members and nonmembers of the organization.[82]

Compliance with GCPs

The objective of a BIMO inspection at a clinical trial site is to assess, through audit procedures, if the clinical records adequately and accurately substantiate data submitted to the FDA to demonstrate safety and efficacy in support of an FDA-regulated product marketing application to determine that the rights and well-being of human subjects was adequately protected during the course of the research and to verify compliance with applicable FDA regulations and guidelines.[83] The objective of a BIMO inspection of a sponsor and/or CRO is to assess how sponsors assure the validity of data submitted to them by clinical investigators, and verify their adherence to applicable regulations.[84]

There are three classifications of BIMO inspections of a clinical investigator: study-oriented inspections; investigator-oriented inspections; and bioequivalence study inspections.

The study-oriented inspection is conducted by the FDA field office personnel and is usually assigned by FDA headquarters on the basis of a pending sponsor application to market a new drug, device, or biologic, rather than as per an FDA-defined schedule. When FDA reviewers are considering a marketing application or supplement for approval, they will choose clinical trial sites for inspection. The selection of a clinical trial site(s) for a study-oriented inspection is usually based on the amount of data contributed by the clinical trial site (the highest enrolling sites will most commonly be considered for inspection).

Once a site has been selected, the FDA field office will contact the investigator to arrange an inspection date. In general, the FDA will try to schedule the inspection within 10 business days of contact. On arriving at the

[81] See: http://www.livinglinks.net/biotech.html (definition attributed to Society for Clinical Data Management).

[82] Society for Clinical Data Management. Available at: http://www.scdm.org.

[83] Compliance Program Guidance Manual. Bioresearch Monitoring: Clinical Investigators. October 1, 1997. Available at: http://www.fda.gov/ora/compliance_ref/bimo/7348_811/default.htm.

[84] Compliance Program Guidance Manual. Bioresearch Monitoring: Sponsors, Contract Research Organizations and Monitors. February 21, 2001. Available at: http://www.fda.gov/ora/compliance_ref/bimo/7348_810/part_II.htm.

clinical site, the FDA field investigator will present the investigator with a Form FDA 482 "Notice of Inspection" along with their credentials.

FDA investigators are trained to conduct the inspection using the CPGM for clinical investigators, which outlines the minimal scope of the inspection.[85] The investigator will first obtain facts about the study conduct through interviews with the investigator, study coordinator, or responsible party at the clinical site to understand:[86]

- Who did what
- The degree of delegation of authority
- Where specific aspects of the study were performed
- How and where data were recorded
- How test article accountability was maintained
- How the CRA communicated with the clinical investigator
- How the CRA evaluated the study's progress

The FDA investigator will audit the study data, comparing what was submitted to the Agency with all supporting documentation. The FDA investigator will request a clinical trial subject's medical records, which may come from a doctor's office, hospital, nursing home, laboratory records, outpatient clinic records, or other sources.

An investigator-oriented inspection may be conducted when a single investigator's data may prove crucial to a product's approval, if the investigator has participated in many studies or if the investigator has conducted a study outside of his specialty. An investigator may also be targeted for a "for cause" inspection if a study sponsor, patient, or any anonymous "whistle-blower" contacts the FDA with a complaint about the investigator's conduct. An investigator-oriented inspection may also be conducted to investigate any unusual findings or trends noted in the data submitted to the agency. The conduct of an investigator-oriented inspection is much the same as a study-oriented inspection with the exception that the FDA investigator may dig deeper into the data audit and may audit data from more than one study.

The bioequivalence study inspection may be conducted on the basis of a pending NDA or abbreviated NDA (ANDA) for which a bioequivalence study is critical to product approval. Bioequivalence studies often support the approval of generic versions of innovator drug products or the approval of new formulations of marketed drugs. Bioequivalence studies have both a clinical component and an analytical component, thus bioequivalence study inspections differ from study and investigator-oriented inspections in that there is often participation from an

---

[85] See: http://www.fda.gov/ora/compliance_ref/bimo/7348_811/Default.htm.

[86] See: http://www.fda.gov/oc/ohrt/irbs/operations.html#inspections.

FDA chemist who can assess the validity of the analytical methods used to indicate bioequivalence.[87]

The vast majority of all BIMO inspections are study oriented. An FDA investigator will generally take two to four days on site to conduct a study-oriented inspection. At the conclusion of the inspection, an exit interview will be held with the clinical investigator, where all findings will be discussed and clarified. If deviations from applicable regulations have been noted during the inspection, the FDA investigator will issue a Form FDA 483 "Inspectional Observations," to the clinical investigator. Note that deviations from guidance documents are not considered inspectional observations and should not be included on a Form FDA 483; although deviations from the FDA guidance may be included in the FDA investigator's written report submitted to the FDA headquarters for evaluation, the EIR.[88]

After the FDA headquarters evaluates the field investigator's establishment inspection report, the FDA headquarters issues a letter to the clinical investigator categorizing the field investigator's findings. The letter can be one of the following three types as described in the FDA Information Sheets[89]:

NAI A notice that no significant deviations from the regulations were observed. This letter does not require any response from the clinical investigator.

VAI A letter that identifies deviations from regulations and good investigational practice. This letter may or may not require a response from the clinical investigator. If a response is requested, the letter will describe what is necessary and give a contact person for questions.

OAI A letter that identifies serious deviations from regulations requiring prompt correction by the clinical investigator. Receipt of an OAI letter may lead to other regulatory actions by the FDA, such as the issuance of a warning letter, requiring the sponsor to throw out the investigator's data, trigger a sponsor inspection, or other regulatory actions up to and including disqualifying the investigator from clinical research, injunction, and criminal prosecution.

---

[87] See: http://www.fda.gov/ora/compliance_ref/bimo/7348_001/Default.htm#PART%20I%20-%20BACK-GROUND.

[88] See: http://www.fda.gov/ora/compliance_ref/bimo/7348_811/48-811-3.html.

[89] FDA Information Sheets – Guidance for IRBs and Clinical Investigators – FDA Operations. Available at: http://www.fda.gov/oc/ohrt/irbs/operations.html#inspections.

BIMO inspections of sponsors and/or CROs occur less frequently than investigator inspections. These inspections are generally unannounced, meaning they greet the company receptionist flashing their credentials and an FDA Form 482 Notice of Inspection, and the frantic telephone calling begins from there.

EIRs are now routinely supplied by the FDA after the report has been evaluated by the FDA headquarters. Redacted copies of EIRs are available through FOI and should be requested by whomever was audited, and the sponsor. Accessing the EIR can provide additional insight to an FDA investigator's inspection strategy and expectations and can prove to be a useful learning tool to design future trials to be conducted in a manner that fulfills current FDA expectations.

Sponsor Audits

Auditing is defined in ICH E6 as a systematic and independent examination of trial-related activities and documents to determine whether the evaluated trial-related activities were conducted, and the data were recorded, analyzed, and accurately reported according to the protocol, sponsor's SOPs, GCP, and the applicable regulatory compliance.[90] Study sponsors are required by regulation to monitor the conduct of a clinical trial; however, auditing is not specifically mentioned. Although not required by FDA regulation, clinical site and vendor (CRO) audits have become an industry standard and are recommended by ICH GCP guidelines. The auditor should be an independent reviewer who is removed from the actual day-to-day conduct of the study, so that they can provide an unbiased opinion on the setup and conduct of the study.

Audits are often conducted according to the same principles that the FDA Bioresearch Monitoring Program follows. The decision to audit a study is usually based on what phase of study is being conducted, whether or not the data is intended to support a regulatory application, the complexity of the study, and the level of risk to the study subjects. The number of investigator sites to be audited for the trial is determined either by a preexisting sponsor policy, e.g., 10% of phase II study sites are audited, 20% of phase III study sites, or on the basis of other factors such as trial duration. The selection of investigator sites to be audited is generally based on enrollment (high enrollers are more likely to be audited), problems discovered by CRAs, AE reporting (abnormally high or low AE rates), the presence of an investigator's financial interest in the sponsor company, or previous experience with the investigator.

SUMMARY

A successful Regulatory Affairs professional recognizes the importance of ensuring their company's compliance with regulations while at the same time

---

[90] International Conference on Harmonization E6 1.6.

working to meet submission timelines and business objectives. One must keep abreast of an ever-changing GxP environment by constantly monitoring the evolution of new regulations and guidance documents. The Regulatory professional is the conduit and gatekeeper in the data flow process from GLP, GMP, and GCP activities to the FDA and other global health authorities, and while you are not expected to be an expert in all stages of drug development, having an understanding of the GxPs, how they are enforced, and the consequences of noncompliance is essential.

INTERNET RESOURCES

GxP References

Freedom of Information: ORA documents frequently requested by the public through the Freedom of Information Act. Available at: http://www.fda.gov/foi/foia2.htm.

Compliance Program Guidance Manuals (CPGM): Compliance programs and program circulars (program plans and instructions) directed to field personnel for project implementation. Available at: http://www.fda.gov/ora/cpgm/default.htm.

Revisions, Drafts, and Updates to ORA compliance references: A chronologic listing of updates to the FDA Office of Regulatory Affairs compliance references. Available at: http://www.fda.gov/ora/compliance_ref/revisions.htm.

Public Use Forms and How to Obtain Them: Access page to current versions of FDA forms. Available at: http://www.fda.gov/opacom/morechoices/fdaforms/fdaforms.html.

Guidance Documents: A link to various guidance documents that outline the Agency's and/or other regulatory authorities thinking on a variety of topics. There are links to CDER, CBER, CDRH, CFSAN, CVM, and ORA. Available at: http://www.fda.gov/opacom/morechoices/industry/guidedc.htm.

Application Integrity Policy: Regarding the integrity of data and information in applications submitted for FDA review and approval. Available at: http://www.fda.gov/ora/compliance_ref/aip_page.html.

Electronic Records; Electronic Signatures, 21 CFR Part 11: Background information and updates on the rule that allows the use of electronic records and electronic signatures for any record that is required to be kept and maintained by other FDA regulations. Available at: http://www.fda.gov/ora/compliance_ref/part11/Default.htm.

Public Health Service (PHS) Administrative Actions Listings: Individuals who have had administrative actions imposed against them. The list is maintained by the PHS Office of Research Integrity (ORI). Available at: http://silk.nih.gov/public/cbz1bje.@www.orilist.html.

Bioresearch Monitoring Program: BIMO main page providing links to regulations and CPGMs as well as to lists of inspections and lists of firms/individuals who have been disbarred/disqualified/have made assurances. Available at: http://www.fda.gov/ora/compliance_ref/bimo/default.htm.

From Test Tube To Patient Protecting America's Health Through Human Drugs: A Special Report From the *FDA Consumer Magazine* and the FDA Center for Drug Evaluation and Research providing the general public with an overview of FDA's oversight during of the drug development lifecycle. Available at: http://www.fda.gov/fdac/special/testtubetopatient/default.htm.

FDA's Warning Letters and Responses Search Engine. Available at: http://www.fda.gov/foi/warning.htm.

FDA Industry Portal: Information for FDA regulated industry. Available at: http://www.fda.gov/oc/industry/.

GLP References

21 CFR 58: Good Laboratory Practice for Nonclinical Laboratory Studies. Available at: http://www.accessdata.fda.gov/scripts/cdrh/cfdocs/cfcfr/CFRSearch.cfm?CFRPart=58.

Bioresearch monitoring Good laboratory Practices: GLP references and Guidance. Available at: http://www.fda.gov/ora/compliance_ref/bimo/glp/default.htm.

FDA Guidance: Good Laboratory Practices, Questions and Answers. Available at: http://www.fda.gov/ora/compliance_ref/bimo/GLP/81GLP-qanda.pdf.

OECD Series on Principles of Good Laboratory Practice and Compliance Monitoring: Link to all 15 guidance/advisory documents and position papers regarding GLPs. Available at: http://www.oecd.org/document/63/0,2340,en_2649_34381_2346175_1_1_1_1,00.html.

Society of Quality Assurance Regulatory Reviews: GLP Q&A by Topic. Available at: http://www.ovpr.uga.edu/qau/indes2.html.

FDA Preamble to the GLPs. Available at: http://www.ovpr.uga.edu/qau/prefda1.html.

Bioresearch Monitoring Good Laboratory Practice compliance program 7348.808. Available at: http://www.fda.gov/ora/compliance_ref/bimo/7348_808/default.htm.

GMP References

Field Management Directives: The primary vehicle for distributing procedural information/policy on the management of Office of Regulatory Affairs (ORA) field activities. Available at: http://www.fda.gov/ora/inspect_ref/fmd/default.htm.

Guides to Inspections of...: Guidance documents written to assist FDA personnel in applying FDA's regulations, policies and procedures during specific types of inspection or for specific manufacturing processes. Available at: http://www.fda.gov/ora/inspect_ref/igs/iglist.html.

IOM: Investigations Operations Manual: Primary procedure manual for FDA personnel performing inspections and special investigations. Available at: http://www.fda.gov/ora/inspect_ref/iom/default.htm.

Inspection Technical Guides: Guidance documents that provide FDA personnel with technical background in a specific piece of equipment or a specific manufacturing or laboratory procedure, or a specific inspectional technique, etc. Available at: http://www.fda.gov/ora/inspect_ref/itg/itgtc.html.

Human Drug CGMP Notes: a periodic memo for FDA personnel intended to enhance field and headquarters communications on CGMP issues. Available at: http://www.fda.gov/cder/dmpq/cgmpnotes.htm.

Questions and Answers on Current Good Manufacturing Practices. Available at: http://www.fda.gov/cder/guidance/cGMPs/default.htm.

Center for Devices and Radiologic Health: Medical device GMP reference information. Available at: http://www.fda.gov/cdrh/comp/gmp.html.

Medical Device QSIT Inspection Guide. Available at: http://www.fda.gov/ora/inspect_ref/igs/qsit/default.htm.

Compliance Policy Guides (CPG): Contains FDA compliance policy and regulatory action guidance for FDA staff. Available at: http://www.fda.gov/ora/compliance_ref/cpg/default.htm.

Regulatory Procedures Manual (RPM): Contains FDA regulatory procedures for use by FDA personnel. A reference document for enforcement procedures, practices and policy guidance. Available at: http://www.fda.gov/ora/compliance_ref/rpm/default.htm.

International GMP References

Pharmaceutical Inspection Convention and Pharmaceutical Inspection Co-operation Scheme (PIC/S): International group dedicated to developing harmonized GMP standards and guidance documents. Available at: http://www.picscheme.org/index.php.

European Union GMPS. Available at: http://ec.europa.eu/enterprise/pharmaceuticals/pharmacos/gmp_doc.htm.

World Health Organization (WHO) GMPs: WHO is the directing and coordinating authority for health within the United Nations system. Available at:

http://www.who.int/medicines/areas/quality_safety/quality_assurance/
production/en/index.html.

GCP References

E6 Good Clinical Practice: ICH Consolidated Guideline. Available at: http://
www.fda.gov/cder/guidance/959fnl.pdf.

FDA Office of Good Clinical Practice: Homepage with links to all GCP regs/
guidance/hot topics, etc. Available at: http://www.fda.gov/oc/gcp/.

GCP Regulatory Activities: Provides links to lists of all disqualified investigators, warning letters, listing of all investigators who've been inspected by
FDA. Available at: http://www.fda.gov/oc/gcp/clinenforce.html.

Office for Human Research Protections (OHRP): Under Department of Health
and Human Services, references on protecting the rights of human research
subjects. Available at: http://www.hhs.gov/ohrp/.

Declaration of Helsinki and Belmont Report: OHRP webpage providing a link to
these documents. Available at: http://www.hhs.gov/ohrp/international/.

Pharmaceutical Research and Manufacturers of America: Principles on Conduct
of Clinical Trials and Communication of Clinical Trial Results. Available at:
http://www.phrma.org/clinical_trials/.

GCP Questions E-Mail Messages: An FDA webpage providing links to email
Q&A. Available at: http://www.fda.gov/oc/gcp/redactedEmails/default.htm.

Clinical Research Training: A course developed by the National Institutes of
Health to train its own investigators. It may be accessed by others to enhance
their knowledge of clinical research. Available at: http://www.nihtraining.com/
crtpub_508/index.html.

Online training on human subject protection: Provided by the Office for Human
Research Protections. Topics include HHS regulation & institutional responsibilities, investigator responsibilities & informed consent, and human research
protections program. Available at: http://ohrp-ed.od.nih.gov/CBTs/Assurance/
newuserreg_1.asp.

Proposed Regulations and Draft Guidances on Good Clinical Practice and
Clinical Trials. Available at: http://www.fda.gov/oc/gcp/draft.html.

9

FDA Regulation of the Advertising and Promotion of Prescription Drugs, Biologics, and Medical Devices

Karen L. Drake

*Cubist Pharmaceuticals, Inc., Lexington,
Massachusetts, U.S.A.*

INTRODUCTION

The Food and Drug Administration (FDA) has been regulating food and drugs since 1906, when Congress enacted the Federal Food and Drugs Act. In 1938, the Federal Food, Drug, and Cosmetic Act (FD&C Act) was enacted and gave the FDA authority over the safety of drugs and food additives and established the enforcement processes now followed by the FDA.

In 1962, Congress enacted the 1962 Drug Amendments, or the Kefauver–Harris Amendments named after the two congressional representatives who sponsored the bill. The law required that all drugs be shown to be safe and effective, and it broadened the FDA's authority over other aspects of drug manufacturing and marketing. The FD&C Act Section 502(n) gives the FDA specific authority over the advertising of prescription drugs, and the provision is also applied to biologic products, medical devices, and prescription animal drugs (1).

Since 1962, the FDA has issued a number of regulations under the FD&C Act Section 502(n), which can be found in Title 21 of the Code of Federal Regulations (CFR). These regulations specifically address prescription drug advertisements, what needs to be included in such advertisements, the definition

267

of types of advertising (e.g., reminder advertisements and price advertisements); and the requirements of presenting product information relative to its safety and efficacy (2).

The FDA regulations for advertising and promotion have had very few revisions since their enactment. The regulations were written at a time when medical journal advertising and industry sales representatives calling on physicians were the primary ways in which drug products were promoted to physicians. In today's world, the FDA policies for the regulation of advertising and promotion have been created on a case-by-case basis or through FDA guidance documents, rather than a formal rulemaking process.

In essence, the FDA's view is that any product-related material issued by a pharmaceutical or biotech company is subject to FDA regulation of such material, and industry has generally accepted this view. Companies are reluctant to challenge the broad authority of the FDA's jurisdiction. To ensure a successful risk assessment of their marketing materials and activities relative to the regulations, companies remain current on the FDA's regulatory thinking by monitoring the agency's activity in this area, reviewing regulatory correspondence (e.g., warning letters[1] issued to companies when in violation of the regulations), and guidance documents.

The following sections will describe the regulation of prescription drugs, biologics, and medical devices.

REGULATION OF THE ADVERTISING AND PROMOTION OF PRESCRIPTION DRUGS

Within the Center for Drug Evaluation and Research (CDER) is the Division of Drug Marketing, Advertising, and Communications (DDMAC). DDMAC has the responsibility for regulating prescription drug advertising and promotion. The regulations that set forth the rules applicable to prescription drug advertising and promotion also include promotional labeling.[2]

The regulations also address specific requirements for the content of labeling; e.g., the label must have the name and place of business of the manufacturer, packer, or distributor (3). More general rules for labeling include the prohibition against making labeling claims that are false or misleading regarding

---

[1] Regulatory communications from the FDA to a company are usually in the form of a notice of violation (NOV) letter, sometimes referred to as an "untitled" letter, or a warning letter. NOV letters are usually sent first and may involve minor health or safety issues. Warning letters involve serious health issues or occur when similar NOVs have been submitted to the same company.

[2] Brochures, booklets mailing pieces, detailing pieces, file cards, bulletins, calendars, price lists, catalogs, house organs, letters, motion picture films, film strips, lantern slides, sound recordings, exhibits, literature, and reprints and similar pieces of printed audio or visual matter descriptive of a drug and references published for use by medical practitioners, pharmacists, or nurses, containing drug information supplied by the manufacturer, packer, or distributor and which are disseminated by or on behalf of its manufacturer, packer, or distributor (Code of Federal Regulations Title 21 Section 202.1(1)(1)).

another company's product (4). While the labeling regulations do not contain provisions relative to advertising, the general position of the FDA is that the advertising regulations apply to promotional labeling.

PROMOTING PRESCRIPTION DRUGS—GENERAL POLICIES

Prior Approval and Preclearance of Promotional Materials

Except in certain circumstances, the FDA cannot require preclearance of advertising and promotional materials (5). This includes launch materials[3] and direct-to-consumer (DTC) advertising.[4] If such materials are submitted for a DDMAC review, the submission is done on a voluntary basis. However, most companies *do* submit their launch and DTC materials (at first use) for prior approval or preclearance for two reasons: (*i*) there is considerable time, money, and effort spent on a company's part to create these materials; therefore, if the materials are submitted to DDMAC at first use, rather than obtaining DDMAC's prior approval, the company runs the risk of DDMAC requiring them to pull the materials if they are found to be in violation of the regulations; (*ii*) by obtaining DDMAC's prior approval, the company will have a very good sense of the acceptance of their promotional claims and how DDMAC views them relative to the regulations, before creating more materials within a certain marketing campaign.

DDMAC will review advertising and promotional materials at a company's request and will try to accommodate requests for rapid approval of time-sensitive materials (6). Comments from DDMAC to the company are always in writing, and DDMAC may change its decision about an advertisement after approving it. These situations are rare; however, if they do happen, the agency notifies the company of the change in opinion with a change-of-opinion letter and provides a reasonable time for correction before taking any regulatory action.

When Is Preclearance Required?

If a company has committed serious or repeated violations of the advertising and promotion regulations, the FDA can require preclearance of the company's advertising and promotional materials. The preclearance requirement remains for six months to two years.

The regulations also require preclearance of all promotional materials for drugs approved under the FDA's accelerated approval process.[5]

---

[3] Launch materials are generally defined as initial marketing materials created at the time when a drug is new to the market or has been approved for a new indication.

[4] DTC materials are advertising and promotional materials intended to be seen or used by a consumer and mention directly or indirectly a specific product.

[5] Certain drugs for life-threatening conditions can qualify for accelerated review and the process requires all promotional materials to be precleared prior to dissemination.

The "Fair Balance" Requirement

Fair balance in advertising and promotional materials is regulated at 21 CFR Section 202.1(e) (6).[6] It is one of the most important requirements for advertising and promotional materials and is one of the most frequent requirements violated by companies. As such, it is very often the subject of regulatory correspondence citing violations of the regulations (7).

21 CFR Section 202.1(e)(5)(ii) states "fair balance must be achieved between information relating to side effects and contraindications and information relating to the effectiveness of the drug." The efficacy and safety claims must be presented in "balance" with the risks of the drug. Risk information must have a prominence and readability reasonably comparable to the presentation of effectiveness claims. For example, efficacy claims on a piece cannot be in 14-point, bold black font, and the risk information appear at the bottom of the piece in 8-point light-color font. Fair balance applies to the content as well as the format of the material. DDMAC looks at typography, layout, contrast, headlines, paragraphing, white space, and any other techniques apt to achieve emphasis (8).

The fair balance requirement does not appear in the FD&C Act or in the regulations governing labeling; it only appears in the prescription drug advertising regulations. Certain ways in which an advertisement may not meet the fair balance requirement include

1. failure to provide balanced emphasis of side effects and contraindications;
2. failure to be clear where the risk information appears when multiple pages are involved; and
3. failure to refer readers to the risk information in a multiple-page advertisement, if located on a different page (9).

The decision regarding whether or not advertising materials meet the fair balance regulations is considered subjective. Many companies and industry organizations have long requested a better definition of fair balance, and DDMAC has indicated that a guidance document is under development.

The Brief Summary Requirement for Prescription Drug Advertisements Directed to Physicians

The brief summary requirement relates to advertisements (e.g., an advertisement in a medical journal) and in essence comprises certain major sections from the product's package insert. All advertisements must be accompanied by a "true statement of information relating to side effects, contraindications, and effectiveness" (10). Side effects, warnings, precautions, and contraindications are the four categories of risk information required for the brief summary and are taken directly from the product labeling.

---

[6] Every promotional piece must meet the fair balance requirement.

The brief summary of the product labeling is usually printed on the adjacent page from the advertisement. Including the brief summary in an advertisement does not relieve the company from providing fair balance on the page or pages that contain product benefit information. The instruction to "see the full prescribing information" does not mitigate the requirement that the benefits of a product must be fairly balanced by providing the appropriate risk information in a reasonable prominence (11).

In 1994, the FDA issued an industry-wide letter in which they stated that "wrap-around" advertisements (presenting advertising on the front cover and the brief summary on the back cover) do not comply with the brief summary requirement. The brief summary must appear adjacent to the advertisement (12).

Advertisements Exempt from the Brief Summary Requirement

21 CFR Section 202.1(e)(2) specifies that certain advertisements are exempt from the brief summary requirement. The four categories of such advertisements are reminder advertisements, help-seeking advertisements, advertisements for bulk-sale drugs, and advertisements for prescription-compounding drugs.[7]

Reminder advertisements. These advertisements do not make product claims; therefore, they are exempt from providing risk information in the form of fair balance or a brief summary. Reminder advertisements are typically materials like pens, notepads, or giveaways for physicians such as medical textbooks. The materials can only contain the proprietary or established name of the drug, the established name of each active ingredient in the product, and other types of information that do not represent the benefits of the product (13). Reminder advertisements cannot be used for products that have "black box" warnings.[8]

Help-seeking advertisements. Help-seeking advertisements are used by a company to inform consumers of a disease state, or symptoms of a particular condition, and to encourage them to seek the advice of a health care practitioner if the consumer has the particular symptoms. Help-seeking advertisements do not refer to the drug product used to treat the condition or symptoms.

There is a draft guidance titled "Guidance for Industry: Help-Seeking and Other Disease Awareness Communications by or on Behalf of Drug and Device Firms" that the FDA issued in February 2004. In the guidance, the FDA explained the types of communications that constitute help-seeking advertisements. The guidance explicitly warned against attempting to use the help-seeking advertisement in combination with reminder advertisements or any advertisement that contained a product claim that would cause a connection by

---

[7] Advertisements for bulk-sale drugs and prescription-compounding drugs are beyond the scope of this discussion.

[8] "Black box" warnings are imposed by the FDA to highlight a major risk(s) of a drug.

the consumer between the disease or symptom conditions discussed in the help-seeking advertisement and the product used to treat the condition or symptoms.

Product Name and Placement

The advertising and promotion prescription drug regulations are very specific about the requirement for product name and placement. 21 CFR Section 201 and Section 202 set out the major requirements of the regulations as follows:

1. Brand name drug advertisements must reference the generic name of the drug.
2. The established name should be placed directly to the right or directly underneath the proprietary name.
3. There should be no intervening matter that would in any way detract from the established name.
4. The generic name must be cited every time the brand name is featured; it is not necessary for the generic name to appear in running text.
5. The generic name must be a font size that is at least half the type size of the brand name and must have a comparable prominence to the brand name.

The type size, prominence, and juxtaposition requirements also apply to broadcast advertisements, audio-visual promotions, and electronic media such as the Internet and CD-ROMs.

Submission of Promotional Materials to DDMAC

The FDA regulations state "specimens of mailing pieces and any other labeling or advertising devised for promotion of the drug product" must be submitted to DDMAC "at the time of initial dissemination"[9] (for promotional labeling) or "initial publication"[10] (for advertising) (14). A specific form titled "Transmittal of Advertisements and Promotional Labeling for Drugs for Human Use" (Form FDA 2253) must be completed in its entirety and submitted with all advertising and promotional materials at their first use. Failure to submit materials at first use may result in regulatory action against the company.

DDMAC has limited resources for reviewing materials; they receive thousands of submissions annually and do not review all materials that are submitted. They reserve the right to request the medical reviewers of each division to assist in the review of materials to address scientific and medical content.

---

[9] "Initial dissemination" is generally defined as when the material is sent to or shown to a health care provider or health care audience.

[10] "Initial publication" is generally defined as the date on which the advertisement first appears in print in one or more publications.

Product Claims for Prescription Drugs

Within the regulations for advertising and promotion of prescription drugs, guidance documents, letter to industry, and public pronouncements, the FDA has expressed its view on how companies can promote their products. Tension continues to exist between the FDA and companies as to the "how" in terms of a company promoting its product and being able to do so in a way that differentiates its product from the competition.

Unapproved Products and Unapproved Uses for Approved Products

When a drug is under investigation (i.e., not yet approved for an indication), or is an approved drug being reviewed for a new use, claims of safety about the drug are expressly prohibited (15). The primary concern of the FDA regarding preapproval promotion is that a health care provider may form an opinion about the drug's use on the basis of claims by the company before the drug's approval, and that opinion may be incorrect, relative to the future approved use. The incorrect opinion on the part of the health care provider could lead to incorrect use of the drug.

The FDA does have two exceptions regarding preapproval promotion.

1. "Institutional ads" in which a company states that it is conducting research in a certain therapeutic area to develop a new drug, and the proprietary or established name of the drug cannot be mentioned in the advertisement; and
2. "Coming soon" advertisements, which state the name of the product, but make no representation about the new product relative to its safety, efficacy, or intended use. A drug with a potential "black box" warning cannot be the subject of a coming soon advertisement.

Once a company has chosen either an institutional advertisement or a coming-soon advertisement, they cannot change to the other type (16).

Accelerated Approvals—Relationship to Advertising and Promotion

As of 1992, certain drugs that treat life-threatening conditions (e.g., AIDS or cancer) can qualify for accelerated review. Essentially, these types of drugs are given priority for review and can be approved in a much shorter timeframe than the typical new drug application review.

While accelerated review can make a positive difference in terms of getting a product to market faster, thereby potentially helping patients with life-threatening illnesses sooner, there are restrictions on a company in how it handles its advertising and promotional materials.

The accelerated approval regulations require that a company submit copies of its promotional materials intended for dissemination during the first 120 days after approval as part of DDMAC's preapproval review process (17). This is different from the product launch review process in which a few core promotional materials intended for use at the beginning of the launch are submitted to DDMAC for review. In addition, after the first 120 days of the launch period, the regulations require the company to continue to submit materials for preapproval, and they must do so 30 days before the material is intended to be disseminated.

The process for preapproval of promotional materials continues until the FDA informs the company otherwise, and it is very common for companies to never receive this notice from the FDA. If the agency determines that pre-approval is no longer necessary for the safe and effective use of a product, they will lift the preapproval requirement (18).

Off-Label Promotion

Much like the concept of fair balance, off-label promotion is one of the most frequent topics of regulatory action taken by the FDA against a company. Off-label promotion occurs when a company promotes its product for an indication for which the product is not approved.

The most widely known case involving the concept of off-label promotion is the Washington Legal Foundation (WLF) case that began in October 1993, in which the WLF—a D.C.-based public interest group—filed a citizen's petition with the FDA, challenging the agency's policy on off-label promotion as being in direct conflict with the First Amendment and the right to free speech.

The case was in the court system for more than seven years. During that time Congress enacted the FDA Modernization Act of 1997 (FDAMA), which included a provision (Section 401) for the dissemination of off-label information. On the basis of the FDAMA and the agency's implementing regulations at 21 CFR Part 99, which allowed for a "safe harbor"[11] for companies to disseminate off-label information, and after several communications between the FDA and WLF, the FDA's position regarding the dissemination of off-label information is more clearly understood. Most companies would say they do not agree with the FDA's position and feel it is their obligation and right to disseminate any and all information about their product to have informed and educated health care practitioners and consumers.

---

[11] Under 21 Code of Federal Regulations Title 21 Subpart B Section 99.101, information about the safety, efficacy, or benefit of a drug for a use not described in the approved labeling may be disseminated and shall (*i*) be about a drug already approved; (*ii*) be in the form of an unabridged reprint, peer reviewed by experts and scientifically sound; (*iii*) not pose a significant health threat; (*iv*) not be false or misleading; (*v*) not be derived from clinical research conducted by another manufacturer; and (*vi*) not be letters to the editor, abstracts, phase 1 publications, publications containing little substantive discussion(publications regarding observations of fewer than four people are not scientifically sound and not allowed to be disseminated).

Under 21 Code of Federal Regulations Title 21 Subpart C 99.201 before disseminating information under Section 99.101, a company must submit the materials to the FDA 60 days prior, any clinical trial information the company has, a bibliography of the articles that are being disseminated, and commit to a timeframe in which the company plans to conduct studies to obtain approval for the unapproved indication.

In addition to FDA violations, off-label promotion also crosses over into the jurisdiction of the Department of Justice and the Office of Inspector General. This occurs if a doctor prescribes a product for a treatment that the product is not indicated for, on the basis of off-label promotional claims made by a company. If the product is reimbursed, by the government or private insurer, they have essentially paid for a product that otherwise would not have been prescribed but for the company's off-label promotion. The most notable example of this was the Parke-Davis (Pfizer) case in which the drug Neurontin® was promoted for the off-label use as first-line monotherapy treatment for epilepsy; the actual indication is for *adjunctive* therapy in the treatment of epilepsy. Parke-Davis was charged with engaging in a fraudulent scheme to promote the sale of prescription drugs for off-label uses, thereby causing the submission of false claims to the government for Medicaid benefits and reimbursement. The result was that Pfizer (who then owned Parke-Davis) was liable for over $430 million in fines and was subjected to very negative publicity. Since the Neurontin case, there have been other companies charged with similar offenses and the resulting fines have been larger than what Pfizer had to pay.[12]

In addition to the large fines, companies who engage in and are charged with these types of violations are often held to a Corporate Integrity Agreement (CIA), which is an agreement between the violating company and the government, that outlines the restrictions on the company's promotional activities, additional compliance measures that must be instituted, and the consequences of not following the CIA.

Comparative and Superiority Claims

Comparative claims occur when a company implies, suggests, or represents that its product, when compared with a competitor product, is comparable or superior to the competitor product. The FDA reviews such claims with the same standards as they review efficacy and safety claims in a product's approved label.

When such comparative claims are made, either as comparable or superior, there must be substantial evidence to support the claim. Substantial evidence is generally based on two adequate and well-controlled clinical studies that compare one drug with another in head-to-head clinical trials, and the comparison must be clinically and statistically significant (19). Unsubstantiated superiority claims made by a company about its product when compared with a competitor product are often the subject of regulatory communications from DDMAC to a company. For example, in 2005, Pfizer was sent a warning letter for making unsubstantiated superiority claims about its product Zyrtec®, by stating in their promotional materials that Zyrtec was more effective in treating allergies than other allergy products, when in fact Pfizer did not have the data to support such a claim (20).

---

[12] Serono, Inc. paid over $700 million and Purdue Pharma paid ∼$500 million.

Pharmacoeconomic Claims

Pharmacoeconomic (PE) claims relate to the cost-effectiveness of a company's product and often do so in terms of a competitor's product. Most companies do not conduct formal well-controlled PE trials in which their product is compared with that of a competitor's.

Often, PE claims are the result of a scientific approach of cost-modeling. The standard of two well-controlled clinical trials to obtain PE data is not necessary, unless a company wants to tie clinical efficacy of a product to the cost-effectiveness position. In that case, the company would have to conduct trials to be able to make claims that suggest that because of a product's efficacy, it is more cost-effective than a competitor's product.

Quality-of-life Claims

Quality-of-life (QOL) claims are those that position the company's drug in a favorable light relative to a patient's daily life activities. It is difficult to obtain such data in a clinical trial because having QOL as a primary endpoint of a study is viewed as too broad.

DDMAC has informally advised companies that measurement instruments, when adequately validated, may be appropriate to adequately support QOL claims. In a draft guidance published in February 2006,[13] the FDA takes the position that patient-reported outcomes (PRO) instruments may be effective endpoints in clinical trials. A PRO is a measurement of any aspect of a patient's health status that comes directly from the patient (i.e., without the interpretation of the patient's responses to a physician or anyone else). At this time, it is not clear when the guidance will be finalized.

"New" and "Now Available" Claims

While there is no official regulation or guidance for the use of these terms, the generally accepted timeframe for a company to use these terms is six months from product launch (21).

Promotion to Health Care Professionals

The FDA regulates virtually all contact between a manufacturer of prescription drugs and a health care provider. Field force visits by sales representatives to hospitals and doctors' offices, promotional speaking events, and medical conferences, all come under FDA's watchful eye, as does any other venue that is or could be perceived as a place or event in which promotional activity occurs.

---

[13] FDA Guidance for Industry: Patient-Reported Outcome Measures: Use in Medical Product Development to Support Labeling Claims. FDA, Rockville, MD, February 2006.

Drug Detailing

Potentially, any materials used by or oral statement made by a sales representative is subject to the advertising and promotion regulations. Generally, conversations between a sales representative and health care provider are difficult to monitor, making it difficult for the FDA to learn of violations. However, there are a few ways in which the FDA receives information about violative advertising and promotional activities.

First, health care providers can contact the FDA to report improper activity by a sales representative. Second, competitors of drug products will report inappropriate activity to the FDA. Finally, many FDA employees are practicing physicians and will report inappropriate behavior. The FDA takes these reports seriously and usually conducts an investigation.

Most companies have internal processes and procedures to ensure, to the best of their ability, that their sales representatives are adequately trained on the "dos and don'ts" of promotional activity. The FDA's position is not "who" makes a promotional oral statement or hands out a promotional piece; rather, it is the "what" that the FDA monitors, and they do not distinguish between sales representatives or other company representatives when monitoring and regulating promotional activities. This includes Medical Science Liasions (MSLs)—a group typically found within a Medical Affairs department of a company—who are typically responsible for working in the field with sales representatives to discuss the science behind a product.

Medical Conferences and Exhibits

Promotional exhibits sponsored by prescription drug companies and accompanying promotional materials found at medical meetings or conferences are subject to the advertising and promotion regulations. Several warning letters have been issued to companies exhibiting at medical conferences.[14]

Unsolicited Requests for Information

Often, companies will receive requests for information from physicians through the company's sales representatives or Medical Affairs department. Most requests are for scientific information about the company's product(s), and the response will likely contain off-label information (e.g., Doctor X asks if a drug prescribed at 4 mg/kg for a certain indication can be given at a different dose for a different indication for which the drug is not approved). The FDA does not consider the responses to such questions to be promotional as long as the

---

[14] In a January 31, 2005 letter to GlaxoSmithKline, the FDA cited the company for not prominently displaying the risk information for the products on display. In May 2001, DDMAC issued 12 untitled letters for promotional activities at the American Society for Clinical Oncology, mostly for promotion of unapproved uses and investigational drugs. Available at: www.fda.gov/warningletters.

company maintains documentation concerning the nature of the requests and does not show a pattern of repeated dissemination of information.

In 1994, the FDA published its current policy on responses to unsolicited requests in a *Federal Register* notice:

> [C]ompanies may . . . disseminate information on unapproved uses in response to unsolicited questions for scientific information from health care professionals. Scientific departments within regulated companies generally maintain a large body of information on their products. When health care professionals request such information, companies can provide responsive, nonpromotional, balanced scientific information, which may include information on unapproved uses, without subjecting their products to regulation based on the information. This policy permits companies to inform health care professionals about the general body of information available from the company" (22).

Generally, the policy is designed to allow for the exchange of scientific information without subjecting the company to potential violations when discussing off-label information about a company's product.

Exchange of Scientific Information—Including CME

It is typical for prescription drug manufacturers to sponsor Continuing Medical Education (CME) events and events in which scientific information is exchanged (e.g., a poster presentation of a disease state at a medical conference). The FDA supports such exchange of information and does not regulate it; however, if the agency perceives that a manufacturer is unduly influencing[15] such activities or exchange of information, especially by using the activity as a way to disseminate off-label information that otherwise could not be lawfully disseminated, the agency will step in and review the activity under the advertising and promotion regulations.

Most companies today have internal programs that follow the Accreditation Council for Continuing Medical Education (ACCME) guidelines regarding CME events and exchange of scientific information. The ACCME has strict accreditation requirements that CME providers must adhere to in order to hold an event and provide the educational materials for an event. Likewise, manufacturers who support CME events (primarily financial support) must keep an arm's-length approach to their collaboration with CME providers and cannot in any way influence the selection of presenters for an event or the subject matter for an event (23).

---

[15] "Unduly influencing" refers to a manufacturer providing the content of a CME event, or strongly suggesting a specific speaker for a CME event who will talk about the manufacturer's product in an off-label way and not provide fair balance by discussing other treatment options.

Single-Sponsor Publications

When pharmaceutical companies sponsor publications that bear any contextual relationship to a company's drug product, the publication is subject to the regulations as promotional labeling. These types of publication require disclosure by the sponsoring company of any support provided by the company (e.g., "This publication was funded by Company X"), an accompanying package insert, and if the publication deals with multiple products, each product must be presented in a fair an objective manner (24).

Use of Spokespersons

A company may use spokespersons, including celebrities, to promote their product(s).

If the spokesperson is a celebrity, the company must disclose the affiliation between the celebrity and the company, and the discussion or presentation, including a TV or radio advertisement, cannot go beyond the product's label.

Many companies use physicians to speak on the company's behalf about their product(s). These physicians are typically under contract with a company and present promotional programs to physician audiences. The presenting physicians are subject to the same regulations as any other member of a company and must present information in an appropriate regulatory manner. Presenting physicians can be held accountable by the FDA if their actions violate the advertising and promotion regulations.[16]

DTC Advertising

DTC advertising is subject to the advertising and promotion regulations and to the laws and regulations of the Federal Trade Commission (FTC).

In addition to the defined materials under the advertising and promotion regulations, DTC advertising and promotion consists of radio, TV, and Internet materials. DTC materials that are not sponsored financially or influenced in any way by a drug company are not subject to FDA regulation (e.g., a pharmacy price advertisement).

Broadcast and Print Media

A primary difference between broadcast materials and printed material is the presentation of the risk information. For print advertisements, the brief summary of risks must accompany the advertisement, and it may be written in consumer-friendly language (25). For broadcast advertisements, the brief summary does

---

[16] See www.fda.gov/warningletters/gleason.

not have to accompany the advertisement; however, there must be clear information about where the consumer can access the prescribing information.[17]

DTC advertising must contain the critical risk factors of the drug, the indication(s) and contraindications in consumer-friendly language, not be false or misleading, and provide information as to where to obtain the package insert.

The FDA does not preclude the use of DTC advertising in any therapeutic area; however, the Drug Enforcement Administration has opposed the advertising of controlled substances (e.g., opiates, narcotics) via DTC advertising (26).

Press Releases, Video New Releases, and Materials for the Financial Community

Generally, the FDA considers product-specific press releases, video new releases (VNRs), and materials for the financial community to be subject to the advertising and promotion regulations. For press releases and VNRs, it is generally a good idea to submit "major announcement" types of materials to the agency prior to public release (e.g., approval of a new indication) so that the agency can be prepared for questions or communications they may receive regarding the major announcement.

For routine press releases or VNRs, there is no need to preclear the materials; instead the material can be submitted at initial dissemination via the process for submission of materials to DDMAC.

When a company has material financial information, it must meet the requirements of the Securities and Exchange Commission (SEC) for reporting such information. The FDA has not taken action against a company for reporting information (including product-related information) exclusively to the financial community. This is because it is not the intent of the company in this instance to promote the product; rather, it is to make investors aware of the most current financial status of the company and its product(s).

However, red flags can be raised. For example, if a company issues a press release announcing dramatic study results and the financial content is minimal, the FDA may perceive that the company, under the guise of disseminating important financial results per the SEC regulations, is really intending to get clinical news out about its product.

A precedent-setting case occurred in April 1986 when Upjohn Co. issued a press release regarding positive study results for its drug Minoxidil®, a hair growth product. At the time, Minoxidil was not approved by the FDA. Upjohn was issued a warning letter stating that they had violated the misbranding

---

[17] Providing access to the full prescribing information has four components: a toll-free number, reference to a print advertisement containing the brief summary, recommending asking a health care professional for the information, and an Internet address directing the consumer to the package insert.

provisions of the FD&C Act (27) by promoting a drug for an unapproved use. Upjohn contended that the press release was "financial and was released to meet the SEC requirements." However, the FDA stated that the release contained highly detailed reporting of study results, and this reporting went beyond the SEC requirements and was deemed promotional labeling under the regulations (28).

In 2004, the FDA and SEC agreed to collaborate to assist one another in protecting the public and investors. The FDA provides technical and scientific support to the SEC and has established a centralized procedure for FDA staff to use in referring to the SEC statements by pharmaceutical companies to the investment community that may be false or misleading.

Industry Organizations

While drug, biologic, and medical device companies are regulated by the FDA, certain industry organizations have established voluntary guidelines that deal with promotion to health care professionals, CME, gift-giving to health care providers, and promotion to consumers.

The Pharmaceutical Research and Manufacturers of America (PhRMA) has adopted the "Code on Interactions with Health Care Professionals," the "Code of Pharmaceutical Marketing Practices," and the "Guiding Principles on Direct-to-Consumer Advertising."

For medical devices, AdvaMed has approved a "Code of Ethics on Interactions with Health Care Professionals," which took effect on January 1, 2004. It provides guidance in seven areas in which device sales representatives interact with health care professionals. In addition, in 1994, the Hearing Industries Association adopted a "Code of Principles for the Advertising and Promotion of Hearing Health Products."

REGULATION OF THE ADVERTISING AND PROMOTION OF BIOLOGIC PRODUCTS

The Center for Biologics and Research (CBER) implements the regulations of the two laws governing biologic products: the FD&C Act and the Public Health Service (PHS) Act. The procedures for the review and monitoring of biologics are almost identical to CDER. In addition to the regulations in 21 CFR Section 202, biologics are also regulated under 21 CFR Section 600 and Section 601.

General Policies

As a practical matter, the same substantive rules that apply to prescription drug advertising and promotion also apply to biologics advertising and promotional activities and materials. CBER applies the same basic criteria for approval of advertising and promotional materials as CDER. In the CBER Procedural

Guidance Document, there are four main criteria listed for the approval of advertising and promotional materials:

1. Materials cannot be false or misleading.
2. Materials must be consistent with the approved package insert.
3. Materials must contain fair balance.
4. Materials must include proper prescribing information (e.g., brief summary).

In addition, the generic name of the product must be used in advertising, in type size at least half the type size of the brand name, and must be used each time the brand name is featured. And, like prescription drug reminder advertisements, biologic product reminder advertisements do not require fair balance.

Like CDER, CBER issues notice of violation (NOV) letters and warning letters for violations of the regulations.

REGULATION OF THE ADVERTISING AND PROMOTION OF MEDICAL DEVICES

The FDA and the FTC regulate the advertising and promotion of medical devices. The FDA, via the Center for Devices and Radiological Health (CDRH), regulates the advertising and promotion of "restricted"[18] devices, and the FTC regulates the advertising of all other devices.

Medical device approval is regulated under 21 CFR Section 801 and medical device investigational device exemptions are regulated under 21 CFR Section 812.

DIFFERENCES BETWEEN POLICIES FOR DRUGS AND DEVICES

CDER's policies have provided a basis for the development of CDRH guidelines; however CDRH pays close attention to CDER policies and ensures that the differences between drugs and devices are clear when setting CDRH guidelines and policies.

CDRH does view many of CDER's advertising and promotion policies to be applicable to devices. However, CDRH also recognizes that devices have important characteristics that are different from prescription drugs.[19] This

---

[18] A device is deemed by the FDA to be "restricted" if it is sold, distributed, or used only with a licensed practitioner's oral authorization or when specific conditions established by the agency are met. Devices are decreed restricted in a case-by-case basis by either regulation, such as has occurred with hearing aids, or as a condition of premarket approval.

[19] Devices are mechanical instruments requiring a different level of education for health care professionals to use them; devices are subject to ongoing modifications; devices present a different level of investment.

translates into differences between drug advertising and promotion and restricted device advertising and promotion.

1. Restricted device advertising and promotion have no regulations. They do, however, have regulations specific to labeling (i.e., type size, prominence, etc.) under 21 CFR Section 801.
2. CME for devices is often intended as training for technicians or doctors on the use of the specific device, whereas CME for physicians is typically for a broader subject matter such as a category of drugs for a therapeutic indication.
3. Preapproval promotion rules for devices are different than those for drugs.[20]
4. There is less public and congressional focus on the advertising and promotion of devices, unlike the advertising and promotion of drugs, which is constantly under the scrutiny of government agencies, consumer-interest groups, and the general public.

CDRH does not require the routine submission of most advertising and promotion materials and relies heavily on competitor complaints to monitor companies and exert regulatory action. Device companies can request pre-clearance of their materials; however, comments from CDRH are considered advice rather than official clearance. Labeling that is part of a premarket approval is reviewed during the market application approval process (30).

GENERAL PROMOTION OF DEVICES

Currently, CDRH is focusing on the promotion of marketed devices for unapproved uses and the promotion of devices that are the subject of premarket notifications (510(k)s). CDRH's policy on these issues is based on the FD&C Act, which states that promotion of an unapproved use renders a device misbranded (31).

Pharmacoeconomic Promotion

There are no specific regulations regarding PE promotion of medical devices, and the CDRH has informally stated that companies may promote or discuss price as long as the information is truthful and accurate.

Investigational Device Advertising

During the investigational stage of device development, CDRH prohibits any type of commercialization of the device, unless it is advertising that is seeking to recruit clinical investigators or enroll patients in a study (32).

---

[20] If a device is pending approval, the manufacturer may advertise it, provided that the manufacturer discloses the current regulatory status (e.g., pending approval) but cannot take orders for the device or claim safety or efficacy or make comparative claims.

DTC Promotion of Medical Devices

DTC marketing of medical devices has been on the increase in recent years. For example, contact lenses are considered a device, and it is common to see advertisements on television for such devices. In February 2004, CDRH issued a draft guidance titled "Consumer-Directed Broadcast Advertising of Restricted Devices," which spells out guidelines for device manufacturers who choose to market their products to the consumer. For the most part, the guidance mirrors CDER's "Guidance for Industry: Consumer-Directed Broadcast Advertisements" issued in 1999.

Similarities Between CDER Policies and CDRH Policies on Advertising and Promotion

In other areas of advertising and promotion, CDER policies and CDRH policies are quite similar, with CDRH basically following CDER policies. This applies to educational and CME events, press releases and public relations materials, materials for the financial community, single-sponsor publications, device detailing by sales representatives, medical conferences and exhibits, and Internet advertising.

FDA Enforcement—Violation of the FD&C Act or FDA Regulations for Advertising and Promotion of Prescription Drugs, Biologics, and Medical Devices

Primary Enforcement Tools

The types of enforcement mechanisms most often used by the FDA are the warning letter and untitled letter (NOV). These letters require specific remedies to correct the alleged violations of the FDA regulations, the FD&C Act, or the PHS Act.

While the number of enforcements has decreased since 1999, there has been an increase in alleged violations for certain types of claims, particularly omission or minimization of risks (i.e., fair balance) (33). In 2000, DDMAC began publishing the violative materials along with the issued letter. The agency views this available material as instructive for industry in general.

Untitled Letters

NOV Letters typically deal with the least violative advertising and promotional activities. Generally, the violation does not jeopardize the public health and can be easily remedied. There is typically a requirement that the dissemination of the violative materials is immediately ceased.

When determining whether to send an NOV letter or warning letter, the FDA considers whether there are public health implications associated with the alleged violation, the regulatory history of the company regarding previous violations, and whether there is evidence that the violation is part of a larger promotional campaign.

Warning Letters

Warning letters are issued for more serious violations of the regulations or FD&C Act. They are issued from the respective center[21] and require a reply from the company within 15 business days. Failure to respond and comply with the letter may result in further regulatory action, including judicial action such as seizure and injunction.[22] These letters are sent to the chief executive officer of the company. Doing this holds the top company official accountable for the violation and the remedies.

Companies do have the right to appeal a warning letter. The appeal must be made to the appropriate Center. Warning letters become public information after they are issued.[23]

Remedies for Warning Letters

When seeking remedies, the FDA considers the seriousness of the violation and the regulatory history of the company. Remedies can include the following:

1. Discontinuation of dissemination of the violative materials
2. "Dear Health Care Professional" letters
3. Corrective advertising
4. Appropriate communication to sales representatives to discontinue use of violative materials
5. Submission of a corrective action plan by the company

"Dear Health Care Professional" Letters

These letters are sent to health care professionals involved in the purchase, use, or prescribing of a company's product(s), alerting them that the company's promotional materials are false and/or misleading. Typically, the letters are required to appear in the venue in which the violative materials appeared. For example, if the violative material is a sales detail aid, the letter would be mailed directly to the associated health care professionals. If the violative material is a journal advertisement, the letter has to appear in the journals or publications in which the violative advertisement appeared, for the time period in which the advertisement appeared.

---

[21] Center for Drug Evaluation and Research, Center for Biologics and Research, or Center for Devices and Radiological Health.

[22] Seizure is a civil enforcement action brought in federal District Court and if upheld, the company's product is "seized" and not allowed in interstate commerce until the case is resolved. Injunction actions must be brought in federal court, and if the FDA is successful they can enjoin a company from disseminating all promotional materials and possibly the related product until the case is resolved.

[23] See www.fda.gov/foi/warning.

Corrective Advertising

These advertisements are reviewed and approved by the FDA and must run in the same publication in which the violative advertisement appeared (much like a "Dear Health Care Professional" letter). The advertisement must clearly show that it is a corrective advertisement and is FDA mandated. In addition, the advertisement must be explicit about the violations that the FDA found in the advertisement and adequately explain how the corrective advertisement addresses the violations. It is important that the corrective advertisement look and feel like the violative advertisement so that they are "linked" when they appear side by side in a publication.[24] Corrective advertisements can also be run for violative television advertisements made via broadcast DTC advertisements.

CONCLUSION

When considering the abundance of advertising and promotion regulations for prescription drugs, biologics, and medical devices, it may seem as if companies can say very little about their products without the concern of a regulatory communication from the FDA. However, it is safe to say that a company has significant ways to legally disseminate its advertising and promotional materials for its product(s) as long as the company adheres to the regulations and remains current on FDA policies and guidance documents.

The primary concern must always be for public health, and while the regulations for advertising and promotion of a company's product(s) may seem cumbersome and unduly burdensome, it is clear that regulation of marketing practices must exist to guard the public from false and misleading information.

It is also important, however, that companies continue to be allowed to disseminate scientific information about their product(s) to keep the health care community and patients informed of the current state of drugs, biologics, and medical devices and to be able to freely disseminate this information without fear of overregulation by government agencies.

The balance between public health and safety and the right of a company to disseminate information about its product(s) continues to be a balance that may be viewed as difficult to achieve.

---

[24] For example, DDMAC issued a warning letter to Cubist Pharmaceuticals in August 2004 for a violative medical advertisement. The original advertisement showed a man's bicep holding a mallet with the heading "STRIKE FAST" in capital letters. The corrective advertisement ran in the same medical journal for a period of nine months and in a prominent box stated "IMPORTANT COR-RECTION OF DRUG INFORMATION, CUBICIN" above the "Dear Health Care Professional" letter, correcting the violation.

REFERENCES

1. U.S.C. Title 21 Section 502(n).
2. Code of Federal Regulations Title 21 Part 202.
3. Code of Federal Regulations Title 21 Section 201.1(a).
4. Code of Federal Regulations Title 21 Section 201.6(a).
5. U.S.C. Title 21 Section 352(n).
6. Code of Federal Regulations Title 21 Section 202.1(j)(4).
7. www.fda.gov/foi/warning.
8. Code of Federal Regulations Title 21 Section 202.1(e)(7)(viii).
9. Code of Federal Regulations Title 21 Section 202.1(e)(7).
10. Code of Federal Regulations Title 21 Section 202.1(e)(1).
11. Code of Federal Regulations Title 21 Section 202.1(e)(3).
12. FDA Industry-wide Letter: Current Issues and Procedures. FDA, Rockville, MD, April 1994.
13. Code of Federal Regulations Title 21 Section 202.1(e)(2)(i).
14. Code of Federal Regulations Title 21 Section 314.81(b)(3)(i).
15. Code of Federal Regulations Title 21 Section 312.7(a).
16. FDA Industry-wide Letter: Pre-approval of Rx Drug Ads. FDA, Rockville, MD, August 19, 1986.
17. Code of Federal Regulations Title 21 Section 314.550.
18. FDA Guidance for Industry: Accelerated Approval Products – Submission of Promotional Materials. FDA, Rockville, MD, March 1999.
19. Code of Federal Regulations Title 21 Section 202.1(e)(6)(i).
20. www.fda.gov/foi/warning/2005/zyrtec.
21. www.fda.gov/cder/ddmac/faqs.
22. 59 Fed. Reg. 59,820,59,823 (1994).
23. www.accme.org.
24. Code of Federal Regulations Title 21 Section 202.
25. Code of Federal Regulations Title 21 Section 202.1(e)(i).
26. FDA Guidance for Industry: Consumer-Directed Broadcast Advertisements, September 1999; FDA Draft Guidance for Industry: Using FDA-approved Patient Labeling in Consumer-Directed Print Advertisements. FDA, Rockville, MD, March 2001.
27. U.S.C. Section 352(a).
28. www.fda.gov/foi/warning/upjohn 1986.
29. 58 Fed. Reg. 42340: Formation of CBER Advertising and Promotion Labeling Branch, April 1993.
30. Code of Federal Regulations Title 21 Section 814.20(b)(10).
31. Food, Drug, and Cosmetic Act Section 502.
32. Code of Federal Regulations Title 21 Section 56.111(a)(3).
33. www.fda.gov/foi/warning.

_____ **10** _____

Electronic Submissions—A Guide for Electronic Regulatory Submissions to FDA

Shylendra Kumar and Yolanda Hall

Datafarm, Inc., Marlborough, Massachusetts, U.S.A.

Vahé Ghahraman

*Regulatory Operations and Technology, Dyax Corporation,
Cambridge, Massachusetts, U.S.A.*

INTRODUCTION

Since the last edition of this book, there have been numerous new developments in the electronic submissions (e-submissions) arena across the world, specifically in the International Conference on Harmonization (ICH) regions (United States, European Union, Japan, and Canada). Several initiatives, some independent and some directly related to e-submissions, have been either implemented or are at the point of being finalized for implementation.

Depending on the regions of your operation, the electronic common technical document (eCTD) is becoming a major part of your working daily life in the near future, if it isn't already. In Europe (except for the United Kingdom, Netherlands, Belgium, and Germany, who already require either eCTD or another form of e-submission) there is a commitment that state agencies should be ready to accept eCTD submissions with no requirement for an accompanying paper by the end of December 2009. In the United States, eCTDs are already

289

being accepted and will effectively become the only electronic format for submission to CDER from January 2008. In Japan, it is optional and in Canada, hybrid eCTD submissions (part paper CTD and part eCTD) have been accepted since June 30, 2006. Although a deadline has not yet been established by Health Canada, there are plans to accept full eCTD submissions in the near future.

Since November 2005, the FDA has implemented new requirements for preparation and submission of product labels for drugs and biologics. These new requirements termed as "structured product labeling and physician labeling rule" or SPL-PLR allows the FDA to standardize the content and the format of product labels provided by sponsors.

Spearheaded by Clinical Data Interchange Standards Consortium (CDISC) and HL7 and other stakeholders, major efforts are being spent to standardize the data structure and elements in clinical and nonclinical studies for creation of study data.

Submission of medical images as part of the drug's effectiveness review for the approval of new drugs or biologics is also gaining momentum. This is especially the case for studies involving biomarkers with image-driven endpoints. An ongoing and major initiative involving sponsors, CROs, the FDA, medical imaging technology vendors, and other stakeholders, aims at standardizing the process of acquiring, collecting, independently reviewing, and submitting these images to the agency.

Overall, this process of evolving technology for e-submissions is an ongoing phenomenon. The technology and business requirements forces agencies to consider changes in their systems, guidelines, and processes to make drug development more efficient and cost effective. For example, the FDA in collaboration with HL7 is focusing on a new standard called regulatory product submission (RPS). The idea behind this new initiative is to have a single standard for all submission types regulated by the FDA. The eCTD is focused only on human drugs and biologics and does not cover devices, veterinary, food, and agriculture product submissions. The goal of the RPS is to streamline these processes by providing one standard for any type of submission.

Even if the FDA introduces this new standard, it will probably require several years to phase out the current standard, which is eCTD. Since eCTD is an international initiative, it is our belief that the eCTD is here and will be the globally recognized submission format for next several years (or, until our next edition!).

PREAMBLE

The documentation required in an application for marketing approval of a new drug is intended to accurately present the drug's whole story, how the drug is formulated—its components and composition; how it is synthesized, processed, manufactured, and packaged; results of the animal studies; and how the drug behaves in the human body. The Food and Drug Administration (FDA) requires samples of the drug that represent the different levels of dosage available to the public, along with associated labeling. Full reports of a drug's studies in all phases must be submitted so that the FDA can evaluate the data. The review team at the agency—chemists, pharmacologists, physicians, pharmacokineticists, statisticians, and microbiologists need access to this information in order to evaluate the safety, efficacy, and benefits of the drug in order to complete the review process.

Traditionally, most of the new drug/biologic applications were submitted to the agency in paper form that commonly ran into thousands of pages. In order to accommodate copies required for all review team members, archiving, and internal record keeping, the sponsor had to create multiple copies of the dossier. After shipping to the agency, these documents needed to be recorded, archived, and sent to the appropriate divisions for review. The handling of such enormous volumes of documents was at best a formidable and time-consuming task, and often resulted in delays in the review process. As one FDA official stated, "a typical drug application has so much paper that we need a forklift to transfer it"(1).

After more than 15 years of collaborations with the industry and experiencing the potential benefits of the computer-assisted marketing applications, in 1999, the FDA released several guidance and specification documents on full e-submissions related to new drug application (NDA) and biologics license application (BLA) (2–4). In November 2001, FDA released the draft guidelines for an electronic abbreviated NDA (eANDA) (5). Subsequently, in February 2002, Center for Biologics Evaluation and Research (CBER) released a new guidance document for electronic investigational new drug application (eIND) (6) where pilot submissions by sponsors were strongly encouraged. In November 2000, another milestone for e-submission was reached by the finalization of the CTD, which aimed at harmonizing the global dossier submissions in different regions. In February 2002, the final guidelines (7) for an eCTD were published.

The increased influx of e-submissions specifically those in eCTD format have substantiated the following list of advantages, comparing a paper submission to its electronic counterpart.

- Enhanced quality and organization of the dossier
- Expedited review process by providing
  - Easy access to documents and data
  - Faster navigation
  - Flexibility
  - Capability to copy and paste information
- Improved and more efficient communication and correspondences between the agency and the sponsor, especially when there are questions and inquiries
- Elimination of the need for compiling and shipping of thousands upon thousands pages of documents
- Reduction (and often elimination) of the need for storage and archiving of huge volumes of paper

The process of electronic regulatory submission is a dynamic one and it is still in its evolving stages. New concepts for streamlining and expediting the drug development process, along with advancing technological tools and the establishment of new regulations and requirements are among a variety of factors that contribute to the evolution of this fast-changing field.

This chapter presents an overview of the regulatory process that started close to three decades ago and led to the introduction of e-submissions as an alternative to the paper format for submitting a new drug application. The chapter also presents a brief history and background of the e-submissions activities within the different divisions of the FDA. Furthermore, the type of submissions for which currently the FDA accepts marketing applications in electronic format have been described. Finally, the specific requirements for planning of an e-submission to regulatory agencies have been outlined and the process for electronic regulatory submission have been described in detail and specific recommendations are made in every step for managing the process. As eCTD is becoming more and more widespread, the need to implement it across the regions for sponsors is becoming a high priority. The last section of this chapter outlines considerations and practical recommendations for implementation of eCTD capabilities.

The information presented and the procedures recommended here are based on several years of hands-on experience gained by the authors, and should be viewed as a guide and a roadmap for the electronic regulatory submissions process from a practical perspective. The reader should refer to the sources listed at the end of this chapter for more specific, detailed, and up-to-date information on this subject.

It should also be noted that to conform to the scope and the objective of this publication, the current chapter focuses primarily on the marketing applications submitted to the FDA, and specifically to Center for Drug Evaluation and Research (CDER) and CBER. The process of e-submission in the other two major divisions of the FDA, namely Center for Devices and Radiological Health (CDRH) and Center for Veterinary Medicine (CVM), however, is not as advanced as the former ones. Currently, there are considerable efforts to prepare these two divisions to accept full e-submissions.

OVERVIEW OF REGULATIONS

Before the 1900s, prescribing and taking drugs was risky business for doctors and patients alike. Little was known about drugs, no scientific standards existed, and sometimes medicines caused illnesses along with severe side effects rather than curing or preventing them. The Food and Drug Act of 1906 established the first steps, in a series of many to follow, for the implementation and publishing of controls of prescription drugs. It prohibited interstate commerce in misbranded and adulterated foods, drinks, and drugs. Subsequently, several Acts were passed that helped shape the current FDA drug review process. This new review process assured that drugs are safe and effective. It was lauded for years for the scientific and manufacturing quality it ensured in our drugs. However, for decades, the review process drew criticism for taking too long. Getting beneficial drugs on the market quickly was just as much a part of the FDA's public health mandate as keeping unproven and dangerous drugs off the market. Early in the 1990s, the FDA started reforming the drug review process to speed the delivery of new drugs to consumers while preserving high standards of quality and safety.

To obtain added resources for reform, the FDA, Congress, and the pharmaceutical industry negotiated the Prescription Drug User Fee Act (PDUFA) (8) of 1992. These much needed financial resources, by way of the user fees, derived from the drug companies, thus enabling the agency to hire additional scientists to review marketing applications for drugs. As part of the negotiations, the FDA for its part agreed to phase in ambitious performance goals such as reviewing priority new drugs in six months or less and standard new drugs in a year or less. The FDA also standardized policies, improved communications, and streamlined many burdensome rules and regulations. Influenced by the positive results, the PDUFA that was originally chartered for five years was extended in 1997 by the FDA for additional five years (PDUFA II) (9).

Subsequently, in 1997, Congress passed the FDA Modernization Act (FDAMA) (10)—*To amend the Federal Food, Drug, and Cosmetic Act and the Public Health Service Act to improve the regulation of food, drugs, devices, and biological products, and for other purposes.*

Following the success of PDUFA II, PDUFA III was approved by Congress in June, 2002. PDUFA IV (11) is the most recent proposal and was submitted to Congress by the FDA in October of 2008. This latest version, if adopted, would significantly broaden and upgrade the agency's drug safety program, increase resources for review of television drug advertising, and facilitate more efficient development of safe and effective new medications for the American public (12).

This act embraced some of the most sweeping changes to the Food, Drug, and Cosmetic Act in 35 years. The act contained changes in how user fees are assessed and collected. For example, fees were waived for the first application for small businesses, orphan products, and pediatric supplements. The act codified the FDA's accelerated approval regulations and required the agency to provide guidance on fast-track policies and procedures. In addition, the agency was required to issue guidance for NDA reviewers (1).

In 1997, the CDER and the CBER, at the FDA jointly embarked upon a major undertaking to revamp the whole regulatory submissions process by mandating the acceptance of submissions in electronic format starting 2002.

More Efficient Drug Development was one of the goals set forth by the FDA's reinvention goals in 1997 and was later revised in 1999 (1). It stated, "By the year 2000, reinvent the drug development and review process, thereby lowering the development costs and, more importantly, reducing by an average of one year the time required to bring important new drugs to the American public. The FDA will accomplish this through early and frequent consultation with product sponsors, implementation of an automated application filing process and an electronic document management system, and reauthorization of an enhanced user fee program."

On March 20, 1997, the agency published the electronic records; electronic signatures regulation (21 CFR Part 11) (12), that *"provides criteria under which FDA will consider electronic records equivalent to paper records, and electronic signatures equivalent to traditional handwritten signatures."* In September 1997, CDER released the guidance for industry for archiving submissions in electronic format. This guidance document provided details on submitting records and other documents in electronic format. According to this guidance, the electronic archival document submission should (*i*) display a clear, legible, easily viewed replica of the information that was originally on paper; (*ii*) provide the ability to print an exact replica of each page as it would have been printed in a paper submission, including retaining fonts, special orientations, table formats, and page numbering; (*iii*) include a well-structured index and the ability to easily navigate through the submission; (*iv*) offer the ability to electronically copy text and images; and (*v*) serve as a substitute for paper copies.

In summary, the FDA's expedited drug approval initiative, through the adoption of e-submissions is aimed at

- assisting the reviewer community in meeting PDUFA goals,
- providing reviewers with intuitive, standard presentations and tools,
- establishing e-submissions standards and guidance,
- providing the ability to manage all submission types,
- enabling the FDA to meet their PDUFA, FDAMA, and MDUFMA (Medical Device User Fee and Modernization Act) mandates and time-lines,
- decreasing administrative processing time, and
- decreasing processing time to facilitate reviewer access to regulatory submissions through the use of electronic routing and the secure transmission of regulatory documents.

Realizing the new trend and encouraged by the potential benefits of e-submissions, many sponsor companies and contract research organizations (CROs) have opted to implement this process from the very beginning. The FDA started to receive more and more submissions in electronic format. As a result, the reduction in paper volumes increased 20% during 1997–1998; 30%, during 1998—1999, and 50% during 1999–2000 (13).

According to CDER 2002 "Report to the Nation" (14), "The number of new drug applications submitted electronically continues to grow. Last year's e-submissions were double the number submitted in the previous year. Overall, we had more e-submissions last year than in the previous four years combined." This trend was presented by Levin (2002) (15) in Figure 1.

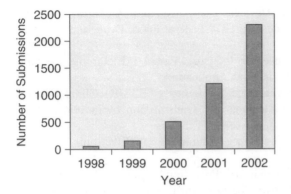

Figure 1 Number of electronic NDA submissions to CDER.

"The number of participating companies and the number of applications with electronic components continues to grow. About 70% of newly filed new drug applications have an electronic component and two-thirds are completely electronic. About 17 percent of new or expanded use applications have an electronic component with 85 percent being completely electronic (14)."

MILESTONES IN THE IMPLANTATION OF E-SUBMISSIONS

- September 1992—Prescription Drug User Fee Act (PDUFA)
- March 1997—Electronic Records; Electronic Signatures Act (21 CFR Part 11)
- September 1997—the FDA extended the PDUFA (PDUFA II)
- November 1997—the FDA Modernization Act (FDAMA)
- January 1999—Guidance for Industry: Providing Regulatory Submissions in Electronic Format—General Considerations
- January 1999—Guidance for Industry: Providing Regulatory Submissions for NDA
- November 1999—Guidance for Industry: Providing Regulatory Submission to the CBER in Electronic Format—BLA.
- January 2001—Guidance for Industry: Providing Regulatory Submissions in Electronic Format—Prescription Drug Advertising and Promotional Labeling
- May 2001—Guidance for Industry: Providing Regulatory Submissions in Electronic Format—Postmarketing Expedited Safety Reports
- March 2002—Guidance for Industry: Providing Regulatory Submissions in Electronic Format—IND
- June 2002—the FDA extended the PDUFA II (PDUFA III)
- October 2002—ICH M2 Expert Working Group (EWG)—Electronic Common Technical Document Specification Published by the FDA in April 2003

- October 2002—Medical Devices User Fee and Modernization Act (MDUFMA) (16) – amended the 1938 Federal Food, Drug, and Cosmetic Act.
- September 2003—Guidance for Industry: Part 11, Electronic Records; Electronic Signatures—Scope and Application
- September 2005—ICH; Guidance for Industry: E2B(R) Clinical Safety Data Management: Data Elements for Transmission of Individual Case Safety Reports
- April 2005—Providing Regulatory Submissions in Electronic Format— Content of Labeling
- April 2006—Guidance for Industry: Providing Regulatory Submissions in Electronic—Format—Human Pharmaceutical Product Applications and Related Submissions Using the eCTD Specifications
- October 2006—The following guidelines were withdrawn by the FDA:
  - Regulatory submissions in electronic format; new drug applications (1999)
  - Providing regulatory submissions in electronic format—ANDAs (2002)
  - Providing regulatory submissions in electronic format—annual reports for NDAs and ANDAs (2003)

The next section presents a history and background of the e-submissions activities within the different divisions of the FDA.

HISTORY AND BACKGROUND

The overall effort of implementing a process for regulatory submissions expressly, the computer-assisted new drug applications (CANDA) or product license applications (CAPLA) have been the focus of both CDER's and CBER's activities since the 1980s. Initially, each division embarked on the effort separately, until the 1997 consensus unified the effort and standardized these processes to include all types of submissions. Currently, some efforts have begun at CDRH and CVM to allow e-submission of specific applications. A brief history of each division's undertakings is presented in this section.

In a parallel development, a process of standardization and harmonization of global dossier submissions, under the auspices of the ICH is gaining momentum. A brief background on the formation of the ICH and the harmonization process, manifested through the development of the CTD and the eCTD, is presented at the end of this section.

CDER

The advent of desktop computers along with the multitude of the software applications that followed have mobilized the life sciences industry in general, and drug development process in particular. Starting in early 1980s, a new philosophy evolved around a concept called CANDA that was described by the FDA as basically "any method using computer technology to improve the transmission, storage, retrieval, and analysis of data submitted to the FDA as part of the drug approval process" (17).

The CANDA process, initially embraced by CDER, went through several iterations and testing during the period between 1984 and 1988. The first prototype of a CANDA system was developed in 1984 by Research Data Corporation for Abbott Laboratories to assist them in the clinical review of two NDAs (18) submitted to the Cardio-Renal Division. In September 1988, convinced by the benefits of the new process from their four-year survey results, the FDA officially established the CANDA process by providing the basic guidelines (19), thus allowing pharmaceutical companies and interested parties to submit sections of their NDA electronically.

The success and dynamics of CANDA brought a new wave of changes and excitement both to the FDA and the life sciences industry. As with any major change, it also created its own challenges and pitfalls. CANDAs were originally envisioned to include only submission of documents and data related to a new drug. However, often-times the process involved loading all custom software applications along with the documents and data, associated with a new drug, into computer systems and shipping them to the FDA for review. The main problem for such practice was the incompatibility of the systems that were used to produce a submission (on the sponsor side) and those used at the FDA for review purposes. Typically, the industry had access to more advanced systems than the FDA, thus calling for the sponsor to supply the entire system.

Although the new process was a better alternative to paper submission, soon after the implementation of CANDA, the FDA was faced with a major dilemma. Because of the fact that standard formatting was not defined for the submission of CANDAs, the agency was flooded with submissions of varying formats that were created using different technologies and software applications that accompanied each new drug dossier. This required that FDA reviewers receive training on variety of different hardware and software systems, which further complicated the review process and ultimately created new bottlenecks that, to some extent, impeded the perceived automation gains.

The status of the CANDA initiative and its level of industry acceptance was described in detail in two reports (20,21) published by PAREXEL/Barnett in 1992 and 1995. These reports detailed the projected future technical issues related to this process in terms of establishing a standardization scheme. The publication of CDER CANDA guidance documents in 1992 (first edition) (22) and 1994 (second edition) (19) further clarified the agency-industry communications related to CANDA submissions.

The CDER's submission management and review tracking (SMART) initiative in 1995 targeted the verification and enhancement of the review technologies and strategies that the agency had been evaluating over the previous decade (23). An important objective of SMART was to minimize, or eliminate altogether, the hardware, and software system(s) provided by the sponsors for the review process, thus limiting the items provided to the agency to electronic documents and information, exclusively. Another objective of the initiative was to advocate the implementation of CANDA as an ongoing process during the life cycle of drug development and not necessarily toward the end of the spectrum.

In March 1997, the FDA laid the foundations for e-submissions to replace the entire paper-based submissions (12). Specifically, the final rules for accepting electronic records and electronic signatures (21 CFR Part 11) were published in the *Federal Register*, which set the standards for electronic records for the FDA and its regulated industries. This proved to be a major improvement to the existing process, which had previously accepted e-submissions only as a supplement to the earlier paper submissions. In addition, for the first time, the sponsor companies were allowed to use the portable document format (PDF) for their submission documents (24), an option that in 1999 became the de facto standard.

In a parallel effort, in early 1997, the FDA and industry asked Congress, during the PDUFA reauthorization process, to mandate the agency to develop a paperless, e-submissions system for *all types* of applications (25).

In September 1997, CDER published the "Archiving Submissions in Electronic Format—NDAs" guideline that specifically focused on providing directions and requirements for submission of the CRT and CRF sections of the application, to accommodate the archival copy. In April 1998, CDER issued a new guidance that provided information for submitting a complete electronic format NDA for the archival copy (18).

In 1997, CDER and CBER joined efforts to streamline the whole regulatory submissions process by mandating the acceptance of regulatory submissions in electronic format, starting in 2002. As a result, during 1999, the FDA released several guidance and specification documents (2–4) on full e-submissions related to the NDA and BLA that are still in effect today. In November 2001, CDER released the draft guidelines for the eANDA (5) for marketing generics, which became final in June 2002 (26).

CBER

In the late 1980s, observing and learning from the CDER's experience, CBER initiated its own CAPLA process. One important observation and conclusion made by CBER was the need to provide some standards for CAPLA submissions, which was lacking in CANDAs. In July 1990, CBER issued a brief guidance document for the sponsors and manufacturers of new biological products, outlining the information to be provided to the agency when a CAPLA was planned. In this document titled "Points to Consider: Computer-Assisted Submissions for License Applications"(27) the FDA provided the first standards for the formatting and content of any such submission. It also described the CAPLA review (CAPLAR) process at CBER. The first official CAPLA, however, was submitted before the document was released. In 1989, Genentech submitted the first CAPLA to the Division of Cytokine Biology, which included the summary reports, line listings, SAS datasets, and clinical data tables, and summaries as the electronic components (28).

In 1991, CBER adopted a new approach for the review of CAPLAS, by developing a single reviewing system, thus eliminating the need for training reviewers on several different systems. Before the end of 1991, CBER had developed the first set of concrete objectives for a complete e-submission process. McCurdy (1993) presents a very detailed description of the CBER's 1991 "system-based" initiatives and what followed, in a book published by PAREXEL (29).

In June 1998, CBER published draft guidelines for CRTs, CRFs and for biologic license applications/product license applications/establishment license applications (BLA/PLA/ELA) (18). Subsequently, as mentioned earlier, in 1999, CBER joined efforts with CDER to finalize the general guidelines for e-submissions. The final guidelines (4) for an eBLA were released in November 1999.

In February 2002, CBER released a new guideline (6) for the eIND, where sponsors were encouraged to submit pilot applications to assist the FDA with troubleshooting and enhancing the review process.

In recent years, with the passing of the PDUFA II and the FDAMA in 1997, CBER's goals for the review of the above submissions changed (29). The acts mandated expedited review of license applications and INDs. To fulfill these mandates, the agency created the Electronic Regulatory Submission and Review (ERSR) Program. Within CBER, the ERSR's electronic document room (EDR) and electronic secure messaging (ESM) systems help to address some of the requirements for these mandates.

ESM assists in fulfilling the ERSR goals of enabling secure, electronic correspondence between CBER and its industry partners. A secure communications channel between CBER and industry enables the submission of electronically signed and encrypted regulatory amendments in a fully automated fashion. ESM was made available in October 2002 to industry by CBER as a pilot project accepting only amendments to BLA with the goal to expand this service to other divisions within the FDA (30).

- Scope—delivery/receipt of regulatory documents and correspondence
- Limitation—limited to sponsors with electronic submissions
- Focus—Receipt of regulatory submissions to preexisting electronic application
- Performance enhancement—In the case of regulatory documents sent from sponsors on the West Coast via secure e-mail to CBER are received by the application regulatory project managers (RPM) in less than 12 minutes.

In addition to electronic delivery, ESM provides the following:

- Electronic signature
  - Digital signatures fully compliant with 21 CFR Part 11
  - Adobe and VeriSign certificates, with future plans for additional vendor support
- e-routing
  - Provides fully electronic workflow for the routing of IND and BLA submissions.
  - Presents simple electronic forms (paper-based forms presented as electronic formwork) to RPMs. These forms allow RPMs to perform direct data entry of regulatory information into corporate databases.
  - Notifies reviewers of new submissions.

CDRH

In March 1996, the CDRH published its first e-submission-related guidance document (31). This guide presented an outline for a manufacturer to follow in preparing an abbreviated report, or abbreviated supplemental report, for Cephalometric devices intended for use with diagnostic X-ray equipment.

A recent initiative at CDRH is the proposed reengineering of the FDA medical device registration and listing (L&R) system (32), where the goal is to develop a simplified, more efficient system, meeting the needs of the FDA, industry, and the public. The first grassroots meeting of the FDA and industry representatives was held in May 1999, where the goals and the objectives of this initiative were reiterated and a course of action was proposed.

Currently, CDRH is accepting medical device applications in electronic format (33). The Office of Device Evaluation (ODE) is currently developing formal guidelines regarding e-submissions. Until they are finalized, CDRH is requesting the industry to give prior notification of their desire to submit an application in electronic form. This lead time is required to discuss any special considerations with the sponsor prior to development of the documents.

CVM

The CVM has developed and implemented methods to accept electronic files as legal, original submissions for review (34). Specifically, after the publication of the FDA's final rule on electronic records and electronic signatures (21 CFR Part 11) in March 1997, a pilot project was developed for this purpose.

This project was intended to increase the efficiency of the review process of the investigational new animal drug file (INAD), the new animal drug application (NADA), the investigational food additive petition (IFAP), and the food additive petition (FAP) by providing for the e-submission of notices of claimed investigational exemption (NCIE). The purpose of the pilot project was to determine the practicality and feasibility of e-submission and review as an alternative to the current paper-based processes.

The pilot began September 8, 1997, with 12 companies participating, and an interim review (35) was concluded after three months. In March 1998, the center extended the pilot to increase participation to additional industry while the final notice was prepared for the e-submission docket.

The center then drafted guidance and planned to expand the e-submission capability into other reporting-type submissions. After meeting Government Paperwork Reduction Act requirements, guidance documents were posted on the center's Web page and their availability published on the *Agency Electronic Submissions Dockets* in February of 2001. These actions increased the scope of the project to include requests for a meeting or teleconference and agendas, notices of final disposition of slaughter for human Food purposes, and notices for final disposition of animals not intended for immediate slaughter. Several guidelines on e-submissions are planned for publication by CVM in the near future.

ICH and Global Submissions

Around the time when NDA and BLA specifications were being developed, a new concept was being cultivated by the global regulatory agencies to *standardize* and *expedite* the process of submitting marketing application(s) to different regions. The efforts that ensued culminated in the formation of the International Conference on Harmonization for Registration of Pharmaceuticals for Human Use, or ICH, in 1990 to oversee and implement such an initiative.

The ICH is a unique project that brought together the regulatory authorities of Europe, Japan, and the United States and experts from the pharmaceutical industry in the three regions to discuss scientific and technical aspects of product registration to reduce the requirements and eliminate the duplications involved during the research and development of new medicines. The next few paragraphs, adapted from the ICH Web site (36), summarize the process by which the ICH and its EWG were formed. In addition, they describe the implementation *steps* and the *current status* of the CTD and eCTD.

The European Community, pioneered harmonization of regulatory requirements in the 1980s, as the European Union (EU) moved towards the development of a single market for pharmaceuticals. The success achieved in Europe demonstrated that harmonization was feasible. At the same time, there were multilateral discussions between Europe, Japan, and the United States on possibilities for harmonization. It was, however, at the World Health Organization (WHO) Conference of Drug Regulatory Authorities (ICDRA) in Paris in 1989 that specific plans for action began to materialize. Soon after, the authorities convened to discuss a *joint regulatory-industry* initiative on international harmonization and ICH was conceived. It was eventually established in April 1990 in Brussels.

CTD

At the first Steering Committee meeting of the ICH, the *terms of reference* were agreed upon. It was decided that the *topics* selected for harmonization would be divided into three categories namely: safety, quality, and efficacy to reflect the three criteria that are the basis for approving and authorizing new medicinal products. It was also agreed that six-party EWGs should be established to discuss scientific and technical aspects of each harmonization *topic*. Eleven such *topics* were identified for discussion at the First International Conference on Harmonization. One of the topics considered in the agenda was the creation of a CTD for preparing the marketing dossier in different regions. The ICH adopted a *harmonization process*, for each *topic*, which included the following five steps:

Step 1—Consensus building
Step 2—Start of regulatory action
Step 3—Regulatory consultation
Step 4—Adoption of a tripartite harmonized text
Step 5—Implementation

The compiled text of the draft CTD reached step 2 of the ICH process at the Steering Committee Meeting in July 2000. A final CTD was completed in November 2000 (step 4). A schematic illustration of CTD and its modules are shown in Figure 2. The EU and Japan regulatory authorities require submission in CTD format starting July 2003.

eCTD

The eCTD reached step 2 in June 2001 and after reaching step 4 in February 2002, the final eCTD specification document was published. The ICH defines the eCTD as "'an Interface for Industry to Agency' and the desired method for the 'transfer of regulatory information' while at the same time taking into consideration the facilitation of the creation, review, life cycle management and archival of the e-submission. The eCTD specification lists the criteria that will make an e-submission technically valid. The focus of the specification is to provide the ability to transfer the registration application electronically from Industry to a Regulatory Authority" (7). Figure 3 shows the number of eCTD submissions received at the FDA (37).

One of the major differences of the eCTD compared with the paper CTD was the incorporation of the XML (extensible markup language) technology and introduction of an XML backbone file to serve as an overall table of contents (TOC). Another difference was the inclusion of all the regional specific requirements into a separate module (module 1). Table 1 shows a high-level comparison of paper and eCTDs. The common modules of the eCTD (modules 2 through 5) were finalized in September 2002 during the Washington D.C. meeting. An illustration of the eCTD modules is presented in Figure 2. The final European Union regional module (module 1—European Union) reached step 5

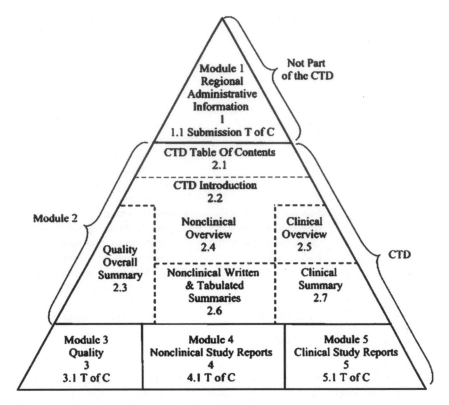

Figure 2 Schematic illustration of the CTD format.

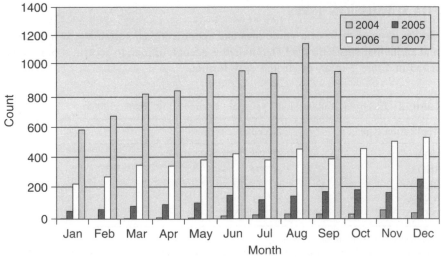

Figure 3 eCTD submission received at the FDA as of September 30, 2007. *Source*: From Ref. 37.

Table 1 Comparison of CTD and eCTD Submission Formats

Item	CTD	eCTD
Submission format	Paper	Electronic
Specifications/ guidance	• Regional modules are not addressed • It describes only modules 2 to 5	• ICH M2 EWG has produced a specification for the eCTD that is applicable to all modules • Module 1 specifications addressed by regional authorities (European Union, United States, Japan)
Submission life cycle	It does not cover details related to amendments or variations to the initial application	Covers the entire lifecycle of a product: Initial applications, Subsequent amendments, supplements and variations
File formats	N/A	PDF, XML and some regional-specific files (e.g., SAS datasets, Word, WP, Excel, etc.)
Overall table of contents	In paper format	In XML backbone format

in March 2003. The draft U.S. regional module (module 1—United States) was released in July 2003; and the Japan regional module (Module 1—Japan), originally scheduled for release before July 2003, was initially released on May 27th 2004, and was replaced by an updated release on June 29th, 2005.

FDA SUBMISSION TYPES

On the basis of the recent guidelines and specifications, pertaining to reviewing and archiving, currently the FDA divisions accept, or plan to accept, submissions listed in Table 2 in an electronic only format.

Table 2 Electronic Submission Types and Formats post January 2008

Application type	Acceptable format
NDA	**eCTD**
SNDA	**eCTD**
BLA	eCTD/eBLA[a]
ANDA	eCTD
IND	eCTD/eIND[a]

[a]Applicable to CBER submissions only.
Abbreviations: NDA, new drug application; SNDA, supplemented new drug application; BLA, biologic license, application; ANDA, abbreviated new drug application.

The detailed contents and directory structures of these submissions are presented under the section "eCTD Electronic Submissions."

PLANNING A REGULATORY SUBMISSION

Traditionally, the sponsor companies started thinking about a plan for e-submission only as they approached the end of the drug development spectrum. This often created tremendous amount of distress, panic, and complications for the people that were responsible (normally from regulatory affairs group) for preparing the electronic version of the dossier. Learning from their own experience, or observing their peers' experience, many sponsors realized the benefits of developing an early plan and a strategy for the marketing approval of their product. It is highly recommended that the sponsor start the planning activities as early as phase 1 to facilitate better control of the overall submission process. Several requirements should be addressed when planning a regulatory submission.

Table 3 provides a checklist of the most common requirements for the planning stage. The checklist will aid in planning the e-submission capabilities and identify the needs of the sponsor to decide on a future course of action for proceeding with the submission process. The following section describes some of the general requirements in more detail.

Regulatory Requirements

There are several documents that the sponsor should acquire and maintain for reference purposes during the course of any submission. They include the FDA guidance documents; minutes of FDA meeting(s); and other specific and relevant documents/guidelines.

Currently, the majority of the FDA guidance documents are intended to assist the applicant/sponsor during the preparation of regulatory submissions in electronic format to CDER and CBER.

The guidance documents on e-submissions, discusses both the general issues, and the topics specific to each submission type. For the common parts, they discuss issues, such as acceptable file formats, media, and submission procedures that are applicable to all submission types. In some cases, the guidance for one center differs from that of the other due in part to differences in procedures and computer infrastructures. The FDA diligently works to minimize these differences wherever possible. For the specific parts, the guidance documents delineate the directory structure; file and folder naming convention for the submission items; and specific formats that need to be followed for creating item level TOC or elements. In later sections of this chapter, we will discuss the details associated with each item in different submissions and will make specific recommendations on the formatting of the involved documents.

The agency guidance documents on electronic regulatory submissions are updated regularly to reflect the evolving nature of the technology involved and

Table 3 Checklist of Items for Planning an Electronic Regulatory Submission

Item	Sub item(s)	Status
Regulatory requirements	• Type and scope of the submission • FDA guidance documents • Minutes of FDA meeting(s) • Other specific documents/guidelines	
Personnel resources	• eSubmission team ➤ Project leader/project manager ➤ Team leaders ➤ Process area specialists • Roles and responsibilities • Work flow	
Tools and technologies	• Software ➤ Adobe® Acrobat® ➤ Office productivity tools (e.g. Word Processor, Spreadsheet, etc.) ➤ Scanning software ➤ SAS® and SAS® Viewer ➤ XML Editor ➤ Other necessary software applications specific to company • Hardware ➤ Industry-standard desktop PCs/servers ➤ Scanner(s) ➤ Large screen monitors ➤ CD/DVD RW drives ➤ Highspeed printer(s) ➤ Copier(s) • 21 CFR Part 11 compliance and system validation • EDMS or file server with defined storage, version control, backup and security • Publishing system or Acrobat plug-in tools	
eSubmission process	• Process checklist • Submission process ➤ Authoring ➤ Publishing (*see next bullet*) ➤ Final compilation ➤ Overall quality assurance ➤ Submission ➤ Validation	

Table 3 Checklist of Items for Planning an Electronic Regulatory Submission (*Continued*)

Item	Sub item(s)	Status
	• Publishing process	
	➢ Scanning	
	➢ PDF conversion	
	➢ Bookmarking and hypertext linking	
	➢ Document information fields	
	➢ Pagination	
	➢ Document level quality control	
	➢ Compilation	
	➢ Quality assurance	
	➢ Optimization	

the experience of those using this technology. Thus, it is strongly recommended that the people involved in the e-submissions visit the FDA Web site for up-to-date information. For a list of guidance documents on e-submissions that have been developed or are under development, see the Reference section of this chapter.

In addition to regional guidances, ICH specifications, deference to the minutes of any FDA meeting (e.g., pre-NDA, pre-IND, etc.) remains critical. These documents not only outline and specify the agreements reached with the review division, in terms of providing the quantity and substance of the information and its format, they document authorized deviations from the standard guidelines.

Recommended General Considerations for PDF Files

This section describes key components from general recommendations for publishing PDF files (extracted from "Providing regulatory submissions in electronic format—general considerations," January 1999) (2) which will assure creating PDF files with formats that are compliant with the agency requirements for review and archival purposes. It will be beneficial here, to provide a brief overview on PDF. The following two paragraphs are extracted from the Acrobat white paper on PDF (2003) (24) and is intended to provide some background information to the reader.

What is PDF?

"The term Portable Document Format, or PDF, was coined to illustrate that a file conforming to this specification can be viewed and printed on any platform—UNIX®, Mac OS, Microsoft® Windows®, and several mobile devices as well—with the same fidelity. A PDF document is the same for any of these platforms. It consists of a sequence of pages, with each page including the text, font specifications, margins, layout, graphical elements, and background and text colors. With all of this information present, the PDF file can be imaged accurately for the screen and the printing device. It can also include other items such as metadata, hyperlinks, and form fields.

PDF is a publicly available specification, regardless of the fact that Adobe created it and advances the specification through subsequent releases. Many people confuse PDF, the data format, with Adobe Acrobat, the software suite that Adobe sells to create, view, and enhance PDF documents. In 1993, the first PDF specification was published at the same time the first Adobe Acrobat products were introduced. Since then, updated versions of the PDF specification continue to be available from Adobe via the Web. The current version of PDF specification at the date of this publication is version 1.7 and is available at http://partners.adobe.com/asn/developer/acrosdk/docs.html. All of the revisions for which specifications have been published are backward compatible, that is, if your computer can read version 1.4, it can also read version 1.3 and so on. Since Adobe chose to publish the PDF specification, there is an ever-growing list of creation, viewing, and manipulation tools available from other vendors."

Version. The PDF files must be capable of being read by Acrobat Reader version 4.0 with a search plug-in, without the necessity for additional software.

Fonts. All the fonts used should be embedded in the PDF files to ensure that those fonts will always be available to the reviewer. Three techniques that help limit the storage space taken by embedding fonts include the following:

- Limiting the number of fonts used in each document
- Using only True Type or Adobe Type 1 fonts
- Avoiding customized fonts

The agency believes that Times New Roman, 12-point font is adequate in size for reading narrative text. Although sometimes tempting for use in tables and charts, fonts smaller than 12 points should be avoided whenever possible. We recommend the use of a black font color. Blue font may be used for hypertext links.

Page orientation. Pages should be properly oriented before saving the PDF document in final form to ensure correct page presentation.

Page size and margins. The print area for pages should fit on a sheet of A4 (210 × 297 mm) and letter (8.5″ × 11″) paper. A sufficient margin (at least 2.5 cm) on the left side of each page should be provided to avoid obscuring information if the reviewer subsequently prints and binds the pages for temporary use. For pages in landscape orientation (typically tables and publications), smaller margins (at least 2.0 cm at the top and 0.8 cm left and right) allow more information to be displayed legibly, on the page (see Fonts). Header and footer information can appear within these margins, but not so close to the page edge to risk being lost upon printing.

Source of electronic document. PDF documents produced by scanning paper documents saved as image files are usually inferior to those produced from an electronic source document. Scanned documents are more difficult to read and do not allow search or copy and paste text for editing. They should be avoided if at all possible.

Methods for creating PDF documents and images. For creating PDF documents a method should be selected that produces the best replication of a paper document. Documents that are available only in paper should be scanned at resolutions that will ensure the pages are legible both on the computer screen and when printed, while limiting the size of the PDF file. It is recommended scanning at a resolution of 300 dots per inch (dpi) to balance legibility and file size.

Hypertext linking and bookmarks. Hypertext links and bookmarks are techniques used to improve navigation through PDF documents. Hypertext links can be designated by rectangles using thin lines or by blue text or using invisible rectangles for hypertext links in a TOC to avoid obscuring text.

In general, for documents with a TOC, bookmarks, and hypertext links should be provided for each item listed in the TOC, including all tables, figures, publications, other references, and appendices. In general, including a bookmark to the main TOC for a submission or item is helpful. Make the bookmark hierarchy identical to the TOC.

Hyperlinking throughout the body of the document to supporting annotations, related sections, references, appendices, tables, or figures that are not located on the same page are helpful and improve navigation efficiency.

Use relative paths when creating hypertext linking to minimize the loss of hyperlink functionality when folders are moved between disk drives. Absolute links that reference specific drives and root directories will no longer work once the submission is loaded onto our network servers. The guidance stipulates that the Inherit Zoom magnification setting should be applied to bookmarks and hyperlinks, so that the destination page displays at the same magnification level that is being used by the reviewer.

Page numbering. Only individual documents should be paginated. If a submission includes more than one document, it is not needed to provide pagination for the entire submission.

It is easier to navigate though an electronic document if the page numbers for the document and the PDF file are the same. To accomplish this, the initial page of the paper document should be numbered page 1.[1]

Document information fields. Recommendations for the document information fields (DIFs) will be provided in the regional guidance for the specific submission type.[2]

Open dialog box. The Open dialog box sets the document view when the file is opened. The initial view of the PDF files should be set as Bookmarks and Page. If there are no bookmarks, the initial view should be set as Page only. Set the Magnification and Page Layout to default.

Security. No security settings or password protection should be included for PDF files. Printing, changes to the document, selecting text and graphics, and adding or changing notes and form fields should all be allowed.

Indexing PDF documents. There are no current plans in the ICH regions to use full text indexes. Refer to regional guidances for index requirements for non-eCTD e-submissions.

Use of Acrobat plug-ins. It is acceptable to use plug-ins to assist in the creation of a submission. However, the review of the submission should not require the use of any plug-ins, in addition to those provided with Acrobat Reader.

Electronic Signatures

The FDA has developed new procedures for archiving documents with electronic signatures. Until those procedures are in place, a paper copy that includes the handwritten signature must accompany documents, such as certifications, for which regulations require an original signature.

Personnel

For any project, a submission team should be assembled and the roles and responsibilities of the members clearly identified, at the initiation phase. These items are discussed subsequently.

---

[1] Please refer to section "Pagination" for more details.

[2] Please refer to section on "Document Information Fields" for more details.

Submission Team

The submission team is typically a composite representation of the following individuals and skill sets:

- Project leader
  Generally the regulatory director, project manager, or submission manager
- Team leaders
  Typically one person from each of the following disciplines:
  - Regulatory affairs and dossier publishing
  - Nonclinical
  - Clinical/medical
  - Chemistry and manufacturing
  - Biostatistics and data management
  - Information technology (IT)
  - Quality assurance
  - Marketing and risk management
- Process area specialists
  Authors, reviewers, quality assurance (QA) specialists, publishing specialists, scanning specialists, etc.

Roles and Responsibilities

The team members' roles and responsibilities will vary according to the submission filing type. In the instance of filing an eCTD dossier, these functions will be defined at the document, element, and XML levels. When filing an eCTD submission, the assignments should beat both the item and document levels. Regardless of the submission type, it is important to clearly define the roles and responsibilities of the submission team before initiating the work. The sample template shown in Table 4 can be used to define team-level responsibilities along with appropriate timelines.

Work Flow

The preparation of any e-submission involves a team-based process encompassing multiple tasks and steps. This process requires collaboration between individuals from different departments within an organization and other client representatives (e.g., CROs, contractors, consultants, etc.) that contribute to different parts of a project. For instance, a document from its inception goes through several stages before it is finalized and fully ready to be included in a submission. A typical scenario may include authoring, quality control (QC), scanning, publishing, compiling, validating and final QA, and preparing for media transmittal. Extrapolating this process to many documents that are handled by several people simultaneously makes management of the dynamics of

Table 4 A sample of eSubmission Checklist

Element/task	Deliverable components	Responsible group	Target date
Module 1	Cover letter, forms, labeling, administrative information etc.	Regulatory/publishing	
Module 2	Summaries	CMC/nonclinical/clinical/ regulatory/publishing	
Module 3	Quality	CMC/regulatory/publishing	—
Module 4	Preclinical	Nonclinical/regulatory/ publishing	—
Module 5	Clinical	Clinical/medical writing/ data management/ regulatory/publishing	
Security and network backup		IT	
Media preparation	CD-ROM or Tape	IT/regulatory/publishing	
Overall QC of the submission media	Quality assurance report	Regulatory, QA, publishing	
Overall submission management	Submission timeline and overall inventory	Regulatory, program management	

this process quite challenging. In order for these functionalities to work smoothly and in a timely fashion, a process flow for guiding the team members is a must.

Tools and Technologies

Any e-submission project requires a set of specific hardware and software tools and technologies. Depending on the long-term goals of a company and the scope and size of each project, these requirements may vary significantly from one project to another. Thus, for a given project, these requirements should be identified and efforts extended to meet those requirements. Hence, a minimum level of compliance with these requirements should be established to ensure the e-submission capabilities for a mid-size project. Table 3 shows a list of tools and technology items essential for the e-submission process. A description of each item follows.

Software

The following is a recommended list of software:

- Adobe® Acrobat® 5 or later
- Acrobat® plug-ins (provided by third party vendors)

- Office productivity tools (e.g., word processor, spreadsheet, etc.)
- Scanning software
- SAS® and SAS® Viewer 8.2 or later (for data management and statistical programming groups) to produce version 5 XPT compliant files
- XML editor (or an application capable of creating XML backbone for eCTD)
- Other necessary software applications specific to company

Hardware

The following is a recommended list of hardware:

- Network system with security, backup and virus-protection capabilities
- Pentium IV—1 GHz or higher processor PCs with a CD/DVD burner, a large (40 GB) hard drive and at least 256 MB of RAM for the scan station
- 18- to 20-inch monitors for scan station and publishing PCs
- High-speed scanner(s) with automatic feeder (duplex option recommended)
- Color scanner/printer (optional)
- High-volume and high-speed printer(s) with PostScript option
- Photocopier(s)

21 CFR Part 11 Compliance and System Validation

In March 1997, the FDA issued final regulations (Part 11) that provided criteria for acceptance by the FDA, under certain circumstances, of electronic records, electronic signatures, and handwritten signatures executed to electronic records as equivalent to paper records and handwritten signatures executed on paper (12). These regulations, which apply to all the FDA program areas, were intended to permit the widest possible use of electronic technology, consistent with the FDA's responsibility to protect the public health.

21 CFR Part 11 regulations address any electronic document or record that is part of a regulated system. These regulations therefore apply to regulatory submissions, as well as all GMP, GCP, GLP, and QA/QC data. They cover issues such as validation, audit trail, legacy systems, copies of records, record retention, security, and electronic signatures. This meant that all systems would be required to maintain prior revisions of data and documents (38). Furthermore, it will also be necessary to keep the record of the changes as to who made a change, when the change was made, and describe what the old and new data is. These rules have compelled companies to rethink their business process as well as to examine their current systems.

Since part 11 became effective in August 1997, significant discussions have ensued between industry, contractors, and the agency concerning the interpretation and implementation of the rule (39). Several concerns have been raised particularly in the areas of part 11 requirements for validation, audit trails, record retention, record copying, and legacy systems. As a result, in February 2003, the FDA issued a new draft guidance, by which it announced that it intends to exercise enforcement discretion with respect to the validation, audit trail, record retention, and record copying requirements of part 11. However, records must still be maintained or submitted in accordance with the underlying predicate rules. It was also mentioned that the FDA intends to exercise enforcement discretion and will not normally take regulatory action to enforce part 11 with regard to systems that were operational before August 20, 1997, the effective date of part 11 (commonly known as existing or legacy systems) while the part 11 is undergoing reexamination.

Electronic Document Management System

The efficient management and publishing of submission content is a requirement—not an option—for the life sciences industry. Life sciences organizations need to securely and efficiently control the flow of submission content, authorize and verify recipients, and track changes, thus ensuring compliance with regulatory agencies.

Electronic document management provides a secure, organized structure for storing and retrieving documents. The system can be designed to match the specific needs of any group or the entire company.

The benefits of an electronic document management system (EDMS) are many fold and the features may include the following (40):

- Access control—Controls access to documents.
- Accessibility—Provides control over all versions of a document and allows quick access to the final version.
- Protects overwriting—Eliminates overwriting of prior versions.
- Edit control—Allows locking documents while being modified so that only one person is able to make changes at any time.
- Audit trail—Allows viewing the name of the person who has modified a document and the time of the modification(s).
- Version control—Allows maintaining prior versions of documents (life-cycle).
- Retrieval—Allows searching for documents based on key attributes.
- Workflow—Create, review, and approve—provides routing documents for review and approval.

The purpose of an EDMS is to provide a repository for the documents as well as the security and tools to review and approve them.

It is important to note that many of the small to medium-sized companies presently lack EDMS because of the high costs associated with implementing and maintaining such an elaborate system. These companies, therefore, operate on the basis of file servers and have to address the requirements regarding the work flow, storage, security, version control and backup within that framework. These items are described in proceeding sections. Although this chapter addresses issues related to both the EDMS and file servers, the emphasis is on the latter case where EDMS is not present.

Publishing Systems

Depending on the level of sophistication and comprehensiveness, there are different publishing tools and systems for regulatory submissions. Brown et al. (2002) (41) have described the following "levels" of sophistication for regulatory publishing systems:

- Level 1—Pen typewriters
- Level 2—Word processing software (SW)
- Level 3—Combination of word processing SW with ability to convert to PDF/XML
- Level 4—Combination of word processing SW, PDF/XML conversion capability, and tools for publishing (e.g., Acrobat plug-ins)
- Level 5—Off-the-shelf publishing software with word processing and PDF/XML conversion capabilities and tools for publishing

The first three levels are considered either outdated or impractical, thus are not used as often as the last two levels, and are not covered here.

Typically, a level 5 solution is considered a complete "start-to-end" publishing system that has many built-in attributes that are essential for any publishing process. While, a level 4 solution provides the basic features required for a publishing process within a very cost-effective framework. The main features of these systems are contrasted in Table 5.

Acquiring, implementing, and maintaining a complete publishing system (level 5), along with training knowledge worker(s) who will use it, requires commitment and a considerable amount of financial and human resources. Many small- to medium-sized companies often cannot afford such costs and consequently resort to level 4 solutions. The following sections are geared towards a level 4 publishing solution.

Selecting a New System

The process of selecting and implementing a new system can be extremely challenging for a company that intends to acquire and/or integrate a new technology into their existing infrastructure. It also requires careful planning along with prudent and calculated projections. Once the feasible solutions are identified, the ramification of such changes and the impact of each alternative solution should

Table 5 Comparison of Main Features of Level 4 and 5 Publishing Systems

Item no.	Attribute description	Publishing system	
		Level 4	Level 5
1	Integrated within an EDMS (i.e., requires EDMS)	No	Yes
2	Provides audit trail (identifying users, document status, version control, and change control)	No	Yes
3	Provides report and other document templates for authoring	No	Yes
4	Allows authentication of digital or electronic records	No	Yes
5	Allows security on files, databases and repositories	No	Yes
6	Automatic indexing (bookmark creation)	Yes	Yes
7	Automatic Hyperlinks to tables, figures, references, and other sections or documents, etc.	Yes	Yes
8	Automatic TOC creation	Yes	Yes
9	Automatic Thumbnails creation	Yes	Yes
10	Automatic Pagination	Yes	Yes
11	Batch PDF processing	Yes	Yes
12	DIFs creation	Yes	Yes
13	Provides ability to modify hyperlinks attributes (color, style, rectangle visible, etc.)	Yes	Yes
14	Provides ability to modify bookmark fonts attributes	Yes	Yes
15	Validates the bookmarks and hyperlinks status and provides their number in a document (or in a submission)	Yes	Yes
16	Provides both paper and e-submissions	Yes	Yes

Source: From Ref. 39.

be carefully weighed. The following are suggested general steps that should executed during the selection and implementation of any new system (38).

- Evaluate the current business process and workflow.
- Identify a set of needs/requirements.
- Identify and compare alternatives.
- Develop a plan for purchase, support, and maintenance.
- Formulate a partial implementation (pilot project) plan.
- Develop a plan and strategy for full implementation and training.
- Validate the system.

Depending on the circumstances of the project, each step may require additional (more detailed) examination during the selection and implementation process.

It is important to note that PDF, featured with navigational review aids such as bookmarks and hyperlinks, is the foundation and the common denominator in all of the e-submissions. As a result, the selection of the PDF publishing system is an extremely important mission. On the basis of previous experience with different submissions, a majority of authors recommend a PDF publishing solution that is modular and is based on open architecture. A flexible system capable of producing quality PDF files can easily accommodate the needs of an eCTD, eIND, eBLA, and eNDA application.

Storage

For companies with an EDMS, the source documents will be stored in a repository, and accessed by authorized personnel. This infrastructure/system offer constant tracking of the document life cycle by maintaining the audit trails and version controls. If a company does not have such a system, the source and the final published documents can be stored and maintained in a file server using an appropriate directory structure under a designated network share. An example of such a directory structure, consisting of seven subfolders: PM, docs-in, publishing, pre-comp, repository, QC and working, final and knowledge base is shown in Figure 4, and described below.

PM. This folder is typically used to share information related to the submission project such as the project plan, and corporate publishing standards. In addition, it may hold the CHECKLIST, meeting agendas and minutes, and other relevant

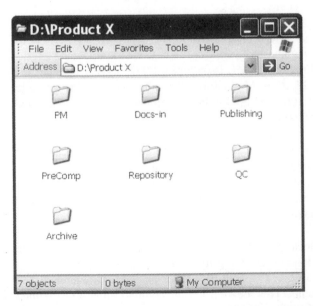

Figure 4 A recommended directory structure configuration when working with file servers.

documents. A Guidance subfolder may also be introduced and will hold necessary guidance documents from the agency to provide the relevant and up-to-date reference information to the team members.

Docs-in. The docs-in folder should be used for environments which do not employ a document management system. Its primary purpose is to provide document version control. As such, the files in this location are to be carefully tracked by the PM and subject matter experts to ensure that the correct version is promoted to the publishing folder. This area will hold the final submission documents and maintain the eCTD directory structure. On completion of the content quality assurance and sign-off, the finalized documents are advanced to the next process.

Publishing. The purpose of this directory is to provide the users with a working area where they can create, and/or modify the required navigational requirements. It also allows them, when necessary, to create additional temporary directories, or create documents with different naming conventions for inclusion in the XML backbone. In addition to publishing the files in accordance with ICH /regional guidance, overall document compliance verification occurs at this stage.

Pre-comp. The pre-comp folder or pre-compilation location is the staging area for documents awaiting compilation into the XML backbone. These files are submission ready and processes should be in place to restrict content-related or navigational changes.

Repository. This is the designated location for the actual eCTD dossier and its related sequences, amendments, and variations. Only the components of the submission, e.g., the ICH/regional XML backbones, DTD, stylesheets, and the files should reside in this location. Maintaining the submission folder structure within this location is critical to maintaining the functionality of the navigational items and overall eCTD compliancy.

QC. This is the location for approval of the final quality assurance of the submission prior to transmitting to the regional authority. The purpose is to quality check and review the submission for completeness. Accessibility to this location should be restricted to subject matter experts, e.g., CMC, medical writing, and those individuals who possess executive privileges.

Archive. This directory location is reserved for storing an archived copy of the submitted dossier(s). Maintaining the integrity of the submission is the primary purpose of this directory location as this is critical for successful life cycle of the submission and its documents. This location and its contents should be deemed as read-only. The archive location should reflect exactly what has been provided to the regulatory agencies and allow the sponsor to view the status of their product from either a cumulative (all files which have been submitted to date) or current view (all files relevant to the product review).

Security

Security is based on the roles and responsibilities defined by the project team. The IT representative is responsible for assigning appropriate privileges to team members in coordination with the team leader and systems administrator. Also, the IT representative is responsible for managing the backup of the project area on a regular basis, based on the standard of operations (SOP) for network security and backup.

Version Control

This is an automatic process for the EDMS, however for file server environments; it becomes the responsibility of the team members to maintain the versions throughout the submission process. Establishing a SOP for version control process (defined during the project initiation) is highly recommended.

THE ELECTRONIC SUBMISSION PROCESS

In order for the publishing process to proceed effectively and smoothly, it is of the utmost importance for the e-submission team members to possess the knowledge of the basic steps involved in any project. As outlined in Table 3, the e-submission process, in general, involves the following steps:

- Inventory of submission items (checklist)
- Authoring
- Publishing
- QA
- Final compilation
- Submission

Figure 5 illustrates a workflow for a typical eCTD as well as a non-eCTD e-submission publishing process.

The following scenario outlines the steps for a typical regulatory publishing process:[3]

1. Create an e-submission team.
2. Define roles and responsibilities of the team members.
3. Identify all the tools and technologies to be used in the project and provide appropriate training and technical support for team members.
4. Identify a workflow for the project.

---

[3] This assumes that there is no EDMS or publishing system in place.

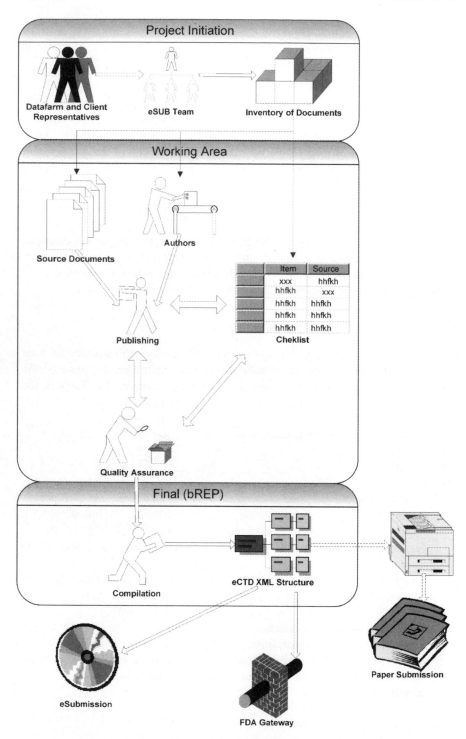

Figure 5 Illustration of steps involved in a typical eSubmission publishing process.

5. Identify a storage location for the project-related files.
6. Compile an inventory of all the documents to be submitted and record them in the checklist.
7. Finalize authoring of each source document and update the checklist accordingly.
8. Perform QA/QC in every step to check and verify the status of documents; update the checklist.
9. Convert all the documents into regulatory compliant format (e.g., PDF document with appropriate navigational items).
10. Compile individual modules of the submission after all the documents are finalized.
11. Perform QA/QC to verify the status of documents; update the checklist.
12. Compile each completed PDF file from the working folder or pre-compilation staging area into the appropriate location in the final folder.
13. Apply the external hyperlinks and bookmarks.
14. Perform QA/QC to verify the status of documents and the associated navigational items; update the checklist.
15. Apply the finishing touch-ups (e.g., common bookmarks, DIFs, pagination) to finalize the submission items; update the checklist.
16. Create the submission media (e.g., CDs, DVDs, tape).
17. Perform the final QA/QC on the submission media to verify the status of submission items and their navigational items.
18. Print from finalized documents for paper submission and perform a QC (if paper submission is required).
19. Ship the submission media to the appropriate regulatory division.

Process Checklist

One of the most critical tools for managing an e-submission project is a checklist in which all the steps in the process have been clearly delineated. This checklist provides an opportunity to compile an inventory of submission documents that are planned for submission to the agency and plays an especially important role in managing the publishing stage. The success of a project will depend on careful and timely maintenance and usage of its checklist. A typical checklist can be a spreadsheet created using appropriate components for a specific submission type and is based on the granularity defined by the guidance and specifications documents for that submission type.

During the initial meetings, the team members should identify and create the inventory. The list may be categorized on the basis of appropriate the FDA form and its corresponding sections for that submission (e.g., 356h for NDA/BLA/ANDA, 1571 for IND). Each document is entered under the appropriate section and under the designated item, and their status will be updated along the entire publishing process. Once the inventory of all source documents is completed, team members will be assigned at the document level. A sample

Title	ICH Recommended File Name	Source Name	Source Format	PDF Conversion	PDF QC	PDF file name	Pre-Compile/Publish Location	Number of Pages	QA & PM Sign-off
m1-regional	*Folder Name Only (m1\us)*								
m1-forms	*Folder Name Only*								
m1-1-1-fda-form-1571	fda-form-1571.pdf								
m1-1-2-fda-form-356h	fda-form-356h.pdf								
m1-1-3-fda-form-3397	fda-form-3397.pdf								
m1-1-4-fda-form-2252	fda-form-2252.pdf								
m1-1-5-fda-form-2253	fda-form-2253.pdf								
m1-1-6-fda-form-2567	fda-form-2567.pdf								
m1-2-cover-letters	coverletter.pdf								
m1-3-administrative-information	*Folder Name Only*								
m1-3-1-applicant-information	*Folder Name Only*								
m1-3-1-1-change-of-address-or-corporate-name	corporate-change.pdf								
m1-3-1-2-change-contact-agent	agent-change.pdf								
m1-3-1-3-change-in-sponsor	sponsor-change.pdf								
m1-3-1-4-transfer-obligation	oblig-transfer.pdf								
m1-3-1-5-change-application-ownership	oblig-transfer.pdf								
m1-3-2-field-copy-certification	field-copy-cert.pdf								
m1-3-3-debarment-certification	debar-cert.pdf								
m1-3-4-financial-certification-disclosure	finan-cert..pdf								
m1-3-5-patent-exclusivity	*Folder Name Only*								
m1-3-5-1-patent-information	patent-info.pdf								

◄ ► ►| \ eCTD \ **Module 1 - US** / Module 2 / Module 3 / Module 4 / Module 5 / Notes /

Figure 6 eCTD process checklist.

document-level publishing process checklist is shown in Figure 6. The project leader and the team leaders should constantly update the checklist to monitor the status of the items and individual documents, and the progress of the project.

Authoring

The essential components of any regulatory submission are the documents with which the submission is built. These documents are created in various departments in the sponsor company and may come from different collaborating partners, CROs, and other consultants. Therefore, it is of utmost importance for an organization to acquire a set of standard tools that will guide and assist those involved in authoring of documents for the life cycle of a drug product. In addition to word processing software, which is a basic requirement, the following are essential elements for any authoring project:

- Standard style and format guides
- General and specific templates—internal (e.g., study protocols, amendments)
- Specific templates based on FDA or ICH requirements (e.g., clinical study reports)

The standard style and format guides will assure that the final documents have all the attributes required for creating automatic TOC, bookmarks, links, and references on the basis of defined heading and TOC styles. This will also become extremely useful when converting the documents to PDF format by transferring the above navigational aids.

Another important tool is development of templates for internal purposes or for submission purposes. Both the FDA and ICH have developed a number of guidelines and specification documents regarding the specific items to be included for different sections of a submission (e.g., clinical study report template). Following these specifications, during the creation of the documents, will assure conformance to the agency requirements and eliminate any delays or confusion.

Publishing

The publishing process, a subset of e-submission process, can involve the following steps when working in a traditional file server setup. These steps show the most common order of the workflow in the publishing process; however, depending on the circumstance of the project, and policies and priorities of the sponsor company, the orders can be altered, combined, deleted or new steps added.

- Scanning
- PDF conversion
- Bookmarking/linking
- Document information fields
- Pagination
- Compilation—document/item level
- Optimization
- Quality assurance
- Full-text indexing (per regional requirements only)
- Validation

Scanning

Occasionally, the source format for a set of documents that should be provided to the agency with a submission is paper only. This could be the case for reference publications; case report forms (CRFs), study protocols and amendments, documents related to chemistry, manufacturing and controls (CMC), etc. Although scanning is generally discouraged by the agency, in some cases it is inevitable. In those cases, the original paper documents should be scanned into PDF and bookmarked and linked on the basis of guidelines provided by the agency. This will ensure compliance with the readability, file size, navigational aids, and other requirements outlined in the guidance documents.

Scanning can be performed and PDF files can be created directly using Acrobat or any other custom software. Some of the more sophisticated scanning tools provide additional capabilities for bookmarking/linking via optical character recognition (OCR), and for process automation, albeit at a cost.

PDF Conversion

The regulatory agencies accept PDF as the format for the transmission of submission files, thus all source documents, regardless of their original format (e.g., electronic, Web page, paper, image) should be converted to PDF before their inclusion in the submission. Acrobat provides two different conversion methods (utilities): PDFWriter and Acrobat Distiller. In general, PDFWriter converts files more quickly and is recommended for simple text only documents. On the other hand, Distiller allows for more control over the process and provides higher quality output and is recommended for documents containing text, figures, and color images.

PDF files can be created from virtually any application by using Acrobat, or similar software. Generally, in office productivity suites, the PDFMaker macro will be available after the installation of the Acrobat and can be used for PDF conversion in those applications.

Bookmarking/Linking

As outlined by the general guidelines of the agency, each PDF document should contain appropriate bookmarks and links to improve the navigation through the documents and the submission as a whole. As noted in the authoring section, following an appropriate style and formats guide for creation of the original electronic documents, will ensure the majority of these navigational items get created automatically during the PDF conversion stage. There are multitudes of Acrobat plug-ins tools that will automate the creation of these navigational items (e.g., common bookmarks, pagination, CRFs, TOCs). It should be noted that no additional plug-in tools should be required for the reviewer at the agency to be able to navigate the documents.

DIFs

When filing a traditional e-submission, the agency requires that the DIFs for every single PDF file be completed with proper information. Before creating the final indexes for different Items in the submission, the DIFs for individual files should be checked to ensure proper indexing and referencing. Reference should be made to individual Items section, in a submission, for detailed description, instructions, and some examples on the information for completing DIFs.

DIF provision is less crucial when filing an eCTD dossier; however, it is common practice to provide the title, subject, and author on each eCTD PDF document.

Pagination

When paginating an eCTD dossier, only the internal page numbers of the document are required (1-n). No additional page/volume numbers running across documents are expected. It is easier to navigate through an electronic document if the page numbers for the document and the PDF file are the same. To accomplish this, the first page of the document should be numbered page 1, and all subsequent pages (including appendices and attachments) should be numbered consecutively with Arabic numerals. Roman numerals should not be used to number pages (e.g., title pages, tables of contents) and pages should not be left unnumbered (e.g., title page.) Numbering in this manner keeps the Acrobat numbering in synchrony with the internal document page numbers.

For all other e-submission types, all the PDF documents should also be appropriately paginated for proper navigation. Occasionally, the agency may request some of items or the entire submission in both electronic and paper format. Therefore, it is strongly recommended that the pagination of the electronic documents should be such that when printing them will produce an equivalent or identical paper submission. Including volume and page number is a typical format used in such scenarios, with each volume containing about 300 to 400 pages. General guidelines should be consulted for more detailed pagination specifications.

Document Level Quality Control

After each PDF document is finalized in the working folder, the following quality control items should be performed to ensure its integrity and compliance with the agency requirements:

- DIFs are complete and accurate.
- Thumbnails are created (non-eCTD application only).
- The file size does not exceed the permitted limit.
- TOC reflects the style and format guides.
- Links and bookmarks are created for required items in the document.
- Magnification option for all bookmarks and links is set to inherit zoom.
- Destination for every (internal) link and bookmark is set properly.
- Links and bookmarks associated with an action is correctly performed.
- Attributes of links are in accordance with the agency's guidelines (e.g, CBER vs. CDER).
- No security level has been applied to the documents

Compilation

The following steps are recommended for compiling the components of an e-submission.

Document level. As the files and their contents are finalized in the working folder, they should be copied via a XML compiler into the final eCTD directory structure. This will allow the submission team members to perform quality control from the ICH technical aspect. For non-eCTD applications, the submission team members should perform additional steps (e.g., full-text indexing, common bookmarking, QC) towards the final preparation. These steps are described later in this section.

Module level. Once all of the files are copied into the final submission folder, the external links should be created across the various modules. Ample time should be allocated for navigational accuracy and bookmark completeness quality check. These steps are applicable for a non-eCTD with the exception of creating bookmarks in the item TOC. Additional attention must be paid to verifying bookmarks for the overall TOC.

Common bookmarks. To facilitate the navigation and review process in a submission particularly within clinical study reports and its appendices, the inclusion of common bookmarks are recommended. When working on non eCTD, applications the agency encourages this practice of creating additional bookmarks in every document to direct the reviewer to the item TOC (e.g., cmctoc, clintoc), overall TOC (e.g., ndatoc, blatoc), and to the roadmap (for CBER submissions only).

Creating Full-Text Indexes

For eCTD applications, full-text index are no longer required. However, for the traditional e-submission, a full-text index is a searchable database of all the text in a document or set of documents. Depending on their versions, either the Acrobat or Acrobat Catalog can be used to create a full-text index of the PDF documents or document collections. Follow the general guidelines for creating indexes for each individual item.

Optimization

The PDF documents go through several publishing steps before becoming final. The size of the files may increase because of the way they were saved. Optimization allows decreasing the file size to an optimum level, without compressing it. Therefore optimizing all PDF for fast Web viewing is a requirement that allows the reviewers faster access to opening the documents. It is also recommended to save the PDF down to Acrobat version 1.4 or Adobe 5 as this may also enhance the viewing capability. Along with optimization, the options for creating thumbnails, and file open can be selected on a library of PDF files at once. Note, creating thumbnails is a recommended activity for the traditional non-eCTD application.

Scanning for Viruses

Normally, all networked computers have some sort of virus scanning software installed in them that is periodically updated by the IT division. Regardless, after all the files in the working directory are finalized and are copied to the final directory, it is a good habit to perform a virus check to ensure that the files submitted to the regulatory agency are clean.

When submitting an eCTD application, the sponsor is required by ICH to provide "a statement that the submission is virus free with a description of the software used to check the files for viruses."

Overall QA

Although initial QC is required in every step of the publishing process, as instructed by the process checklist, a thorough review should be performed to ascertain the validity and correctness of the submission documents, and their various properties. Specifically, the following should be verified:

- DIFs are complete and accurate.
- Thumbnails are created, (non-eCTD application only).
- Full-text indexes have been created for all the required folders (non-eCTD application only).
- The file sizes do not exceed the permitted limit.
- Common bookmarks are present both on the document/item and the submission levels.
- Magnification option for all bookmarks and links is set to inherit zoom.
- Destination for every link and bookmark is set properly.
- Links and bookmarks associated with an action is correctly performed.
- Attributes of links are in accordance with the agency's guidelines (e.g, CBER vs. CDER).
- For external links and bookmarks, the destination path is correct, and there is no reference to a network drive (i.e., absolute path).
- No security level has been applied to the documents.

Creating Submission Media and Final QC

After checking all of the items in the above checklist, depending on the size of the submission, a CD/DVD(s) or a tape containing all the submission documents should to be created. Any commercially available application can be used for creating the submission media. If more than one disc is used, they should be named properly and accordingly (e.g., CD-001, CD-002). Also, the submission number (e.g., N123456 for NDA) should be used for the media (e.g., CD-ROM) title. Once the media is created, a final QC should be performed, preferably on a PC that is not connected to the network, to ensure that the media is functioning correctly and that the reviewer can access all of the files, and there is no reference to the network drive for bookmarks and links.

After the validity and the integrity of the media are tested, it should be sent to the appropriate division in the agency for review. It is important to include the FDA contact name with the package.

eCTD SUBMISSIONS

The eCTD (42) is the electronic delivery structure of the CTD, and defines the creation and transfer of e-submissions from industry to regulatory agencies.

The specification for the eCTD is based upon content defined within the CTD issued by the ICH M4 EWG. The CTD describes the organization of modules, sections, and documents that focus on the authoring process. The structure and level of detail specified in the CTD has been used as the basis for defining the eCTD structure and content. Additional details have been incorporated into the eCTD specification.

The contents of the eCTD are as follows:

- Documents (mainly PDF, regional file formats such as Word, Excel, Word Perfect, SAS XPT, SPL, PIM)
- XML backbone (replaces CTD TOC)—viewable through Web browsers
  - CTD XML file
  - Regional XML file
- Util folder—contains XML backbone–dependant files
  - Document type definitions (DTDs) for ICH and regional modules
  - Stylesheets
  - Other regional specific files

  ICH M2 EWG provides specifications regarding the following:

- DTDs
- Procedures and specifications on modules
- Change management

Why eCTD?

eCTD provides the capability to provide regulatory submissions written in the CTD format to multiple regions simultaneously thus eliminating preparing multiple dossiers for each region. Also, eCTD both eliminates paper and allows more control on managing the workflow dynamics within "multiple dossiers."

- CTD limitations
  - The CTD does not cover the full submission. It describes only modules 2 to 5.

- The CTD does not describe the content of module 1.
- The CTD does not cover details related to amendments or variations to the initial application.

- eCTD advantages
  - eCTD specifications, produced by the M2 EWG, are applicable to all modules.
  - eCTD covers the entire lifecycle of a product.

    - Initial applications
    - Subsequent amendments, supplements, and variations

  - eCTD allows easy navigation of the entire life cycle of an application for viewing and for review.

Process

The process of publishing for an eCTD remains the same across submission formats. Although, there are some structure and compilation tasks that vary among submission formats but on the whole, the majority of the content still requires PDF with navigational features. The only major difference in eCTD compared with other formats of submission is the introduction of the XML file.

Depending upon the format of the submission selected, the following examples, shown in Table 6, may apply.

XML Backbone

The XML backbone is the TOC of an eCTD submission. It holds more information about documents than a typical paper (e.g., NDA, CTD) or an electronic TOC (e.g., eNDA, eBLA). Often this backbone is explained using a *tree* analogy, as shown in Figure 7.

Table 6 Comparison of XML Used for Table of Contents in Different Submissions

Submission format	Specific requirements	Contents	Data
eNDA	TOC in PDF	PDF	SAS^{R} v5 Transport file
eBLA	TOC in PDF & Roadmap	PDF	SAS^{R} v5 Transport file
eIND	TOC in PDF & Roadmap	PDF	SAS^{R} v5 Transport file
eCTD	TOC in XML	PDF	SAS^{R} v5 Transport file (may be XML in the future)

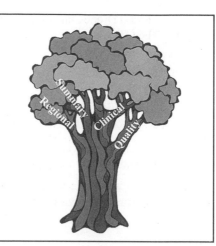

- Backbone is like a Tree trunk
  — Supported by Web browsers

- Sections or modules are branches
  — e.g., module 3 (quality)

- Documents are the leaves
  — e.g., list of manufacturers

Figure 7 A tree analogy of eCTD XML backbone.

Element/Leaf Attributes

In addition to the XML backbone, there are other unique features of the eCTD. One of those features is the format and structure granularity. The ICH specification offers specific recommended folder and file-naming conventions, which industry is cautioned to follow. It is therefore extremely important for sponsors to correctly interpret the specifications when it comes to naming and compiling the elements into the XML in order to create a valid and compliant eCTD dossier. For example, the XML backbone is capable of managing multiple drug products, drug substances, manufacturers, excipients, and indications. Both ICH and regional guidance provide examples and clarification instructing industry as to how to represent such values within the XML backbone.

An element is also commonly referred to as a parent or sub-folder of the five eCTD modules. They are as follows:

Module 1—Administrative information and prescribing information
Module 2—CTD summaries
Module 3—Quality (chemistry, manufacturing, and controls)
Module 4—Nonclinical (safety)
Module 5—Clinical (efficacy)

Nested under these five main elements are numerous predefined subsections that will eventually hold the documents of the submission. Figure 8 illustrates the nesting of subsections for module 2. In certain instances, the sponsor may create unique sub-section(s) for file or document organizational purposes. These undefined subfolders are called node extensions. Refer to the current regional

Module 2	2.1	The TOC is only called for in the paper version of the CTD; there is no entry needed for the eCTD	
	2.2		
	2.3 Note 1	Introduction	
		2.3.S Note 2	2.3.S.1
			2.3.S.2
			2.3.S.3
			2.3.S.4
			2.3.S.5
			2.3.S.6
			2.3.S.7
		2.3.P Note 3	2.3.P.1
			2.3.P.2
			2.3.P.3
			2.3.P.4
			2.3.P.5
			2.3.P.6
			2.3.P.7
			2.3.P.8
		2.3.A	2.3.A.1
			2.3.A.2
			2.3.A.3
		2.3.R	
	2.4		
	2.5		
	2.6	2.6.1	
		2.6.2	
		2.6.3	
		2.6.4	
		2.6.5	
		2.6.6	
		2.6.7	
	2.7	2.7.1	
		2.7.2	
		2.7.3 Note 4	
		2.7.4	
		2.7.5	
		2.7.6	

Key
Documents rolled up to this level are not considered appropriate
One document may be submitted at this level

Figure 8 eCTD Module 2.

and ICH guidance before performing this activity, as node extensions may not be acceptable to all regional authorities.

Generally speaking, when an application contains more than one manufacturer, the drug substance folder should be repeated, but with an indication of each manufacturer concerned included in the folder name, the first instance, e.g., "drug-substance-1-manufacturer-1" and the second "drug-substance-1-manufacturer-2."

Where there is more than one drug substance (e.g., ranitidine hydrochloride and cimetidine), then the first drug substance has a folder named "ranitidine-hydrochloride" and another named "cimetidine."

Where there is more than one drug product (e.g., powder for reconstitution and diluent) then the first drug product has a folder named "powder-for-reconstitution" and another named "diluent."

The management of multiple indications should be handled thusly; the folder name should always include the indication being claimed, for example, "asthma" (abbreviated if appropriate). Where there is more than one indication (e.g., asthma and migraine), then the first indication has a folder "asthma" and the second has a folder named "migraine." ICH eCTD Specification V 3.2 February 04, 2004 (7a) (Tables 7–9).

Adding documents or files occurs once the overall directory structure or XML backbone has been established. According the specification, special attention is given to the leaf attributes. These are values that describe the metadata associated with the PDF file once it has been added to the XML backbone.

Table 7 eCTD Description of Attributes

Attribute name	Description
Leaf	Location in the XML backbone that corresponds to a file.
ID	A unique identifier for this location in the XML instance.
xml:lang	The primary language used by the files in this entire section of the submission.
checksum	The checksum value for the file being submitted.
checksum-type	The checksum algorithm used.
modified-file	Attribute that provides the location of a document that is being modified (i.e., replaced, appended or deleted) by the leaf element.
Operation	Indicates the operation to be performed on the "modified-file."
	Select one of the following valid values:
	• new
	• replace
	• append
	• delete
	See the section "Life Cycle"
application-version	The version of the software application that was used to create a file.
xlink:href	Provide the pointer to the actual file. Use the relative path to the file and the file name.

Most commercially available compilers will manage and automatically populate these required attributes, allowing the sponsor to focus on the submission content and overall navigability.

It is recommended that the reader frequently visit the Web sites mentioned in the "References" section of this chapter to obtain the latest information.

Life Cycle

The eCTD is capable of containing initial submissions, supplements, amendments, and variations. There are no uniform definitions for these terms in the three regions, but amendments and supplements are terms used in the United States and variations apply in Europe.

Once the regulatory body receives the first, or original, eCTD instance, the life cycle of the dossier and its contents commences. With each modification to the original dossier, a new eCTD submission or sequence is required. The variations, supplements, and amendments are used to provide additional information to an original regulatory dossier.

For example, if a new manufacturer for the drug substance were being proposed, this would result in submission of an amendment or supplement to the FDA and a variation to Europe. When regulatory authorities request additional information, the information is also provided as a variation, supplement, or amendment to the original submission. Therefore, the regulatory agencies should have a way to manage the lifecycle of the submission.

In addition to the submission life cycle, documents (leafs) have their own life cycle in the form of operators. In the eCTD construct, there are four such operators.

The sponsor is responsible for determining and managing each individual file in a submission. Understanding operational attributes is the key to successful management. Defining and establishing document business logic should take precedence after submittal of the original application. There are currently two

Table 8 eCTD Lifecycle Operators

Operator	Definition
New	The file has no relationship with files submitted previously.
Append	There is an existing file to which this new file should be associated. (e.g., providing missing or new information to that file). It is recommended that append not be used to associate two files in the same submission (e.g., splitting a file due to size restrictions).
Replace	This means there is an existing file that this new file replaces.
Delete	There is no new file submitted in this case. Instead, the leaf has the operation of "delete," indicating that the file in a previous submission is no longer relevant and should not be considered by the reviewer.

Table 9 eCTD Lifecycle Business Logic Scenarios

Business logic	Current display	Cumulative view
Scenario #1	Structure.pdf (replace, sequence 0002)	Structure.pdf (new, sequence 0000) Structure.pdf (amend, sequence 0001) Structure.pdf (replace, sequence 0002)
Scenario #2	Structure.pdf (new, sequence 0000)	Structure.pdf (new, sequence 0000)
	Structure.pdf (replace, sequence 0002)	Structure.pdf (amend, sequence 0001) Structure.pdf (replace, sequence 0002)

predominate schools of thought regarding the interpretation of replacing an amended document. One business logic states that when replacing an amended file, both the parent (original, sequence 0000) file and its child (the amended file, sequence 0001) are replaced (sequence 0002). The other business logic maintains that the replace operation affects only the amended file (sequence 0001) leaving the original file (sequence 0000) intact and relevant to the reviewer. The table below illustrates the possible scenarios.

The sponsor uses the operation attribute to tell the regulatory authority how they intend the files in the submission to be used. The operation attribute describes the relation between files in subsequent submissions during the life cycle of a medicinal product. In the very first submission, all the files will be new. In the second, third, and subsequent submissions, all the newly submitted files can have different operation attributes because of having or not having a relation with previously submitted files. Therefore one can see the importance of understanding and proper usage of the eCTD leaf operators as the operators are the only means of communicating to the reviewers the documents' relevance to the dossier.

Submission to Agency

In the addition to the traditional methods of submitting applications on physical electronic media formats, the FDA has developed the capability for sponsors to expedite the transmission process via the e-submission gateway (ESG) or Internet protocols. This e-submission process is defined as the receipt, acknowledgment, routing, and notification to a receiving center of the receipt of an e-submission. Each of these terms denotes a step in the process of e-submission delivery, and together, these steps comprise the whole scope of e-submission delivery.

Gateway

The FDA has established the ESG as an agency-wide solution for accepting electronic regulatory submissions. As of May 2, 2006, the ESG replaced the ESTRI (Electronic Standards for the Transmittal of Regulatory Information) as the recommended means of electronically transmitting information via the Internet. The FDA ESG enables the secure submission of regulatory information for review. It is the central transmission point for sending information electronically to the FDA. Within that context, the FDA ESG is only the means for which submissions travel to reach their final destination. The gateway does not open or review submissions; it automatically routes them to the proper FDA center or office. The electronic document room (EDR) is responsible for performing technical validations and releasing the approved application(s) to the reviewer community.

There are three options for sending FDA ESG submissions (43).

1. The FDA ESG Web interface—The FDA ESG Web interface sends submissions via hyper text transfer protocol secure (HTTPS) through a Web browser according to Applicability Statement 2 (AS2) standards.
2. Applicability Statement 1 (AS1) Gateway-to-Gateway—An e-submission protocol that uses secure e-mail for communications.
3. Applicability Statement 2 (AS2) Gateway-to-Gateway—An e-submission protocol that uses HTTP/HTTPS for communications.

Determining the best of these options will be influenced by the types of submissions to be transmitted, infrastructure capabilities, and business requirements. One or more of these options can be selected to submit electronic documents to the FDA. However, a separate registration will be required for each option selected.

ESG was implemented in two phases. Phase 1 supports the receipt of guidance compliant electronic regulatory submissions of up to 100GB in size to CBER, CDER, and CDRH. The FDA ESG also supports the receipt of adverse event reporting system (AERS) reports and AERS attachments. Work on phase 2 has begun with plans to expand ESG capabilities. These plans include receipt of e-submissions targeted for the Center of Veterinary Medicine, Center for Food Safety and Nutrition, and the Office of Orphan Product Designations. The reader should refer to the FDA Web site for the list of electronic regulatory submissions that can be received by the FDA ESG as the list will be expanded as the FDA promulgates additional e-submission guidance documents and extends this capability to new operational units within the FDA.

Secure e-Mail

Secure e-mail, which is also referred to as the Applicability Statement 1 Protocol (AS1) Gateway-to-Gateway, will no longer be available as of January 15, 2008.

The AS1 protocol is restricted to only sending and receiving AERS submissions. Other submission types (including AERS reports) can be sent using the FDA ESG Web interface or the AS2 gateway-to-gateway protocol. Additionally, AS1 Gateway-to-Gateway is only intended for CBER or CDER AERS submissions and attachments.

AERS reports may be in XML or electronic data interchange (EDI) gateway or standard general markup language (SGML) format; however, XML is the preferred format. For more information on preparing SGML submissions, go to: http://www.fda.gov/cder/aerssub/SGML.htm.

All AERS attachments must be in PDF format. For more information on preparing PDF attachments, go to: http://www.fda.gov/cder/guidance/4153dft.pdf (specifically, section III. B, which starts at line 243).

Finally when submitting via AS1 protocol, all submissions must be signed electronically with a digital certificate.

How to Submit

Regardless of the available options, the FDA requires each sponsor (or its designated authority) to set up a test account, and submit a test application. Upon successfully submitting a test application, the sponsor must provide a letter of non-repudiation agreement, obtain a digital signature, select one the submission protocols discussed above for implementation within the production environment. The sponsor must then apply for a production system account, submit a test submission via the production system following the same steps outlined during the testing phase. The FDA approves the sponsor to submit actual data. When the data is submitted via the FDA ESG, the transaction partner or the entity sending submissions/communicating with the receiving and routing component (the FDA ESG) of the community can trace the submission ensuring that it has been received by the gateway and appropriate center. This communication occurs in the form of a message delivering notification, where the ESG sends a notice to the sponsor that the application was received. In like fashion, the intended receiving center generates an acknowledgement to the sender and the FDA ESG when it receives the application (44).

NON-eCTD (Legacy) Electronic Submissions

As the drug development industry and the regulatory agencies advance towards a complete e-submission frontier, new regulations and technologies are used to expedite the process of publishing, review, and approval of marketing/licensing applications.

Currently the FDA divisions accept submission types discussed in the following sections. They present only a summary of the guidelines and specification applicable to these submissions. The reader is strongly encouraged to consult the FDA guidance documents specific to each submission type.

eIND

CBER published the industry guidance document for eIND in February 2002 (6). The FDA intends to update guidance on e-submissions regularly to reflect the evolving nature of the technology and the experience of those using this technology. As the agency develops guidance on electronic IND submissions in the common technical document (CTD) format, they intend to harmonize current guidance on eIND with the eCTD guidance.

The following sections describe some of the specific features of the eIND submission.

eIND Highlights

- Facilitates the submission of INDs in electronic format as well as ensure quick and easy information access for the reviewer.
- Features an IND main folder that is used throughout the life cycle of the application.
- Includes a TOC and bookmark driven navigational construct, which is similar to the structure employed in CBER's electronic marketing application.
- Assigns numeric prefixes to individual PDF file names. The numeric prefix should reflect the amendment number in which the file was submitted for review.
- Facilitates cross-referencing to another IND.
- Features the use of the roadmap.pdf file.

The following are some of the important items to consider while working on a submission. As eIND has specific requirements, it is recommended that the reader refer to eIND guidelines (6) for more details.

Folder and File Names

Guidance provides specific naming convention for the folders (Fig. 9) and subfolders of the submission, TOC files, and the roadmap.

For file names not specifically described, it is recommended that the sponsor use the following naming conventions:

- Include the submission serial number for the file in the initial four numbers of the file.
- Use a descriptive name for the file up to a total of 28 characters. This is a total of 32 characters including the four-digit serial number.
- Use the appropriate three-character extension for the file (e.g., pdf, xpt).
- Be consistent with the file names. For example, if the protocol number is used as part of the name of the original protocol, the same name should also be used for the protocol revision. For example, protocol 1234 provided in amendment number six could be named 0006_1234.pdf. The revised protocol submitted as part of amendment 125 would be named 0125_1234.pdf.

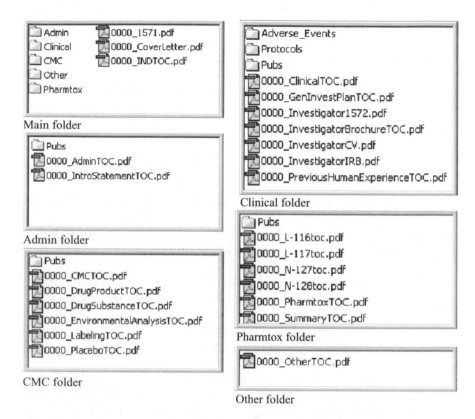

Figure 9 Naming convention and directory structure for an example eIND.

Bookmarks and Hypertext Links

Refer to the common requirements section for details on bookmarks and links. In addition, the reader should be aware of these following specific instructions:

- For a reference list at the end of a document, provide a hypertext link from the item listed to the appropriate PDF publication file.
- Avoid linking items across submission folders.
- Include a bookmark to the roadmap, the submission's main TOC, and the folder's TOC at the highest level of the bookmark hierarchy for documents that are supplied as part of the submission.
  Cross-references to other INDs

At times, IND submissions are supported by a cross-reference to another IND [21 CFR 312.23(b)].

- The utility of the electronic IND submission will be increased if all reference materials are supplied with the IND submission.

- These files should be handled in the same manner as other electronic files submitted to the IND. For example, the files should be generated from an electronic source, rather than from scanned paper documents if at all possible. If the electronic source file is not available, a scanned copy will be acceptable.
- If an electronic IND or other form of documentation already exists in CBER, and the appropriate letters of authorization are supplied, the IND review team will be granted access to those documents.
- If the files chosen for referencing have been provided in electronic format, include the main folder name in which the document resides in place of the volume number required under 21 CFR 312.23(b).
- Provide copies of the appropriate letters of authorization in the admin folder of the submission.

Submission Management

Timely communications with the appropriate center and office staff before the submission of an electronic document are essential. Remember the following important points:

- Sponsor should notify the FDA in writing of their intent to submit an electronic IND at least three months before the target arrival date for the application. Upon receipt and review of the written notification, the division staff will schedule a teleconference to discuss the proposed electronic dossier.
- Sponsor should submit a CD-ROM, containing mock-up text and data, conveying their interpretation of the guidance for review by center staff 45 days before the submission target date.[4]
- Establish the secure e-mail system.

Because the review of an initial IND submission must be completed in 30 days, it is essential that the electronic IND submission function smoothly. The CD-ROM demonstration is a critical part of ensuring that smooth function. The CD-ROM demonstration should facilitate discussions of the planned regulatory submission through the presentations of mock-up text, tables, graphics, and data to CBER from the sponsor. The CD-ROM demonstration will

- present CBER with an opportunity to ensure that documents are presented in a standard format across all electronic IND applications;

---

[4] The sponsor or drug team is required to send a demo only once (i.e., no need to provide demo for subsequent submissions).

- present an opportunity for feedback from the review team on the presentation of regulatory information (e.g., dataset structures, hypertext links, bookmarking, and document quality); and
- present an opportunity for CBER's technical staff to provide feedback on how well the proposed submission structure is consistent with the guidance.

Application Structure

An IND is a compilation of many small submissions collected over an extended period of time. Frequently, during the review of an IND submission, a reviewer will need to refer to earlier submissions. To help reviewers navigate through the entire application, with each new submission a directory that includes a list of not only the files for the current submission but all of the previously submitted files, should be included as well.

This list should be presented in reverse chronological order, by submission, as part of a PDF file called roadmap.pdf. This file is linked to the submission's main TOC, which is in turn linked to the TOC provided in each subfolder. Figure 10 shows a sample roadmap file.

eANDA

This type of submission is used for marketing application approval for generics. The details of the content and format of this application are described in the FDA

ELECTRONIC ROADMAP: I-CureAll

IND Serial Submission Number	IND Submission Date	Submission Content	CD-ROM Serial Number	Link to TOC
I12345, 0002	05-may-2003	Cover Letter 1571 Table of Contents Protocols (Protocol 1234, amendment 1)	CD-2.01	0002_AmendTOC.pdf
I12345, 0001	05-mar-2003	Cover Letter 1571 Table of Contents Chemistry, Manufacturing, & Controls (amended Drug Product and Drug Substance documents)	CD-1.01	0001_AmendTOC.pdf
ABC Pharma I-CureAll, 0000	05-jan-2003	Cover Letter 1571 Table of Contents Introductory Statement General Investigative Plan Investigator Brochure Protocols Chemistry, Manufacturing, & Controls Pharmacology and Toxicology Previous Human Experience Additional Information	CD-0.01 CD-0.02 CD-0.03	0000_INDTOC.pdf

Figure 10 An example roadmap for an eIND.

guidance document "Guidance for Industry Providing Regulatory Submissions in Electronic Format—ANDAs" in June 2002. The submission process for an eANDA closely follows that of an eNDA, except that it is shorter.

Regulations in 21 CFR 314.94 provide general requirements for submitting ANDAs to CDER. Currently, the FDA Form 356h outlines the components required in the submission of an abbreviated new drug application. This form is available on the Internet at (http://aosweb.psc.dhhs.gov/forms/fdaforms.htm). The following general issues should be considered for the e-submission of ANDAs:

- Consistency with NDA guidance—The FDA has tried to make the guidance for ANDA consistent with the NDA guidance, including general issues about refusal to receive or file an application, providing the field copy, electronic signatures, and review aids, if submitted electronically.
- Archival copy—Currently, the agency accepts the archival copy of an ANDA in electronic format. If the sponsor decides to provide an ANDA in electronic format, then the entire submission, and all subsequent supplements and amendments should also be in electronic format. This will reduce confusion and improve review efficiency.
- Review copy—The sponsor is required to submit a review copy of an ANDA in addition to the archival copy. If the archival copy is in electronic format, a separate review copy is not required.
- Supplements and amendments—The recommendations in the guidance apply equally to the original submission, supplements, and amendments to ANDAs.
- Other considerations
  1. Page numbering—Page numbers should be added to individual documents; pagination across all PDF documents is not necessary.
  2. Indexing PDF documents—Creating full text indexes for eANDA is not necessary.
  3. Sending in the e-submission to be archived—The eANDA archival copy, should be sent to the CDER OGD document room (OGDDR).
  4. The type of media that should be used—See general considerations guidance for information on media.
  5. Preparing the media—See general considerations guidance for information on preparing the media.
- Questions on ANDA e-submissions—Questions regarding the preparation of eANDAs should be directed to the e-submissions technical support esub@cder.fda.gov.
- Folders—All documents and data files for the electronic archival copy should be placed in a main folder using ANDA as the folder name. Inside the main folder, there should be six subfolders: *labeling, cmc, hpbio, crt, crf,* and *other.* (see Table 10 for the items and folder organization). Documents and data files that belong to an item should be placed in the assigned subfolder.

Table 10 Items of an ANDA as Described on FDA Form 356h

Item	Description	Folder name
	Cover letter	ANDA
	Regulatory basis of submission	ANDA
2	Labeling	Labeling
4	Chemistry	CMC
6	Human pharmacokinetics (Bioequivalence)	HPBio
11	Case report tabulations	CRT
12	Case report forms	CRF
14	Patent certification	Other
16	Debarment certification	Other
17	Field copy certification	Other
19	Financial information	Other
20	Other	Other

- Cover letter—The cover letter should be included per NDA guidance.
- Basis for the ANDA submission—The information should be provided for the comparison of the generic drug and the reference-listed drug, conditions for use, active ingredients, and route of administration. This information should be presented in a single PDF file named regbasis.pdf and placed in the ANDA folder. This document should have a TOC listing each one of the required items listed above. As part of the comprehensive TOC, bookmarks should be created for each item listed in the TOC.
- FDA Form 356h—The FDA Form 356h should be provided as described in the NDA guidance.
- ANDA TOC (index)—A comprehensive TOC for the submission named *andatoc.pdf* should be created and placed inside the main ANDA folder.

The submission should contain the documents and data files for the appropriate items listed on the FDA Form 356h. The detailed information on how to create each item in electronic format is provided in the guidance to industry (5). These items include the following:

- Item 1—TOC
- Item 2—Labeling
- Item 4—Chemistry, manufacturing, and controls (CMC)
- Item 6—Human pharmacokinetics and bioavailability
- Item 11—Case report tabulations (CRTs)
- Item 12—Case report forms (CRFs)
- Other items—(items 14, 16, 17, 19, and 20, if applicable)

eNDA

In this section the organization and structure of the submission for an eNDA is discussed. It is strongly recommended that the reader refer to guidance document for detailed information.

Organization

- All documents and datasets for the electronic archival copy should be placed in a main folder using the NDA number (e.g., N123456) as the folder name. (The NDA number should be obtained prior to submission).
- Inside the main folder, all of the documents and datasets should be organized by the NDA items, as described on page 2 of the FDA Form 356h.
- Each item has an assigned subfolder where documents and datasets belonging to the item are placed. See Table 11 for the items and folder organization and naming convention.

Folder Structure

Figure 11 shows the main folder and subfolders of an example eNDA submission, N123456, and its contents.

Table 11 Items of an NDA as Described in Form FDA 356h

Item	Description	Folder name
1	Table of contents (Index)	Main folder
2	Labeling	Labeling
3	Summary	Summary
4	Chemistry section	CMC
5	Nonclinical pharmacology and toxicology section	Pharmtox
6	Human pharmacology and bioavailability/bioequivalence section	HPBio
7	Clinical microbiology section	Micro
8	Clinical section	Clinstat
9	Safety update report	Update
10	Statistical section	Clinstat
11	Case report tabulations	CRT
12	Case report forms	CRF
13	Patent information	Other
14	Patent certification	Other
15	Establishment description	Other
16	Debarment certification	Other
17	Field copy certification	Other
18	User fee cover sheet	Other
19	Financial disclosure information	Other
20	Other	Other

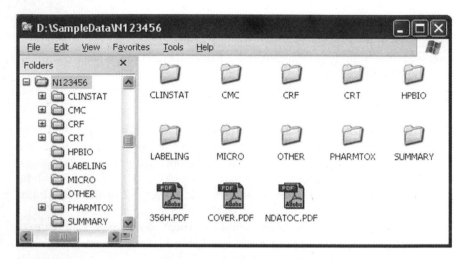

Figure 11 A sample eNDA directory structure.

Comprehensive TOC

Regulations at 314.50(b) require a "comprehensive index by volume number and page number. . . ." The comprehensive TOC, hypertext links, and bookmarks in the electronic version play the same role as the comprehensive index by volume number and page number required in the paper copy. Bookmarks and hypertext links are essential for efficient navigation through an e-submission. For e-submissions, the comprehensive TOC contains three levels of detail and the appropriate hypertext links and bookmarks. CDER may refuse to file a submission that does not contain a comprehensive TOC with hypertext links and bookmarks. The first level of detail simply lists the items in the NDA as shown on page 2 of the FDA Form 356h. Figure 12 presents a sample TOC for the NDA/eNDA.

Required Files/Folders

- This main TOC should be a single page and should be provided as a single PDF file. The file containing the TOC for the original NDA should be named *ndatoc.pdf*. The file containing the TOC for an amendment should be named amendtoc.pdf and the file containing the TOC for a supplement should be named *suppltoc.pdf*.
- The second level of detail contains a TOC for each item (e.g., labeling, CMC, CRT, etc.). Provide the appropriate bookmarks and hyperlinks for each document or dataset listed to the appropriate file.
- The third level of detail is the TOC for each document or dataset. For each document, provide bookmarks for each entry in the document's TOC to the

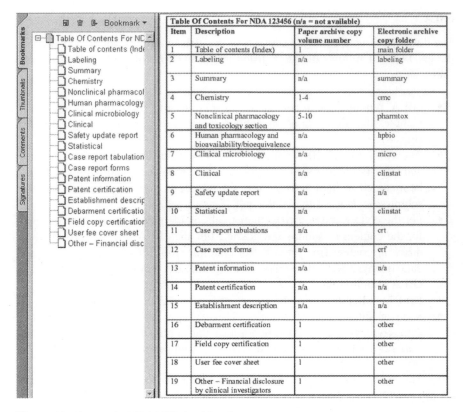

Figure 12 A sample NDA/eNDA table of contents.

appropriate location. For datasets, provide a data definition table (*define. pdf*) as a key to the elements being used in the datasets.

- In cases where a portion of the archival copy is in paper and a portion is in electronic format, the volume number for the paper portion should be indicated. Also, the electronic portion should be placed in the appropriate folder and listed in the TOC.
- Generally, the paper copies for items 13 through 20 are in volume 1, and the electronic copies are in a folder named *Other*. The TOC shows the entire submission including the paper and the electronic portions.
- A hypertext link should be provided from the first-level TOC to the corresponding TOC for each item. These links are essential for establishing a comprehensive TOC for the e-submission.
- Some items, such as item 3 (Summary) and items 13 to 19, are single documents and do not have their own TOC. In such cases, the hypertext link from the first level TOC should go directly to the document.

eBLA

The directory structure and the contents of the eBLA is almost identical to that of the eNDA, as it follows the items listed in the FDA Form 356h, except for the following:

- eBLA requires the roadmap.pdf, similar to that described in eIND. It includes the life cycle of the submission in a reverse chronological order (Fig. 8).
- According to the eBLA guidance (4), "For electronic submissions, Item 8 and Item 10 are identical. Documents describing statistical methods should be included in Item 8. Therefore, for this Item, you only need to link the submission TOC to the clintoc.pdf."[5]
- For the eNDA, the item 10, "Statistical," is identical to item 8, "Clinical," for the content of submission dossier. For the eBLA, the item 10 requires different content from item 8. For example, the statistical/SAS programs, data listings, and other relevant materials are required in this item, for eBLA submissions.
- Item 7, "Microbiology," does not apply to CBER submissions.
- Sponsor should submit a demo CD-ROM, containing mock-up text and data, conveying their interpretation of the guidance for review by center staff prior (six months recommended) to submission target date.[6]

The reader is strongly encouraged to consult the appropriate guidance documents (2,4) for details.

Devices

The CDRH has an e-submissions program, referred to as CeSub (CDRH electronic submissions). CeSub evolved as a result of two very successful pilot programs named "eLaser," and "Turbo 510(k)." The division offers a free software application named CeSub eSubmitter. CeSub eSubmitter can be used for a variety of submission types and is now available for voluntary use by the sponsors and manufacturers in the device and radiological health industries. CeSub eSubmitter allows sponsors to

- electronically complete and submit premarket notification applications [510(k)] to the Office of In Vitro Diagnostic Device Evaluation and Safety (OIVD);

---

[5] Based on our experience, in this item, CBER requires more statistical information, such as analysis datasets, SAS programs, etc. It is highly recommended that the sponsor communicate with the division representatives prior to sending the submission.

[6] The sponsor or the drug team is required to send a demo only once (i.e., no need to provide demo for subsequent submissions).

- electronically complete and submit information for a variety of radiation safety product reports and annual reports for radiation emitting products to the Radiological Health Program; and
- electronically complete and submit the Medwatch 3500A form for medical device adverse event reports.

Refer to CDRH website for most recent information: http://www.fda.gov/cdrh/cesub/

SUMMARY

The FDA had long set the goal of streamlining and expediting the process for drug review and approval. Among the concepts that the FDA explored for achieving its goal was that of switching from paper to electronic media as the format for submitting marketing applications. This proved to be one of the most crucial undertakings in the FDA's strategy.

During the past couple of decades, several events including introduction of PDUFA, FDAMA, Electronic Records and Electronic Signatures Acts, along with publishing of multiple guidance documents on e-submissions helped shape and evolve the current process for e-submissions. This process is a dynamic one and it is still evolving. New concepts for streamlining and expediting the drug development process, along with advancing technological tools and the establishment of new regulations and requirements are among a variety of factors that contribute to the evolution of this fast changing field.

Throughout the years, the process of regulatory submission has evolved, yet its fundamental approach, which is *collect*, *publish*, *compile*, and *submit*, as a general, still applies. The implementation of the e-submission does not change the overall contents of the submissions; it only impacts the submission media (i.e., from paper to electronic). While the directory structure, file naming conventions, and XML backbone (for eCTD) are points of variation for different types of submissions, the core and the common denominator for all the e-submissions is the PDF technology, and it will remain so for a foreseeable future. Hence, the process and the tools used to create the regulatory compliant PDF files are most paramount.

In implementing a solution for e-submissions, one should consider a system that not only satisfies today's needs, but is flexible enough to integrate new technologies and requirements as they become available for tomorrow's needs as well.

ACKNOWLEDGMENTS

The authors would like to acknowledge the contribution of many colleagues and individuals, who through their meticulous review, critique, and advice, made possible the creation and publishing of this manuscript. The authors especially acknowledge Vijaya Hegde, Sharyu Shah, and Jasbir Chohan for their many insightful suggestions and discussions during the preparation of this chapter.

Finally, the authors would like to acknowledge their families for their patience, understanding, and encouragement during this period.

REFERENCES

1. Trenter ML, ed. From test tube to patient: improving health through human drugs. US Food and Drug Administration Center for Drug Evaluation and Research—Special Report, 1999. Available at: http://www.fda.gov/cder.
2. Food and Drug Administration. Guidance for Industry: Providing Regulatory Submissions in Electronic Format—General Considerations, Jan 1999.
3. Food and Drug Administration. Guidance for Industry: Regulatory Submissions in Electronic Format—New Drug Applications, January, 1999.
4. Food and Drug Administration. Guidance for Industry: Providing Regulatory Submissions to the Center for Biologics Evaluation and Research (CBER) in Electronic Format—Biologics Marketing Applications, November, 1999.
5. Food and Drug Administration. Guidance for Industry: Providing Regulatory Submissions in Electronic Format—ANDAs [draft guidance], November, 2001. Available at: http://www.fda.gov/OHRMS/DOCKETS/98fr/010475gd.pdf.
6. Food and Drug Administration. Guidance for Industry: Providing Regulatory Submissions to CBER in Electronic Format—Investigational New Drug Applications (INDs), February, 2002. Available at: http://www.fda.gov/cber/gdlns/eind.pdf.
7. M2 Expert Working Group. Electronic Common Technical Document Specification. International Conference on Harmonisation of Technical Requirements for Registration of Pharmaceuticals for Human Use eCTD specification V 3.0, October 08, 2002. Available at: http://estri.ich.org/eCTD/eCTD_Specification_v3_2.pdf
7a. ICH eCTD Specification V 3.2 February 04, 2004. Available at: http://estri.ich.org/eCTD/eCTD_Specification_v3_2.pdf
8. Food and Drug Administration. Prescription Drug User Fee Act of 1992 (PDUFA), 1992, Available at: http://www.fda.gov/opacom/laws/fdcact/fdcact7c.htm.
9. Food and Drug Administration. Prescription Drug User Fee Act of 1997 (PDUFA II), 1997. Available at: http://www.fda.gov/oc/pdufa2/5yrplan.html.
10. Food and Drug Administration. Prescription Drug User Fees (PDUFA IV), 2007. Available at: http://www.fda.gov/cder/info/industry.htm.
11. Food and Drug Administration. Food and Drug Administration Modernization Act (FDAMA) 1997. Available at: http://www.fda.gov/cder/guidance/105-115.htm.
12. Food and Drug Administration. 21 CFR Part 11 Electronic Records; Electronic Signatures; Final Rule Electronic Submissions; Establishment of Public Docket; Notice. Federal Register 1997; 62(54): 13430. Available at: http://www.fda.gov/ora/compliance_ref/part11/FRs/background/pt11finr.pdf.
13. Levin R. Industry experience with electronic submissions: CDER perspectives. US Food and Drug Administration Center for Drug Evaluation and Research, 2000. Available at: http://www.fda.gov/cder/regulatory/ersr/ersr4.pdf.
14. Food and Drug Administration. Improving public health through human drugs. CDER 2002 Report to the Nation, 2002. Available at: http://www.fda.gov/cder/reports/rtn/2002/rtn2002.htm.
15. Levin R. Electronic submissions to the FDA. Presented at: the Fifth Annual Electronic Document Management Conference, Barcelona, Spain, September 23, 2002. Available at: http://www.fda.gov/cder/regulatory/ersr/2002_09_23_tutorial_talk/tsld001.htm.

16. Food and Drug Administration. Medical Devices and User Fee Modernization Act (MDUFMA) 2002. Available at: http://www.fda.gov/cdrh/mdufma/mdufma2002.html.
17. Dobbs JH. The CANDA: an overview. In: Mathieuy M, ed. CANDA: A Regulatory, Technology and Strategy Report. Waltham, MA: PAREXEL International Corp., 1992:1–12.
18. Ross R, Galle S, Collom W. Regulatory submissions: from CANDA/CAPLA to 2002 and beyond. Drug Inf J 2000; 34:761–774.
19. Food and Drug Administration. CANDA Guidance Manual. 2nd. ed. Rockville, MD: U.S. Department of Health and Human Services, 1994.
20. Mathieu M. ed. CANDA: A Regulatory, Technology and Strategy Report. Waltham, MA: PAREXEL International Corp., 1992.
21. Collins M, ed. CANDA 1995: An International Regulatory and Strategy Report. Waltham, MA: PAREXEL International Corp., 1995.
22. CANDA Guidance Manual. 1st. ed. Rockville, MD: U.S. Department of Health and Human Services, 1992.
23. Flieger K. Getting SMART: drug review in the computer age. FDA Consumer Magazine, October 1994. Available at: http://www.fda.gov/fdac/features/895_smart.html.
24. Mathieu M. New Drug Development: A Regulatory Overview. 4th. ed. Waltham, MA: PAREXEL International Corp., 1997.
25. Adobe Acrobat. PDF as a standard for pharmaceutical electronic submissions—White Paper, 2003. Available at: http://www.adobe.fr/products/acrobat/pdfs/pharmaceutical.pdf
26. Food and Drug Administration. Guidance for Industry: Providing Regulatory Submissions in Electronic Format—ANDAs, July, 2006. Available at: http://www.fda.gov/cder/guidance/5004fnl.htm.
27. FDA Center for Biologics Evaluation and Research. Points to Consider: Computer Assisted Submissions for License Applications. CBER Guidance, July, 1990.
28. McCurdy L. CBER and computer-assisted product license applications. In: Mathieu M, ed. Biologics Development: A Regulatory Overview. Waltham, MA: PAREXEL International Corp., 1993:chap. 15.
29. Food and Drug Administration. Electronic secure messaging v2.0. Working Instructions for Industry–Draft. CBER Electronic Regulatory Submission and Review, May 6, 2002.
30. Fauntleroy MB. E-sub update. Presented at: the BIO Annual Conference, Washington, D.C., June 25, 2003. Available at: www.fda.gov/cber/summaries/bio062303mf_pt1.pdf
31. Food and Drug Administration. A guide for the submission of an abbreviated radiation safety report on cephalometric devices intended for diagnostic use. Center for Devices and Radiological Health (CDRH), March 1996. Available at: http://www.fda.gov/cdrh/comp/guidance/977.html.
32. Benesch BH, Norman JG. Proposed reengineering of the FDA medical device registration and listing (L&R) system. Center for Devices and Radiological Health (CDRH), March, 2003. Available at: http://www.fda/gov/grassroots/gr-meetings.pdf.
33. Food and Drug Administration. Electronic submissions: general information. Center for Devices and Radiological Health (CDRH), 2003. Available at: http://www.fda.gov/cdrh/elecsub.html.

---

34. Food and Drug Administration. Electronic Submissions Project. Center for Veterinary Medicine, 2003. Available at: http://www.fda.gov/cvm/esubtoc.html.
35. Food and Drug Administration. Electronic Submission Pilot Project Report. Three-month report, December 8, 1997. Office of New Animal Drug Evaluation Center for Veterinary Medicine.
36. International Conference on Harmonization. The ICH Harmonisation Process, 2003, Available at: http://www.ich.org/ich4.html.
37. Gensinger G. US update eCTD—The electronic format as of January 1, 2008: what does it mean for the agency? Presented at: the 6th Annual Electronic Submissions Conference eCTD: The Future Is Now, San Diego, November 15, 2007.
38. Prelude Computer Solutions, Inc. Electronic submissions—White Paper Parsippany, NJ: Prelude Computer Solutions, Inc., 2002.
39. Food and Drug Administration. Draft Guidance for Industry on 'Part 11, Electronic Records, Electronic Signatures—Scope and Application. U.S. Department of Health and Human Services, February, 2003. Available at: http://www.fda.gov/cder/gmp/cd0314.pdf.
40. Bartsch GU. Introduction to electronic document management—White Paper. Parsippany, NJ: Prelude Computer Solutions, Inc., 2003.
41. Brown M, Inose C, Ramos C. Regulatory publishing. Regulatory Affairs Journal October, 2002; 13(10).
42. International Conference On Harmonisation. ICH Harmonised Tripartite Guideline—Organisation of the Common Technical Document for the Registration of Pharmaceuticals for Human Use. M4, November 8, 2000. Available at: http://www.ich.org/ICH5C.html#organisation.
43. FDA Electronic Submission Gateway (ESG) User Guide November 20. 2007 http://www.fda.gov/esg/userguide/WebHelp_07_2007/WebHelp_07_2007.htm.
44. FDA Electronic Submissions Gateway (ESG) http://www.fda.gov/esg/default.htm.

11

The Practice of Regulatory Affairs

David S. Mantus

Cubist Pharmaceuticals, Inc., Lexington, Massachusetts, U.S.A.

INTRODUCTION

There are many texts (including this one), journals, Web sites, conferences, and professional societies devoted to the regulation of drugs, biologics, and devices, and interpretations thereof, but very few speak generally to survival and success in the profession of regulatory affairs (RA). The success of regulatory strategy is less dependent on the regulations than on how they are interpreted, applied, and communicated within companies and to outside constituents. The several academic centers providing graduate and certificate training in RA also tend to focus on the hardware of the matter: the laws, regulations, science, technology, and ethics of product development/marketing/regulation. What's missing? The real "fun" stuff consists of those unseen connections between all of these spheres and the balancing act of the persons who manage the connections. It's great to know all the laws and regulations by heart (I don't, not even the regs most applicable to my area!), but what really counts is an ability to interpret and connect, and to adapt this ability based on circumstances. This is what separates *regulation* professionals from *regulatory* professionals. This chapter is an attempt to discuss the practice of RA—the fundamental tools of the trade—without resorting to specific products or classes of products. The chapter is organized in a way that moves from the most general of concepts toward the most practical. To start, a definition of regulatory affairs is provided; a review of education and attitude follows, communications and documentation are then discussed, and the chapter ends with an overview of submissions.

WHAT IS "REGULATORY AFFAIRS?"

Before we can discuss the practice of RA, we have to define regulatory affairs. Too often we define RA by our own limited experience—what it does at our company, in our industry, etc. To broadly define it one must consider every interaction a company can have with a regulatory authority, be that authority national, state/provincial, or local. Then consider every internal department or individual that might need something from, or need to provide something to, a regulatory authority. Then consider the entire life cycle of a product, from conception to marketing (and perhaps, eventual removal), and every type of product that is regulated. The RA group is at the nexus of all of these variables— the conduit between the company and the authorities, over all times, for all products. It's an awesome and incredibly fortunate position in which to be. Figure 1 is derived from several different slides I've used in lectures to encompass the field of RA. It is an imperfect attempt, but gives some sense of scale both across a company and the life cycle of a product.

It's important to remember the broad possibilities of experiences when dealing with colleagues from other companies, with unique perspectives and sometimes narrow views of the field. There are often times when fruitful communications can only be achieved after learning each other's perspectives and explaining one's own position, as shown in the spectrum in Figure 1. What do I

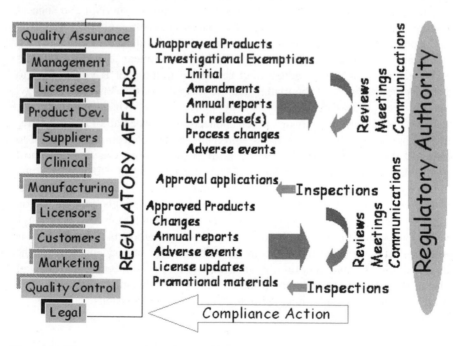

Figure 1 The spectrum of regulatory affairs.

mean by this? Consider your colleagues who are deeply into clinical trial operations. Their goals for the year, their professional ambitions, and their day-to-day activities are all focused on the timely execution of clinical studies. They may be unaware of those manufacturing processes and issues that are either running in parallel or are necessary for timely delivery of clinical trial supplies. Regulatory is uniquely positioned to see the cross-functional dependencies of these issues. Are there other functional departments that have the opportunity to see promotional materials for review, manufacturing batch records, informed consents, and toxicology results all in the same day? What better functional department to assist in managing the interdependencies and to bring to light the gaps in cross-functional plans? In many respects, regulatory is a shadow project management organization—aware and responsible for large, cross-functional networks, but not explicitly identified as project leaders.

BACKGROUND AND TRAINING

Is There a Degree That Matters?

What is the "right" education for an RA professional? When I first entered the field there was no right answer, and this was one of the reasons I entered the field. It does not require any *one* area of technical expertise, but rather the ability to distill multiple technical fields, manage human politics, and write, edit, and collate documents. I have known successful professionals with all manner of degrees (or lack thereof), and I think this diversity is one reason this profession is considered inclusive and has prospered. A trend toward specialization is a bit worrisome—a chemistry degree is not necessary to manage chemistry, manufacture, and controls (CMC) issues, nor is a medical degree necessary to edit or write an investigator brochure (IB). One notable trend is the growth of graduate and certificate degree programs that seek to provide "basic training" in RA. To their credit, most of the programs provide a diverse training across multiple disciplines, in addition to some practical training across industries/product areas.

The open nature of "required training" should encourage more people to enter the RA field. I also hope hiring managers, and managers considering existing employees' career developments don't limit options due to degrees or specific training. A person whose initial training is in devices can succeed in drugs. A person without an undergraduate degree in science can develop CMC sections of submissions.[1] What matters most is an ability to question concepts and data with a critical eye and the courage to ask these questions.

---

[1] This is because an RA professional shouldn't be writing CMC material from scratch! He or she should be a conduit for this information, an editor, and a reviewer. Later sections will expand on this method.

The Importance of Self-Education

At the risk of sounding too much like a self-help book, I believe that the importance of developing one's self can't be overstated. A plethora of courses and workshops across a vast spectrum of technical, legal, and regulatory matters are available. Take advantage of these opportunities—what can't be applied in the short term is liable to be useful in the long term. Such courses also provide a great opportunity for networking. Reading about topics that are less than familiar or intimidating is also recommended. While this *sounds* dull as dirt, there are plenty of authors who've been able to write fairly readable nonfiction books about normally very dry topics. Seek such books out even if they're not your typical read—you'll get a good story *and* learn some things that are useful for work. Some examples include the books of John Allen Paulos.[2] These are well-written tours through the world of mathematics, with few scary formulas and a lot of "back-of-the-envelope" discussions that are useful. Another great book on statistics and decision-making is *Why Not Flip a Coin?* by H.W. Lewis—an easy read and a sometimes scary insight into how decisions are made, especially very important ones that affect millions of lives! These books on specific topics are just examples of the types of reading that you can do on your own time and that both entertains and informs. There are also books about broader topics that can help provide insights useful for regulatory work. Malcolm Gladwell's books *The Tipping Point* and *Blink* are brilliant reviews of trends and change in our society and the nature of decisions based on vast arrays of data made in moments, respectively.[3] Mr. Gladwell has written extensively in the *New Yorker* on a wide array of topics, always using a critical analytical eye, always making it interesting, and always educating. His article "The Art of Failure" is a terrific piece on how things fall to pieces.[4] Another book from my personal reading list is *Complications* by Atul Gawande (interestingly, a friend of Gladwell's), a memoir of a surgeon's training. This last book is mentioned not because it is a technical reference, but because it provides insight into the world of physicians—the folks who study our products, prescribe them, endorse them, and critique them.

All of these books are presented as examples of the type of reading that can provide self-training that can help with regulatory work—help not only with the technical issues that arise but the way one needs to think: broadly, critically, with an open mind, unafraid to ask questions and be questioned.

---

[2] He has a Web page at http://www.math.temple.edu/~paulos/. One example from his book *Innumeracy* discusses diagnostics and specificity. It is a fascinatingly simple study and I've gotten a lot of mileage out of it in discussions and presentations.

[3] He has a great Web site at http://www.gladwell.com/ that includes all of his writings.

[4] *New Yorker*, August 21–28, 2000.

Attitude and Approach

"No." This is the most common word associated with RA and is even more common if you consider it the origin of "not" in the contraction "don't," as in "don't do that," "don't do this," and "don't even think about that." Add "can't" into the equation and you've summed up RA for 99% of the people who work *with* regulatory. In commercial circles, regulatory is sometimes referred to as the "sales prevention group." While the concept of "no" as regulatory's favorite word is a pervasive perception, it is fundamentally wrong, and the fact that products get approved and marketed is evidence. The perception is based on plenty of valid experiences—almost everyone can recall a regulatory person holding up a copy of the Code of Federal Regulations (CFR) and emoting that the proposed action is "in clear violation of subparagraph 345 of paragraph B of section a, subheading iii, chapter 193."[5] The author can reluctantly confess to having said such a thing (or similar) on more than one occasion. The problem is how frequently such a position is taken, and whether any other options exist in terms of opinion and contribution to a project.

Regulatory as Navigator and Architect

One of the most useful analogies for product development (although it can apply to any team moving toward a goal, even if that goal is abstract, such as compliance) is that of a voyage at sea.[6] Think of management (or the board of directors, or investors) as those financing the voyage—providing the ship and supplies with a specific global objective in mind, e.g., getting to point X by date Y. The crew of the ship consists of the various functional groups—the folks who really do the work. I'd like to say that regulatory is the captain, but in the drug, biologic, and device industry this isn't the case. We work in the regulated health care industry, so medical issues (safety and efficacy) are paramount. So imagine clinical (or medical) as the captain of the vessel, chartered with the goal stated above. The question remains, how to get from our point of origin (O) to point X by date Y? The navigator is usually given the job of determining the specific route to follow, and this is a very good analogy for the job of RA. In any navigation problem there are choices—the slow, deliberate, safe route per the chart; the dangerous route over uncharted reefs and rocks; and a middle course, where risks are balanced and timing may be everything (think, waiting for high tide). Even the largest, most resource-rich company shouldn't take the safest, most expensive, and time-consuming path. Every path taken should be a balance of resource, risks, and timing. The "damn the torpedoes" approach is

---

[5] Please don't look this reference up. I made it up in its entirety and any resemblance to regulations past, present, or future is purely coincidental.

[6] I first wrote about this analogy when interviewed in the Regulatory affairs column of *Biotechnology* magazine in the fall of 2000. I honestly can't recall the first time I heard of it.

stereotypical of small companies, but it's usually taken in ignorance rather than using a risk-assessment approach. This navigation analogy works well in considering the function of RA in drug development—laying a strategic and tactical path to the goal. Anyone can plot the safest of courses. It takes skill and experience to plot a course that gets us there in one piece with speed and well-utilized resources.

Another analogy that fits stems from a quote I once heard from a building engineer on a large bridge project. I paraphrase, but he said, "Anyone can build a bridge strong enough to carry a load. It takes skill to build a bridge *just* strong enough to carry a load." The implication is that the goal is a bridge that is affordable and can be built in time, is aesthetically pleasing, and yet carries the load required (Fig. 2). Approval of a drug or device is like that bridge—anyone can get a good drug approved with sufficient time and money. What takes skill is to get it approved in a timely manner with reasonable resources and risk. This is simply a statement of true regulatory strategy—a plan that fits budgets, timelines, and still meets the approval goals.

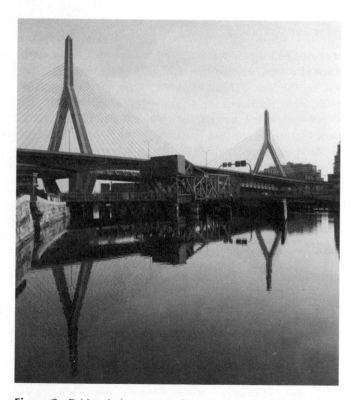

Figure 2 Bridge design as an analogy for drug development. The beautiful Zakim Bunker Hill Bridge—it spans the river, satisfies many audiences (e.g., aesthetes, politicians, commuters), and was completed with a timeline and budget.

Zealotry

Far too often projects, products, even company cultures become "religions" within an organization. A healthy positive attitude is replaced by a blind belief that success, even perfection, will be obtained. Again, while this seems like an extreme observation, many failures in drug development are rooted in an inability to see the obvious, heed prudent advice, and/or recall that we all must obey the rules. Zealotry is a good term for this approach, and it is borne from good intentions based on a strong desire for success and/or a belief in a particular technology/science. In regulated product development, it can be a fatal attitude. I'm not advocating cynicism and despair, simply a healthy dose of skepticism and a reliance on sound data and equally sound advice. Regulatory must often bear the burden of keeping proper perspective. This sometimes makes us easy targets for accusations of "negativism," but in the end a balanced approach is in the interest of the product, the company, and our careers. How do you maintain the balance? Remember that your product is one of many, your company is one of many, and all of us believe we're on *that* project, working at *that* company, which just *has* to succeed! Look over your shoulders, and you see plenty of failed companies and products with very good teams in charge who believed the same things. Saying we're *not* smarter than others sounds like heresy, but usually we aren't smarter. We can be faster at learning, faster at making changes, more responsive, but in general, we have the same brains.

One of the most important times to maintain a balanced (and nonzealous) perspective is in communications with regulatory authorities, such as the Food and Drug Administration (FDA). Another chapter deals with the details of face-to-face meetings, so I will only touch upon the company's *attitude* in these interactions. The FDA has seen plenty of companies claiming to have the best technology, most dedicated clinicians, and the most brilliant management teams. One or two of them have even gotten products approved. But these approvals came based on data, not because the FDA "liked" the company or was in awe of their science. Stick to data, logic, and realistic approaches. It is important to work to understand your FDA counterpart's perspective—what pressures are they facing in terms of other application reviews, congressional oversight, and public opinion? As in any negotiation, understanding the motivations of your partner in negotiation is key to success. In fact, the FDA will usually appreciate a more thoughtful approach, and a more humble attitude will improve the probability of working partnership with the agency.

INFORMATION

Information is often described as the currency of the 21st century, and for RA this has been the case since the earliest days of the profession. Regulatory is the interface between the company/sponsor and the outside world (in terms of regulators/regulatory authorities). As a conduit or a funnel, the regulatory department is a focal point of information, both incoming and outgoing. In order to practice regulatory and succeed, both in objective public measures (e.g., approvals) and internal ones (e.g., recognition and reward), recognizing the power of information and learning to manage it is critical.

What Information Matters?

Other chapters in this book have shown that there are considerable written resources (e.g., books and regulations) to help guide a regulatory professional. However, there are inherent limitations to this information. Published guidance, public presentations, and weekly industry newsletters can't convey mood, body language, and subtexts. They're also available to anyone who can gain access to them, and many are publicly available. While there will be certain "yes or no" answers in these materials, the questions they answer don't require a regulatory person to interpret. Most questions and decisions depend on subtle judgments from regulators, and predicting these judgments, perhaps influencing these judgments requires a mastery of information gathering and management. So the most valuable information is logically the information that is hardest to get— gleaned from informal conversations, e-mails, etc. Also included is information taken from unlikely or difficult-to-find sources. So how does one gather this?

Gathering Information

There should be no need to go over published sources of information, both commercial and governmental.[7] So what are other sources? Any opportunity to see, hear, or talk with a regulator, a more experienced drug development expert, a colleague, or a sworn enemy is an opportunity to gather information. Never be afraid to ask a question, never be afraid to approach a new person who might have information you need, and always be willing to listen. Table 1 provides some basic guidelines for information gathering.

So, what do I mean by novel sources or approaches? A simple anecdote relates to a project I worked on, involving an older chemical entity for which no prior approval appeared to exist. This assumption was based on input from consultants, and even implied in responses to inquiries from the FDA—the Web, the FDA, and Freedom of Information (FOI) had no data on this entity. The assumption was that it was therefore new to the regulatory arena. Then a trip to the library and a review of a more than 30-year-old *Physician's Desk Reference* (*PDR*) helped find the drug—branded and on the market prior to the modern era of regulatory approvals. Included was dosage form information, implied data on pharmacokinetics, etc. This led to a wealth of valuable information to guide the development process and to better inform research on the intellectual property of the compound.

A second anecdote relates to informal conversations with regulators. At a drug development conference recently, a box lunch was provided and served in a

---

[7] If you haven't scoured every square inch of www.fda.gov, do so. It is a treasure trove of information. If it didn't update so frequently, a book could be written about it.

Table 1 Dos and Don'ts of Information Gathering

Do	Don't
Prepare questions ahead of time. Research who you might meet at a conference, dinner, etc. Think about what you might learn!	*Be overly aggressive.* As any good reporter will tell you, people prefer to talk to people who make them comfortable in an exchange that appears two-way.
Make small talk. There is nothing wrong with breaking the ice, finding out more about a person than what you need to know.	*Expect too much.* Regulators in particular know that the information they hold is powerful, and they're not going to tell you that you're approved in the hallway of the Minneapolis convention center.
Look again where others have. Rereading or re-researching sources is OK. You may bring new perspective or a new eye for detail to the matter.	*Assume a source has been checked.* "I assumed someone already checked..." is a very common statement. Never get caught in it.
Look where no one else would. Think of novel sources—this may be academic, former colleagues, old textbooks, or non-FDA government agencies. You have to think of all the ways the information might be important to someone.	*Consider the gathering complete.* You should always be on the lookout for new information. Just because the formal process of searching for data ended doesn't mean you close your eyes.

large ballroom. Such situations usually lead to people distributing to maximize their distance from new people and populating in clusters of familiar faces. I happened to notice the director of an FDA division that our company would probably begin working within the next 9 to 12 months. He was in line for a poorly prepared sandwich. What followed was an informal chat over a meal on general topics related to the state of drug development (not enough truly novel chemical entities), improving communications with industry (more frequent chats and meetings), and how quickly kids grow up nowadays. The company got face time with the FDA, established how follow-up communications with the division work, and the potential for a collaboration started. My new friend/colleague at the agency learned about my company, one new industry person's view of drug development, and perhaps a collaborator on a future conference session.

If it sounds simple, it is. But look around and see how few people execute it.

Communicating Information

What one does with information related to regulatory is as important as the information itself. Who do you tell? Who don't you tell? How do you tell it? The easiest information to share and communicate is *noncritical* information. These are findings and data from public presentations and widely available sources that simply need to be put into a logical and relevant form and shared within the organization. The main issue with such information is getting to the right audience without boring them into forgetting that they're getting useful data. Most companies subscribe to news updates or have internal regulatory information updates via e-mail. However, these updates often have a hard time grabbing attention and actually being used as a resource. One suggestion is to make them playful and user-friendly, using popular Web pages as guides.

What about data you've found from unique sources? Something "dredged up" from an obscure FOI request based on a hunch from a former colleague you met at a conference? I would never suggest hiding these data, but there is no reason to explain openly how they were obtained. Why not keep your regulatory information-gathering secrets secret? The information and your tricks to get it are part of your armamentarium of regulatory tools.

The difficult information to communicate is critical information. This could mean anything vital to the success or failure of a project, specific and important feedback from the FDA, subtle insight that weighs heavily on the future of the company, etc. While it would be simple to just shoot an e-mail off to the entire company, it is neither in the company's interest nor your interest to take that approach. The first thing to do is document the information carefully, so that you fully understand it and its implications. Then think of those individuals who are that combination of "need to know" and "know who else needs to know." At small start-ups this might be the CEO or the president. At larger companies, the head of clinical, a project manager, or a similar middle- to senior-level manager fits the bill. Using these first points of contacts allows the information to pass through appropriate channels. It also allows for the dissemination of the information in the proper context.

One of the most difficult challenges is passing along negative information—bad news. There is a visceral desire to quickly get such information off one's hands, so oftentimes this happens carelessly and winds up feeding "rumor mills" and moving outward without appropriate management. Table 2 provides some hints on handling such information. Don't take this as a cynical approach to regulatory; it is simple realism: just as regulatory is often the recipient of positive approval news, regulatory is the first point of contact when the FDA has to provide negative feedback.

DOCUMENTATION

One of the first things one learns in regulatory and compliance is "if it isn't documented, it wasn't done." Not following this basic principle leads to a large number of compliance failures and can also lead to the downfall of critical development projects. Projects in drug, device, and biologics development can

Table 2 Hints for Passing Along Negative Information

1. Be accurate. Make sure your information is data-rich. If conversations were involved, quote comments verbatim. Avoid adding your own opinions to the information, supply the facts.
2. Think about and research (if necessary) the implications of the "bad news" in terms of resources (costs) and time. You may or may not know the full implication of the information, but if you know a new study costing $500,000 and taking 1 year is the outcome, you might as well share it. It may also be that your first contact—the person you need to tell the information to—is not fully aware of such impacts.
3. Consider an informal, first contact. This should be someone you trust implicitly. Practice your conversation, getting all of the nerves and emotions out. Make sure you're sticking to the first hint!
4. NEVER e-mail this stuff. You may not be fully aware of the ramifications of the information, both legally and in terms of internal politics. E-mail puts the information in written (and therefore documented and available upon discovery) form before you've fully researched all the possible meanings and, perhaps, interpretations.
5. Do your best to suggest alternate paths for success. Just saying "FDA says no" doesn't help the organization. Look for ways goals can still be met. Even if all you can do is to determine what other resources might be available to help extricate the project or company from the situation, suggest it. How much better will it sound to say, "FDA says no, but I'd suggest calling so-and-so at company Z, she's been in this situation before."

take upward of 10 years to complete and cost tremendous amounts of money.[8] The time involved can be upward of five times longer than the average stay in a regulatory job, depending on location and industry.[9] This means projects need to outlast the people who work on them, and the only way they can do this is to have solid documentation to support them. Document progress, document decisions, document information (see above), document failures, document successes. This need to document is important at large companies, where complex dynamics may move a project through the hands of multiple teams, and at small companies, where key decisions may be questioned by advisory boards, investors, potential investors, and potential partners. If you have a well-thought-out defense or opinion on a key issue related to the success or failure of the company or its projects, why not write it down so others can look at it, you can share it, and it outlasts you?

[8] Every few years, the Tufts Center for the Study of Drug Development (http://csdd.tufts.edu/) does a survey that says how much and how long a typical drug takes to develop—the 2002 numbers were seven years (on average) and ~$900 million. Take these numbers with a few grains of salt—they are based on a limited sample size. At a minimum, they give some sense of scale for the biggest and longest projects.

[9] I've been in drug development for 16 years, and am on my fifth job. This seems excessive, but is becoming a more common trend both in biotechnology and the economy as a whole.

The Memo

When I first started nonacademic work at Procter & Gamble, one of the first trainings they provided was in writing a memo. At first I thought it laughable, but since then I believe in the power of the memo. It need not be long, it need not be in one specific format, but it should contain the following elements:

- Your name and initials and/or signature
- The recipient's name
- The date
- A subject line
- Text and references (if necessary)

What power is contained in such a document! Who said what to whom and when! It has the power to document decisions that may have taken years to come to, summarize volumes of data, and correct mistakes. This last "action" is critical to understand. We produce smoothly written standard operation procedures (SOPs), master batch production records (MBPRs), clinical protocols, and policies. It is a very common misperception that in order to "comply," a company must follow the very letter of all of these standard procedures. The reality is that few, if any, actions take place perfectly in line with written procedures. More often than not some level of deviation occurs. The key to deviating *and* complying is to document the deviation. Use a memo! Explain what happened and why those individuals who understand the process and the deviation don't think it's a big deal. It sounds so simple—but read a few warning letters at the FDA Web site to get a sense of how infrequently it's done.

Managing Documents

Volumes upon volumes have been written about document management. I seek only to remind the reader that we have to control the writing, dissemination, filing, and archiving of documents in order for them to be useful. By all means I strongly suggest doing so in the most efficient means possible. Clearly, if resources were no object, this would be a fully electronic document control and management system. I will confess that I am a poor manager of documents. Therefore, I delegate and depend on others to maintain files. The concept of filing is not beyond me; I am merely poorly disciplined at starting and maintaining filing systems. Table 3 provides some useful hints for document management, whether the system is a fully electronic archive or an asbestos-lined fireproof cabinet.

Practical Example: Documenting an FDA Contact

The level of detail and the approach to documenting a contact with a regulatory authority is an ideal example of "good documentation practices." It represents one of the most important functions of RA and should reflect the professionalism and expertise of the person making the record. A generic example follows, and I've tried to add advice and ideas for each section.

RECORD OF CONTACT WITH REGULATORY AGENCY

PRODUCT IDENTIFIER: Product Code or Name	
ORIGINATOR: Your name!	**DATE OF CONTACT:** Date **TIME:** Don't laugh! Multiple calls in one day can get confusing 4 years later.
IND Number: XX,XXX **NDA Number:** **Other File Number:**	**INITIATED BY:** Company Other **TYPE OF CONTACT:** E-mail/Phone/Face-to-face
CONTACT NAME AND TITLE: Get this right, and get every detail. If specific titles don't come up, look them up! Be sure to know where the person stands in terms of decision making. Know the organizational chart of the division/ group!	**AGENCY: Other** **CENTER:** **DIVISION:** **PHONE:** Get actual phone numbers—not general department numbers! **FAX:** **E-MAIL:**
SUBJECT: Why did you talk?	
SUMMARY: Describe in as impersonal a way as possible what transpired. This is not a novel or an attempt at fascinating dialogue. Stick to data. Recording verbatim comments can be incredibly powerful. The specific words people choose say a lot about attitude, and this can then be relayed without editorial or subjective filtering by the reporter. **ACTION(S):** A clear list of actions deriving from this contact needs to be included. **DISTRIBUTION:** **Regulatory File** Be sure to include all appropriate people. Some folks are extrasensitive about being left off the list!	

Abbreviations: IND, investigational new drug; NDA, new drug application.

What are the key concepts? Specificity and objectivity. For this type of document, your opinion shouldn't be reflected. Accuracy and getting specific information is most important. This might take work either before or after the

Table 3 Document Management Ideas

1. Redundancy is OK. It is acceptable and even useful to maintain files in duplicate.
    For example, maintain an IND-specific file, where each submission to the FDA is
    included, along with the FDA feedback and supporting documents. At the same
    time, a chronological file of all the FDA contacts can be kept, which includes
    FDA feedback on an IND submission. In a pinch this redundancy can save you.
2. Use any and all means to keep it simple. Use color code, use multiple cabinets,
    label file folders elaborately. The system has to be able to outlast any one
    person, without an extensive training required for someone else to use the system.
3. Log files. That is to say, keep a table of contents or an index of what is in a file.
    This helps immensely in tracking redundancy (no. 1 above) and in keeping
    a system simple (no. 2 above).

call, but it allows a reader (and a reader who looks at this either 2000 miles away
or 2 years later) the ability to put the contact in perspective.

SUBMISSIONS

Submissions to regulatory authorities are the ultimate "product" created by a
regulatory department, and they also, in terms of content, format, and quality,
represent the company and product. Often voluminous and spanning multiple
technical areas, regulatory submissions are complex documents in every sense—
from an editorial, scientific, and paper-management perspective. At the same
time, these documents represent the ideal opportunity for a regulatory professional to shine—not just in the quality of the final product but in the way the
document is brought together.

Who Writes These Documents, Anyway?

The two extremes to answer this question are both, in my opinion, wrong. At one
end of the spectrum are those folks who believe the regulatory department is
completely responsible for writing all submissions to regulatory authorities. At
the other end are those who would believe all that regulatory does is place a
postage stamp on a document written completely by the technical departments.
The answer is, of course, somewhere in the middle. I will always believe that the
best discussion and presentation of the data will come from those closest to the
data. This means the scientists, engineers, and technicians who produce the data,
do the experiments, etc. At times it can be difficult convincing these folks why
regulatory submissions need to be a priority. It is worthwhile reminding them
that the regulators are the gatekeepers to further development of their projects
and that the regulatory process is a necessary one (even if viewed by some to be
a necessary evil). Another way to encourage inclusion into the regulatory writing
process is to point out that regulatory writing and key contributions to significant

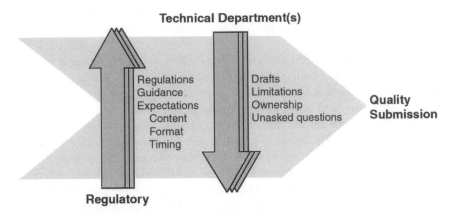

Figure 3 The process of writing submissions.

regulatory milestone submissions (e.g., IND, NDA) are career enhancing and help broaden professional development.

In terms of the writing process, keys to success include recognizing the following:

1. Submission writing is an iterative process.
2. Submission writing is a back and forth process.
3. You need to lower your expectations.

Figure 3 illustrates the first two points. Scientists have usually gained expertise at writing scientific documents such as papers, abstracts, even technical reports. They want (and require) guidance as to what specific data need to be in a submission. Regulatory needs to point to specific regulations and guidelines that provide justification for the work, and guidance as to specific content and format. Expectations as to the quality of the work (e.g., print-ready manuscript vs. handwritten notes) and the timing of drafts are very important to resolve, and to resolve early. At the same time, the technical counterparts to regulatory have their own responsibilities. They need to hit deadlines, be engaged in the process, and deliver quality work. The easiest way to achieve this is to assure *ownership* of the submission or parts of the submission. Ownership implies an individual with responsibility and accountability for the section. This person may not do any writing, but he or she is the one who must be sure that things are delivered. As with expectations from regulatory, gaining concurrence on owners of sections and concurrence on their responsibilities is important to establish early and to communicate upward through management.

The technical owners of submission writing are also responsible (or should be) for making sure unasked questions get asked. That is to say, if key data are not requested by regulatory, or an important issue seems to go unaddressed in the document, the technical group has to mention it. The goal of every regulatory person is to never let this happen, but no one is perfect, and the submission needs to be a true collaboration.

The multiple arrows going up and down on Figure 3 represent the multiple drafts that need to be exchanged as the process continues. These cycles of review, comment, feedback, and rewrite need to be on strict timetables, and regulatory needs to avoid being on the critical path.

The last concept on the list regarding writing was partially facetious: lowering expectations. This refers to reality and the old adage that "the perfect is the enemy of the good." Odds are you are not going to train a technical group to produce "submission-ready" output during the writing process for one submission. The amount of effort this would take leads to diminishing returns when the "polish" on a document can be done within the RA group. I've worked with brilliant scientists who write wonderfully, if they were writing for *Nature* or *Science*. Initially I attempted to alter some of their styles when it came to summary paragraphs that sought to raise more questions instead of simply presenting data. I learned that this was just the way they wrote. It was how they knew to write for journals and editorials and one lowly regulatory submission wasn't going to alter that. Instead of focusing on style I focused on content and data, knowing that the stylistic issues were easy enough to correct in the regulatory edits and reviews and in the writing regulatory owned.

Regulatory Review: Continuity and Connections

Most large regulatory submissions involve multiple technical sections that are written by separate technical groups. As the overall "owner" of the submission, regulatory is responsible to assure the overall quality. This can usually be broken down into the concepts of continuity and connectivity.

Earlier it was implied that regulatory should avoid writing a submission—when it comes to continuity, regulatory must take the lead in writing. Sections of the document need to flow into each other, so the document appears at some level to have one voice. This is particularly important when concepts and data from multiple sections are brought together, as in introductory sections, synopses, and summary conclusions—cut and paste doesn't cut it. The language needs to be fluid, and the order of data logical.

Connectivity is a concept that is seldom recognized overtly by the regulatory community, but is in fact one of our most important responsibilities when it comes to submissions. As the owner of a submission, regulatory is really the only "person" who sees the entire document, and the document is not a linearly attached series of sections—it has multiple internal cross-references and connections. For example, data on preclinical safety connect to clinical protocols in terms of dose ranges and duration of dosing. This same connection is dependent on CMC data showing that the material used for preclinical safety data is truly supportive of the material intended for use clinically. The connections within even a relatively simple document, such as an IND exemption, are multifold and may differ from product to product. Who else is going to check and maintain these connections? Regulatory should have this responsibility and is ideally positioned to manage them.

Presenting Data in Submissions

With the advent of electronic submission production (e.g., Word, Excel, multiple graphics packages), we far too often resort to a quick "cut and paste job" when it comes to presenting data. I would suggest that rather than blindly including graphs and tables of data, it is regulatory's job to look at these data presentations and make sure that the message behind them is clear and that the presentation is suited to the message. If an upward trend in the data is what you want a reviewer to see, a graph is better than a table, for example. Having a y-axis that has a maximum value of 100 when all your data skirt between 0 and 10 may not make sense (of course, if your message is that the data are all well below some threshold, let's say 30, it might make sense!). Edward Tufte has written several books on the inherent value in how data are presented, and I strongly encourage you to read his books and see his lectures.[10] One of the most important concepts is to make sure the data speaks as loudly as possible, and that it speaks the right message without being lost in the noise of the presentation. Bold colors and three- or four-dimensional artwork mean little if a reader cannot grasp the data or the experiments behind the data. A classic example is when multiple experimental points (e.g., subjects in a clinical trial) are compressed into a small number of data points. The goal was clarity, but power is lost—a reader may assume only a few experiments (or a small number of subjects) produced the data. The power of the data is thus diminished.

The Art of Handling Large Documents

Never underestimate the difficulty of handling large volumes of paper or even electronic files. The electronic publishing era is maturing (see the separate chapter on this topic), but the concept still holds. One of the key lessons here is to keep sections of large documents separate, until they really need to be together. This "patience with paper" avoids the need to recollate or edit multiple volumes when only a few pages are in need of work. This concept is at odds with another notion—give yourself enough time to go through the mechanics of printing and copying. When you must move ahead and some small sections (I prefer to restrict them to individual pages) are not ready, use placeholders (colored paper works well) so the pages that need last-minute replacement or fixing can be identified.

---

[10] Tufte's Web site at http://www.edwardtufte.com is almost as good as his books, which are not only educational but works of art. Get them and read them.

Never underestimate the value of individuals who support the handling of large documents (be they electronic or paper). All the content in the world is useless if you can't get 10 copies on a reviewer's desk by Tuesday. Expertise in this area comes from experience. Forget to paginate a document before copying it once, and you remember it forever.[11]

CONCLUSIONS

This was a disjointed roller coaster ride through RA. While not purposeful, this ride is a perfect microcosm of RA: many topics of varying technical detail, connecting the seemingly unrelated, moments of panic, moments of boredom, but never a moment exactly like another. It is this complexity that makes the profession interesting, and it is the position of regulatory at the juncture of so many technical, managerial, and legal disciplines that makes it so vital to the industry. As professionals, we need to go beyond documenting regulations and guidelines, and document how we think, why we do things one way or another, and what has worked. This chapter and this book are intended to be a small start in this direction.

---

[11] Imagine three copies of a document that has to be paginated. Imagine someone (certainly not me!) paginating all three copies and the last page of copy one is 340, while copy two ends at 337 and copy three finishes at 341. A lesson never forgotten.

12

A Primer of Drug/Device Law: What's the Law and How Do I find It?

Josephine C. Babiarz

MS Program in Regulatory Affairs, Massachusetts College of Pharmacy and Health Sciences, Boston, Massachusetts, U.S.A.

INTRODUCTION

Working in a "regulated" environment has many connotations, but to those of us in medical products, the "regulators" always include the Food, Drug, and Cosmetic Act (FDCA), with its tangle of amendments, and the Food and Drug Administration (FDA) itself, which issues innumerable regulations and guidances. You can't be "in compliance" with regulations you've never read or laws you can't find. Hence, this chapter.

In case you're unconvinced, let me give you an example. When a regulation, say the one on informed consent at 21 Code of Federal Regulations (CFR) Part 50, requires that a participant sign and date an informed consent form, the FDA really means that the participant is to sign and date the form. Unless you've read the regulation, you may think, like a lot of nonregulatory people do, that having the participant sign the form was all you needed—that making the participant date the form was irrelevant or clearly less important. So, some folks—woe to them—might use a date stamp to memorialize when a participant signs. These folks are surprised when an FDA inspector writes up a site report, leading to a 483. After all, didn't the participant sign the form? Yes, but the regulation requires that the participant *date* the form. This requirement is very clear *if you read the regulation.* However, if you are looking for informed consent in

21 United States Code (USC), or can't get the current version of informed consent from the CFR, you don't have a chance of finding the regulation, much less reading it. (The pamphlets you pick up at the conferences for free are usually out of date; that's why they are free.) Point made.

So, this chapter will help you know the difference between a law and a regulation and how to find the current ones. Wherever possible, you will be given Internet addresses. Since these can be out of date quickly, there is also information on search engines and finding what you need. You can also find the laws, regulations, and guidances at most public libraries in the United States, using the very same Internet resources we discuss in this chapter. Once you understand the basics, you will be able to skim this chapter for the specific information you need to succeed.

This chapter is organized under topics, with a list of frequently asked questions. Intrepid regulator—forge on! You *can* find it!

1. What is a "law"?
2. Who makes laws?
3. Who interprets laws?
4. What is the difference between a federal law and a state law?
5. What is more important—the state or the federal? What is preemption?
6. Can a nonlawyer make sense out of the laws?
7. Are there any times when state laws control medical products?
8. Where do I find laws?
9. How do I find current laws?
10. What is the difference between the USC and the public laws? How are laws published?
11. What is the difference between the FDCA and the USC?
12. What is an "amendment"?
13. What do all these numbers mean? What is a citation?
14. Why can't I find section 510(k) in the USC?
15. Who enforces laws?
16. What is a "regulation"?
17. What is the difference between a law and a regulation?
18. Which is more important—a law or a regulation?
19. What is the difference between the USC and the CFR?
20. How do I find a current regulation?
21. How do I find older regulations?
22. What is a guidance?
23. Tips for using search engines.

1. What Is a Law?

A law is a rule you have to follow. The laws can also be called "statutes," "public laws," "acts," or "codes." New laws are "enacted" (meaning they are suddenly there and you have to do something about it). Old laws are "repealed" (meaning that they really go away and you don't have to worry about them any more, except to prove that you complied when they were in effect) or "amended" (meaning that they say something a little different now, and you probably need to know what changed).

Most of the laws that concern us will be amended from time to time; we will have examples of amendments and see how they work in question 12, below.

2. Who Makes Laws?

In the United States, laws are passed in two steps: first, the law is written and voted by an elected group of people (the Congress, if it is a federal law, or a legislature, if it is a state law); second, it is signed by the president, on the federal level, or a governor, on a state level. If the president vetoes a law, i.e., refuses to sign it, then the Congress can override the veto by a vote of at least two-thirds of its members. Governors' vetoes can also be overridden.

3. Who Interprets Laws?

There are two branches of government that interpret laws—the executive and the judicial. Because these branches have different jobs, their interpretations are also different.

The executive branch (meaning the president and all agencies controlled by the president, which includes the Department of Health and Human Services (HHS) and inside that department, the FDA) interprets the laws by issuing regulations, which tell people what to do in order to comply with the laws. The executive branch is also charged with enforcing the laws, so if one doesn't follow the regulations, it is easy to get into trouble.

The judicial branch (meaning the courts, including the Supreme Court) also interprets laws, and additionally, interprets regulations to be sure that the regulations issued by the executive branch are consistent with the laws and the Constitution. A court can void a regulation if it decides that the regulation is too vague to be followed, contradicts the law, or gives the executive more power than Congress wrote in the law.

4. What Is the Difference Between a Federal Law and a State Law?

There are two levels of government in the United States—federal and state. On the federal level, the U.S. Constitution establishes the three branches of the government: the Congress, which passes the laws; the executive, which enforces the laws; and the judiciary, which interprets the laws and decides on conflicts between the branches.

The Constitution recognizes that the states each have their own, independent government. The states also have three branches of government, the legislative, executive, and judiciary, which function in the same way as their federal counterparts.

You must comply with all the laws on each level. The Constitution and the courts prevent conflicts between the two levels of government, and each level has its own "turf" so to speak.

5. What Is More Important—The State or the Federal? What Is "Preemption"?

"Preemption" means that the federal laws control, trump, must be obeyed, and any state laws that contradict or conflict with the federal laws are invalid. This *does not* mean that you don't have to worry about any state laws. Read on.

In the United States, because of the Constitution and some early decisions by the United States Supreme Court, the federal government is supreme—a state must enforce federal laws and a state may not pass laws that interfere with any federal law. The state law is "preempted" by federal law.

A perfect example of preemption is in the enforcement of the FDCA. The federal government, acting through the Congress, established certain rules that ALL states must follow. For example, "butter" must have at least 80% by weight of milk fat.[1] Whether you are standing in a Wynn-Dixie in Florida or a Hannaford in New Hampshire, the sticks in the box labeled butter all have at least 80% milk fat. Congress also took on oleomargarine.[2] Whether you are dining out at Wolfgang Puck in Las Vegas or at Penguin Pizza in Boston, margarine must either be in a little carton with a label on it or cut in the shape of a triangle—no exceptions. If perchance your margarine is square, or your butter on a diet, you have "mislabeled" the product, even if state laws allow these changes.

Criteria for marketing a new medical device are also the domain of the federal government, but here, the rules become more complex. Federal law establishes the premarket approval (PMA), the investigational device exemption (IDE), and the 510(k). The FDA has issued certain regulations and application forms, notably the PMA application and the regulations at 21 CFR Part 814 PMA of medical devices and other related regulations. These federal laws and regulations preempt the ability of the Commonwealth of Massachusetts to develop its own state-level requirements to market and sell medical devices. Consequently, Massachusetts cannot require a medical device manufacturer to prove to the satisfaction of the Massachusetts Secretary of Health that any product is safe or effective, as long as that product is under the jurisdiction of the FDCA. That state authority is preempted.

---

[1] See 21 USC 25.

[2] See 21 USC 347(c), Sales in Public Eating Places.

State authority includes the right to determine the basis of personal injury—for example, to sue someone if you purchased a defective car that crashed because the brakes failed. The federal law, specifically the preemption clause named above, means that class III devices that have been approved pursuant to a PMA are generally immune from personal injury state court cases based on product liability.[3] However, note that drugs and biologics are *not* covered under the same preemption doctrines.

The federal law does not do away with all state law requirements, however, or all state requirements of a company that makes devices. Federal law does *not* preempt the ability of Massachusetts to require any company or person doing business in the commonwealth to register with the commonwealth, pay a corporate excise tax to the commonwealth, a property tax to the locality where the business operates, or from collecting sales tax on the sales of any devices in the commonwealth.

In addition, the FDA has accepted certain state regulations on medical products and not overruled them. A query on the FDA's Web site revealed an entire regulation, which lists various state laws that the federal FDCA does *not* preempt: 21 CFR Part 808: exemptions from federal preemption of state and local medical device requirements.[4] So, if you were going to market a medical device from a particular state, or into a particular state, you may want to check this regulation to know about any state laws that you must still meet before you build and ship.

Some people can find these regulations and then decide that the words are unintelligible. So, to demystify this particular one, please continue reading the answer to question 6, which follows.

6. Can a Nonlawyer Make Sense Out of the Laws?

Sometimes it seems that you need a law degree to understand the laws and regulations. As a regulator, however, you must read and understand both the laws and regulations; it goes with the territory. With a few guidelines and a quick "cheat sheet," ordinary people can certainly get the information they need to be compliant.

First, we need an example of a difficult-to-understand law or regulation, and as we all know, they aren't hard to find. There is a wonderful example, right in the regulations, which deals with preemption. Let's start with trying to

---

[3] See Riegel vs. Medtronic, Inc. No. 06-179 (Feb. 2008).

[4] Here is one way to find that regulation—go to the main FDA page (www.fda.gov), and find the text box in the upper left, under "Search," type in the title of the regulation you want, here, it is "Exemptions from Federal Preemption," and hit "Go". My results gave me the regulation on the first hit—"FDA>CDRH>CFR Title 21 Database Search, leading to www.accessdata.fda.gov/scripts/cdrh/cfdocs/cfcfr/CFRSearch.cfm?CFRPart=808.

decipher what Massachusetts laws are not preempted by the federal device requirements.

Quoting from 21 CFR 808.71,[5] the regulation specifies:

> (a) The following Massachusetts medical device re-
>   quirements are enforceable notwithstanding sec-
>   tion 521 of the act because the Food and Drug
>   Administration has exempted them from preemption
>   under section 521(b) of the act:
>
>   (1) Massachusetts General Laws, Chapter 93, Section
>   72, to the extent that it requires a hearing test
>   evaluation for a child under the age of 18.
>   (2) Massachusetts General Laws, Chapter 93, Section
>   74, except as provided in paragraph (6) of the
>   Section, on the condition that, in enforcing this
>   requirement, Massachusetts apply the definition
>   of "used hearing aid" in 801.420(a)(6) of this
>   chapter.

Well, doesn't that little regulation just explain everything! Don't be too frustrated. Yes, it is not written in plain English, and besides that, the regulation doesn't tell you what to do. But, as a regulator you need to read and understand the regulations, so let's see how to make sense of these words.

The federal regulation first names something else, namely, a clause in the Massachusetts General Laws, and even then, the regulation doesn't give you the whole picture, even if you knew what "notwithstanding" meant. (When you see "notwithstanding," substitute "despite anything to the contrary that we say here,"[6] and the regulation will be clearer.) That one word means that this section trumps anything to the contrary in another part of the law/regulation. Since we are talking about whether additional state requirements must be met before selling a product, your ability to find the right answer will save the company money because you found out what had to be done at a state *and* federal level.

First, let's translate that pesky federal regulation into the way we speak. When a clause says, "(a) The following Massachusetts medical device requirements are enforceable notwithstanding section 521 of the act because the Food and Drug Administration has exempted them from preemption under section 521(b) of the act," substitute the words "despite anything to the contrary that we say here"[7] for the word "notwithstanding." So, to translate that regulation: (a) The following *state*-level Massachusetts medical device requirements

---

[5] Supra.

[6] Definition from wordnet.princeton.edu/perl/webwn.

[7] Loc. Cit.

are still good laws that you have to follow, despite anything to the contrary that we the feds, say in section 521 of the *federal*-level law called the FDCA.

Ok, so let's see what section 521 of the FDCA says. It says:[8]

STATE AND LOCAL REQUIREMENTS RESPECTING DEVICES

General Rule

SEC. 521. [360k][9] (a) Except as provided in subsection (b), no State or political subdivision of a State may establish or continue in effect with respect to a device intended for human use any requirement—

(1) which is different from, or in addition to, any requirement applicable under this Act to the device, and

(2) which relates to the safety or effectiveness of the device or to any other matter included in a requirement applicable to the device under this Act.

Exempt Requirements

(b) Upon application of a State or a political subdivision thereof, the Secretary may, by regulation promulgated after notice and opportunity for an oral hearing, exempt from subsection (a), under such conditions as may be prescribed in such regulation, a requirement of such State or political subdivision applicable to a device intended for human use if—

(1) the requirement is more stringent than a requirement under this Act, which would be applicable to the device if an exemption were not in effect under this subsection; or (2) the requirement—

    (A) is required by compelling local conditions, and

    (B) compliance with the requirement would not cause the device to be in violation of any applicable requirement under this Act.

Ok, so now we know that the feds have carved out their turf. A state may not continue to enforce a law or pass a new law that is either different from or in addition to the federal laws governing devices, nor can a state have a law that relates to the safety or the effectiveness of the device or any other device requirement under the FDCA. There are some exceptions—the Secretary of HHS (at the federal level) can make exceptions to this federal law, if the Secretary

---

[8] Food, Drug, and Cosmetic Act, Section 521 ff, as found via the FDA's Web site, at http://www.fda.gov/opacom/laws/fdcact/fdctoc.htm.

[9] To find out what the [360k] reference is all about, see the answer to Question 11, what is the difference between the Food, Drug and Cosmetic Act and the U.S. Code?

decides the state laws are a good idea. For example, an exception can be made if the Secretary decides that the state requirement is more stringent than the federal requirement.

Please note the way this exemption works—the federal Secretary must decide to allow the state law to be enforced (exempted from federal preemption), and then, the exemption only applies to that specific state. By making this exemption, the FDA does not allow these state exemptions across the board.

So, without this provision in the law, there would be no exemption. We can now look at the Massachusetts law to see what it says.

Using Google®, I typed in "Massachusetts General Laws" and was rewarded with several sites. The one I ultimately chose is sponsored by the Massachusetts legislature, but there were a number of free sources I could use. Each of the "free" sources emphasized that they were not the "official" copy of the laws. If I had a few million dollars riding on the outcome of this law, I would pay up and get an official copy, to be sure there were no pesky little typos in the document. But for most purposes, the online access gets me the answer I need.

To understand the FDA's regulation, we must first read the Massachusetts laws that are effected. These laws are in chapter 93, sections 72 and 74.

By scrolling through the table of contents, down to chapter 93, I learnt that it deals with "Regulation of Trade and Certain Enterprises." Section 72 in particular provides:

CHAPTER 93. REGULATION OF TRADE AND CERTAIN ENTERPRISES.

Chapter 93: Section 72. Purchases and sales of hearing aids, prerequisites.

Section 72. No person shall enter into a contract for the sale of or sell a hearing aid unless within the preceding six months the prospective purchaser has obtained a medical clearance.

No person shall enter into a contract for the sale of or sell a hearing aid to a person under eighteen years of age unless within the preceding six months the prospective purchaser has obtained an audiological evaluation. No person except a person eighteen years of age or older whose religious or personal beliefs preclude consultation with a physician may waive the requirement of a medical clearance.

So, in other words, Massachusetts has passed a law that is an additional requirement on the sale of hearing aids, a medical device that is regulated by federal law. WITHOUT THE FEDERAL REGULATION, this Massachusetts law would be preempted by the federal law, because it is an additional requirement on a medical device that is being sold.

Section 74 of the Massachusetts General Laws says:

Chapter 93: Section 74. Sales and delivery receipts; copies of medical clearance and hearing evaluation; customer records.

Section 74. Every person who sells a hearing aid shall accompany such sale with a receipt that shall include: the name, address, and signature of the purchaser; the date of consummation of the sale; the name and address of the regular place of business and the signature of the seller; the make, model, serial number and purchase price of the hearing aid; a statement whether the hearing aid is new, used or reconditioned; the terms of the sale, including an itemization of the total purchase price, including but not limited to the cost of the hearing aid, the ear mold, any batteries or other accessories, and any service costs; a clear and precise statement of any guarantee or trial period; and shall also include the following printed statement in ten point type or larger: "This hearing aid will not restore normal hearing nor will it prevent further hearing loss. The sale of a hearing aid is restricted to those individuals who have obtained a medical evaluation from a licensed physician or otolaryngologist. A fully informed adult whose religious or personal beliefs preclude consultation with a physician may waive the requirement of a medical evaluation. The exercise of such a waiver is not in your best health interest and its use is strongly discouraged. It is also required that a person under the age of eighteen years obtain an evaluation by an audiologist in addition to the medical evaluation before a hearing aid can be sold to such person."

A copy of the medical clearance statement and audiological evaluation, where required, for the hearing aid shall be attached to the receipt.

Upon the date that the purchaser receives the hearing aid, the seller shall provide a delivery receipt signed by the seller and the purchaser which states the date of delivery to the purchaser of the hearing aid.

The seller shall keep records for every customer to whom he renders services or sells a hearing aid including a copy of such receipt, a copy of the medical clearance and the audiological evaluation, a copy of the delivery receipt, a record of services provided, and any correspondence to or from the customer. Such records shall be preserved for at least four years after the date of the last transaction.

So, by applying the language of the regulation to the Massachusetts General Laws, I understand that if I work for a manufacturer of hearing aids, section 72 of the Massachusetts General Laws is *not* preempted, and that it is still valid *to the extent* there has to be a hearing test evaluation for a child under the age of 18 years before the sale. In addition, section 74 is generally valid, as long as the commonwealth uses the federal definition of "used hearing aid" in the state law. You need to know both state and federal law, as well as how to read the regulations, if you want to manufacture and sell medical products.

7. Are There Any Times When State Laws Control Medical Products?

Yes, there are areas where the states exert control over medical products and their development, manufacture, clinical investigations, and other activities, which impact your ability to manufacture and distribute medical products.

Federal law does not address certain really important things like how old you need to be before you can sign a contract (or give informed consent), what medical data privacy rights you have apart from the Health Insurance Portability and Accountability Act (HIPAA), or what is the legal test for a defective medical product, say pill for depression. Legal requirements for disclosures in informed consent are also found on a state level, and the FDA's regulations clearly indicate that federal and state laws *both* govern the document and the process.

In these cases, the federal government adopts the state's definition in enforcing the federal regulation. So, let's say your state says a person can legally sign a contract at 18 years of age. Another state says you have to be 21 years old. Even if your company is located in the state with the 18 years requirement, and you submit your FDA application from your state, and the FDA has reviewed and approved your informed consent form (contract), when you use subjects in a state that says you have to be 21 to sign a contract, you need to have a parent or guardian sign for the 18-year-olds. The FDA does not preempt the local requirement of 21 years. You can have an 18-year-olds sign only in a state that allows 18-year-olds to be bound to contracts. You cannot argue that the federal government preempted the age of consent, where a state says you have to be 21 years old to be bound to a contract.

Pharmacy laws are one of the biggest examples of how each state can and does exert control over medical products. The FDCA provides that certain medical products are available only by prescription from a physician. The FDCA goes on to say that it does not regulate physicians. The states regulate physicians and pharmacists, as well as how certain products are stored, dispensed, and used. As discussed earlier, there are many instances where the federal government is pleased to let the states "work out the details," so to speak.

You should also be on the lookout for certain state laws governing biologics, which can sometimes be cloaked as privacy statutes. These have significant impact on genetic testing, data collection, and product development, which relies on such data.

In conclusion, there is interplay between federal and state laws. The correct answer to the question is that you must comply with all laws that apply to your product. Just complying on a federal level, or on a state level, isn't enough.

8. Where Do I find Laws?

You can find them in a lot of places, which is why saying that the dog chewed your Internet connection or your library is never open after 5 p.m. won't work.

First, if you are going to make a career in medical products, it is worth your while to buy a copy of the relevant FDA-enforced laws. You can buy just the FDA volume, *Title 21*, from a number of publishers. One is available by credit card from the USC Service, Lawyer's Edition, Lexus Law Publishing, at 701, East Water Street, Charlottesville, Virginia. This edition contains not only the laws but also key court cases and the amendment history. You can buy updates each year, which I also recommend.

Why do I think it important to buy the book? Because I find that it saves time and keeps you organized. The Internet gives you access to information in little pieces; it can be very frustrating to use. When you have a text, you can flip easily back and forth between sections, look ahead and behind, and not have to scroll through sections or have pages reload. Additionally, you can write in a book you own and cover it with little tabs that make you look very prepared when you go to a meeting. You can't bring a hard copy of your browser bookmarks to a meeting.

You can also find the laws for free. Most public libraries have copies of the USC, as well as copies of the laws of the state in which the library is located.

You can also find the U.S. laws on the Internet, using the Library of Congress Web site, www.loc.gov/law/guide/uscode.html, which looks like this:

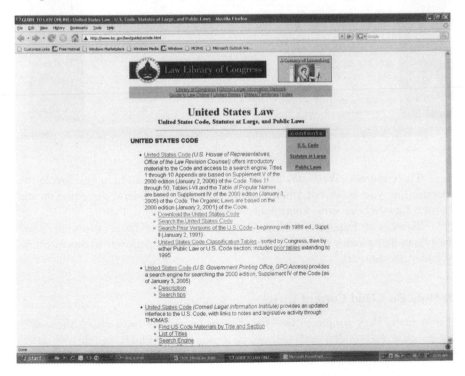

This site links to Thomas, the United States congressional source for information. Thomas' Web address is http://thomas.loc.gov/. A number of law schools have Web sites with useful information, and you can access most of them without paying tuition. One that I like is the Legal Information Institute of Cornell Law School; the Web site is www.law.cornell.edu/, which is referenced below:

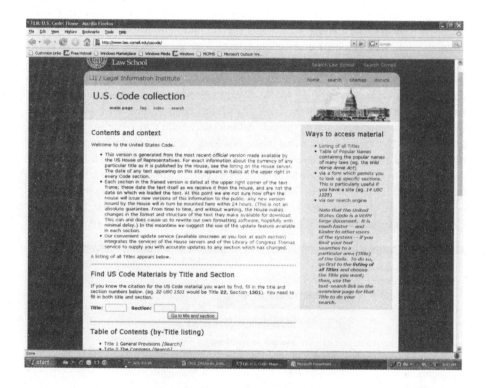

There are also Web sites like Findlaw.com® that can help you locate the specific law you want, but since Findlaw links to the federal government and Cornell Law School sites, you might as well go directly to them.

There is an important trick to finding the laws—and that is to understand the two systems under which the laws are organized. The answer to this question is under question 10.

9. How Do I Find Current Laws?

It is actually very simple to find the current laws. You must check the publication date and understand the source's policy for obtaining current laws. Basically, you want to be sure that any source you check is updated, so you aren't reading something that is old and may not have been updated or is missing the most recent enactments.

For a book, check the title page, with the date of the copyright. If it is this year's date, it is almost current, except for any laws that have passed since the book was published. For an earlier copyright date, check if there is a back "pocket part." If the book is more than a year old, there should be an update, known as the pocket part inserted in the back flap or "pocket" of the book. Because there is an additional cost for the pocket part, and there are recent library budgets cuts, some libraries have cancelled their pocket part subscriptions. But it is always worth a check. You can check for updates using the public laws, discussed in question 10.

For Internet resources, you still have to check the publication date. This isn't the date of your search, at the bottom of the page you print, but is the real date that this compilation of laws was last updated. The compilation date tells you that the compilation does *not* include any laws passed after that date. For example, let's look at the U.S. Government Printing Office's code, available on the Web site www.access.gpo.gov/congress/cong013.html. This Web site itself lets you know that certain editions of the code are current only up to a point. As this goes to press, the latest edition of title 21 (the FDCA) available from the U.S. House of Representatives is supplement IV of the 2000 edition; the supplement is dated January 2005. The code contains the permanent laws as of January 2, 2001. So, while this edition would contain all of FDAMA (the Food and Drug Administration Modernization Act of 1997), this code would not contain laws passed since January 3, 2005. Since Congress has been busy all that time passing laws, you need more than this site has to offer. In particular, you should be interested in the Amendments Act of 2007, which increases most of the filing fees charged by the FDA. You can find this act using Thomas, the Library of Congress megasite named after our third president, which contains legislative information of all types, at http://thomas.loc.gov.

To get the update to this version of the code, you need to use the public laws. Before you can do that, you must understand the difference between the public laws and the code, which is explained in the answer to question 10.

10. What Is the Difference Between the USC and the Public Laws? How are Laws Published?

Really and truly, the USC and the public laws are *both* laws passed by Congress. They are just organized in a different way. The permanent public laws are those laws that Congress works on and passes on a daily basis. The public laws are referenced by the identity number of the Congress working on them. The Congress in session on January 1, 2008 is the 110th Congress, so all of its laws begin with the number 110. For example, it is Public Law 110–85 that increased the user fees paid by pharmaceutical companies and device manufacturers, in addition to other amendments of the FDCA.

As one of my students phrased it, the public laws are like a diary, where each law is recorded on the day it is passed. Congress can pass different laws on the same subject in the same year and in different years, so the only way to find out all the laws passed on a subject using the public laws is to read and search all of the laws. This isn't particularly efficient, which is why the Library of Congress developed the USC.

The USC puts all of the public laws passed on any one subject into one big chapter, or title. The code not only puts all the public laws on one subject together but also edits them to make sense, just as you would revise a term paper that your professor has corrected. If you are asked to add a footnote, or an explanatory section, you add the footnote where indicated, and the explanation in the area that it belongs. You wouldn't do well if you reprinted your error-ridden term paper "as is," and then add a chapter titled, "The Professor thinks I should add this stuff." Same thing with the code. The librarians made the changes called for in the public laws before they published the code. So, the code paragraph numbers and section designations (like a, b, and so on) will be different than those in the public laws, even though the words are the same.

If that explanation was hard to follow, read on to see how the federal government explains it.

The best answer to this question is found on Thomas, the Web site of the U.S. Congress.[10] Here's the inside information:

XIX. Publication

_____ Slip Laws | Statutes at Large | United States Code

One of the important steps in the enactment of a valid law is the requirement that it shall be made known to the people who are to be bound by it. There would be no justice if the state were to hold its people responsible for their conduct before it made known to them the unlawfulness of such behavior. In practice, our laws are published immediately upon their enactment so that the public will be aware of them.

If the President approves a bill, or allows it to become law without signing it, the original enrolled bill is sent from the White House to the Archivist of the United States for publication. If a bill is passed by both Houses over the objections of the President, the body that last overrides the veto transmits it. It is then assigned a public law number, and paginated for the *Statutes at Large* volume covering that session of Congress. The public and private law numbers run in sequence starting anew at the beginning of each Congress and are prefixed for ready identification by the number of the Congress. For example, the first public law of the 108th Congress is designated Public Law 108-1 and the first private law of the 108th

---

[10] Thomas, legislative information on the Internet; http://thomas.loc.gov/home/lawsmade.bysec/publication.html#sliplaws.

Congress is designated Private Law 108-1. Subsequent laws of this Congress also will contain the same prefix designator.

Slip Laws

The first official publication of the statute is in the form generally known as the "slip law." In this form, each law is published separately as an unbound pamphlet. The heading indicates the public or private law number, the date of approval, and the bill number. The heading of a slip law for a public law also indicates the *United States Statutes at Large* citation. If the statute has been passed over the veto of the President, or has become law without the President's signature because he did not return it with objections, an appropriate statement is inserted instead of the usual notation of approval.

The Office of the Federal Register, National Archives and Records Administration prepares the slip laws and provides marginal editorial notes giving the citations to laws mentioned in the text and other explanatory details. The marginal notes also give the *United States Code* classifications, enabling the reader immediately to determine where the statute will appear in the *Code*. Each slip law also includes an informative guide to the legislative history of the law consisting of the committee report number, the name of the committee in each House, as well as the date of consideration and passage in each House, with a reference to the Congressional Record by volume, year, and date. A reference to presidential statements relating to the approval of a bill or the veto of a bill when the veto was overridden and the bill becomes law is included in the legislative history as a citation to the *Weekly Compilation of Presidential Documents*.

Copies of the slip laws are delivered to the document rooms of both Houses where they are available to officials and the public. They may also be obtained by annual subscription or individual purchase from the Government Printing Office and are available in electronic form. Section 113 of title 1 of the *United States Code* provides that slip laws are competent evidence in all the federal and state courts, tribunals, and public offices.

Statutes at Large

The *United States Statutes at Large*, prepared by the Office of the Federal Register, National Archives and Records Administration, provide a permanent collection of the laws of each session of Congress in bound volumes. The latest volume containing the laws of the first session of the 107th Congress is number 115 in the series. Each volume contains a complete index and a table of contents. A legislative history appears at the end of each law. There are also extensive marginal notes referring to laws in earlier volumes and to earlier and later matters in the same volume.

Under the provisions of a statute originally enacted in 1895, these volumes are legal evidence of the laws contained in them and will be accepted as proof of those laws in any court in the United States.

The *Statutes at Large* are a chronological arrangement of the laws exactly as they have been enacted. The laws are not arranged according to subject matter and do not reflect the present status of an earlier law that has been amended. The laws are organized in that manner in the code of laws.

United States Code

The *United States Code* contains a consolidation and codification of the general and permanent laws of the United States arranged according to subject matter under 50 title headings, largely in alphabetical order. It sets out the current status of the laws, as amended, without repeating all the language of the amendatory acts except where necessary. The *Code* is declared to be prima facie evidence of those laws. Its purpose is to present the laws in a concise and usable form without requiring recourse to the many volumes of the *Statutes at Large* containing the individual amendments.

The *Code* is prepared by the Law Revision Counsel of the House of Representatives. New editions are published every six years and cumulative supplements are published after the conclusion of each regular session of the Congress. The *Code* is also available in electronic format on CD-ROM and the Internet.

Twenty-four of the 50 titles have been revised and enacted into positive law, and one title has been eliminated by consolidation with another title. Titles that have been revised and enacted into positive law are legal evidence of the law and may be updated by direct amendment. Eventually all the titles will be revised and enacted into positive law.

11. What Is the Difference Between the FDCA and the USC?

The main difference is the section numbering; the actual substance, the language, is the same. The FDCA is the name of a public law, originally passed decades ago and updated regularly. The USC is the name of the compiled law, and title 21 contains the FDCA, with all its amendments that regulators normally use.

The next section of this chapter explains what an amendment is and how public laws are integrated into the code.

12. What Is an "Amendment"?

An "amendment" is a change to a law or regulation. An amendment is formally approved—that is, passed just as a law, or in the case of a regulation, issued. Let's look at an example of how a public law is actually written, and see how it is integrated into the USC. An easily accessible example is FDAMA, which is specifically known as Public Law 105–115. It was passed in November 1997.

Using Thomas and the public law reference, I was able to obtain a copy of FDAMA, as it was passed. The first section of FDAMA gives instructions as to how to incorporate it into the USC and how to change the relevant sections of the FDCA. The first section of FDAMA reads as follows:

SECTION 1. SHORT TITLE; REFERENCES; TABLE OF CONTENTS.

(a) SHORT TITLE- This Act may be cited as the 'Food and Drug Administration Modernization Act of 1997'.

(b) REFERENCES- Except as otherwise specified, whenever in this Act an amendment or repeal is expressed in terms of an amendment to or a repeal of a section or other provision, the reference shall be considered to be made to that section or other provision of the Federal Food, Drug, and Cosmetic Act (21 USC 301 et seq.).

(c) TABLE OF CONTENTS- The table of contents for this Act is as follows". . .

In (b), we see that FDAMA makes express reference to the FDCA, as it reads in the USC, in title 21. Here, the section in parenthesis refers to the USC citation. A lot of the provisions that follow are simply instructions to the editors of the USC, telling the editors what words and punctuation marks to change. One can only understand the intent and operation of the new law by making these changes and reading the now edited text. Notice that each public law has its own table of contents and section numbers, and that these section numbers aren't the same as those in the code. Each public law follows its own outline numbering system, and the code, because it incorporates all changes from all public laws, has a much larger outline and many more numbers.

For example, FDAMA added the fast track for drug products. The relevant section in FDAMA is section 112, but the part of the code that is affected is different. FDAMA actually reads, at section 112, as follows:

SEC. 112. EXPEDITING STUDY AND APPROVAL OF FAST TRACK DRUGS.

(a) IN GENERAL—Chapter V (21 USC 351 et seq.), as amended by section 125, is amended by inserting before section 508 the following:

SEC. 506. FAST TRACK PRODUCTS.

(a) DESIGNATION OF DRUG AS A FAST TRACK PRODUCT-

(1) 'IN GENERAL—The Secretary shall, at the request of the sponsor of a new drug, facilitate the development and expedite the review of such drug if it is intended for the treatment of a serious or life-threatening condition and it demonstrates the potential to address unmet medical needs for such a condition. (In this section, such a drug is referred to as a 'fast track product'.)

FDAMA refers to the FDCA and changes it first. This is how FDAMA section on fast track products is added to the FDCA[11] (and, by implication, the USC):

SEC. 506. [356] FAST TRACK PRODUCTS.

(a) DESIGNATION OF DRUG AS A FAST TRACK PRODUCT.—

(1) IN GENERAL—The Secretary shall, at the request of the sponsor of a new drug, facilitate the development and expedite the review of such drug if it is intended for the treatment of a serious or life-threatening condition and it demonstrates the potential to address unmet medical needs for such a condition. (In this section, such a drug is referred to as a "fast track product").

The language, as you see, is the same in both versions. The real test is where does one find this language in the code? The FDA has mapped this out for you, by noting the *code* section in brackets, which is put in bold here— section 506 **[356]**.

Looking at section 356 in 21 USC produces the following language:

SUBCHAPTER V—DRUGS AND DEVICES Part A—Drugs and Devices Sec. 356. Fast track products (a) Designation of drug as fast track product (1) In general The Secretary shall, at the request of the sponsor of a new drug, facilitate the development and expedite the review of such drug if it is intended for the treatment of a serious or life-threatening condition and it demonstrates the potential to address unmet medical needs for such a condition. (In this section, such a drug is referred to as a "fast track product".)

The words are the same; it is the classification and numbering system that changes with the source you are using. Only the public laws contain the instructions for actually editing the main body of law, in our case, the FDCA, and by making those changes, impacting the USC itself.

13. What Do All These Numbers Mean? What Is a Citation?

The numbers identify sections and paragraphs of the law and make up the "citation." Happily, Google and many other search engines think of numbers as

---

[11] Taken from the FDA's Web site, http://www.fda.gov/opacom/laws/fdcact/fdcact5a.htm, which shows the sections for both the Food, Drug, and Cosmetic Act and the U.S. Code.

text, so if you type in the citation, in quotation marks, you can often go right to the actual law. This search technique also works for regulations.

The U.S. Office of Patents and Trademarks has published a wonderful graphic and a definition set at its Mumbo Jumbo Gumbo page:[12]

- **What is a (35 USC §123(a)) or a (15 CFR 123(a))?**
- **A **citation** is a listing for a law or regulation which includes the title or chapter number, the name of the collection, and the sections and paragraph numbers.*

USC means United States Code and CFR means Code of Federal Regulations

These citations* are shorthand for the laws and regulations that explain in precise terms what is needed in order for the Federal government to do business. Each is a citation which refers to a particular section of the law or its implementing regulations.

Each law is signed by the President after being enacted by votes of the House of Representatives and Senate. Many new laws are assigned a number in the United States Code which reflects their relationship to similar laws or laws that govern similar programs. The way laws are created follow a formal process which you can learn more about from "How Our Laws are Made."

The Code of Federal Regulations is written to explain in detail how the laws are to be carried out. When a law is written, it usually does not explain in great detail what procedures are to be followed, nor does it include descriptions of the special situations which can arise. This is the job of the regulations, which govern the day-to-day business of the Federal government.

Regulations are actually written by the government agencies responsible for the subject matter of the laws. The United States Patent and Trademark Office writes the regulations concerning patents and trademarks which are found in Title 37 of the CFR.

Below are diagrams explaining how to read these notations:[13]

(This covers the U.S. laws.)

---

[12] See http://www.uspto.gov/web/offices/ac/ahrpa/opa/kids/special/mumbo.htm.

[13] U.S. PTO Web site, supra.

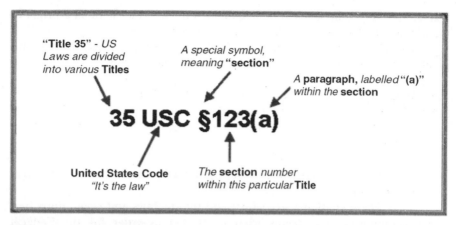

(This covers regulations.)

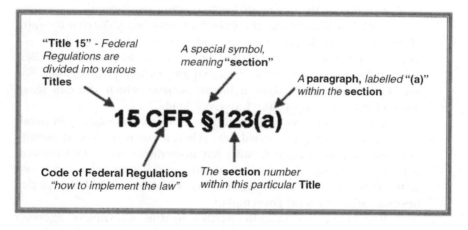

14. Why Can't I Find Section 510(k) in the USC?

Don't panic. "They" have not eliminated that wonderful loophole, known as the "same-as" or "me-too" exemption for devices. The section number by which the provision is known refers to the FDCA. In the FDCA, the numbering system places that section at 510(k). When the amendments were incorporated into the USC, the appropriate numbering system was section 360(k). Again, the FDA Web site assists with the cross-reference. The actual chart of conversions is available at www.fda.gov/opacom/laws/crossref.html; it is accessible from the FDA home page, linking to "Laws FDA Enforces," and from there to "cross-reference."

For the disbelievers, here is the infamous section; the number in brackets indicates the USC section, 21 USC 360. The actual provision reads as follows:[14]

---

[14] See the FDA's Web site, as noted above.

510(k) REGISTRATION OF PRODUCERS OF DRUGS AND DEVICES[1]

SEC. 510. [360]

(a) As used in this section . . . .

(k) Each person who is required to register under this section and who proposes to begin the introduction or delivery for introduction into interstate commerce for commercial distribution of a device intended for human use shall, at least ninety days before making such introduction or delivery, report to the Secretary (in such form and manner as the Secretary shall by regulation prescribe)–

> (1) the class in which the device is classified under section 513 or if such person determines that the device is not classified under such section, a statement of that determination and the basis for such person's determination that the device is or is not so classified, and
>
> (2) action taken by such person to comply with requirements under section 514 or 515 which are applicable to the device.

15. Who Enforces Laws?

At times it seems like everybody does. The fact is that the executive branch of government is charged with enforcing laws. This list includes the Department of Justice, drug enforcement administration (DEA) agents, the federal bureau of investigation (FBI), and state police for criminal matters, and for our purposes, the FDA inspectors for civil matters. However, an FDA inspector may uncover something troublesome and refer a matter out for criminal investigation, so treat all folks carefully.

16. What Is a "Regulation"?

A regulation is a binding instruction issued by an agency (in our case, the FDA) that tells you how to interpret and comply with a law. Regulations are MUST FOLLOWS—that is, if you fail to follow a regulation, and you have an inspection, the FDA inspector must write up your failure on a 483; failures to follow regulations usually end up in the "issued warning letter" section of the FDA Web site, not a good place to be.

Another group of folks who are really interested in regulations and whether or not you comply with them are the lawyers. Any injury to any person caused by any medical product is made far more lucrative if the manufacturer, sponsor, contract research organization (CRO) or other responsible party failed to do what the regulations required them to do. The economics is really simple—injury plus failure to follow regulation equals money from the irresponsible (and hopefully insured) party for the injured, including the legal fees owed to the lawyer to get to the money.

17. What Is the Difference Between a Law and a Regulation?

They come from different branches of government and have different functions. However, each must be obeyed.

Laws come from legislative bodies, like Congress, and set policy in broad terms. Regulations come from the executive branch, and provide details on how laws are to be implemented, or obeyed. The FDA is part of the executive branch of government and is under HHS. HHS is a cabinet agency, whose secretary reports to the president.

Congress sometimes directs the executive branche to issue regulations. That was the case with FDAMA, where Congress decreed that regulations concerning dissemination of information on unapproved products be issued. The FDA did promulgate an initial set of regulations, which restricted the amounts and types of information manufacturers could publish concerning unapproved products. Litigation ensued over the breadth of the regulation, and the courts ultimately decided the regulation was overly broad, in that it infringed constitutional rights of commercial free speech, and so struck down the existing regulation.

While the courts have the power to nullify regulations that are not consistent with the statutes, have been improperly issued (usually meaning that there have been inadequate public hearings), or exceed the agency's authority, these cases are really few and far between. Most of the time, the FDA's regulations are given great deference by a court, and are upheld.

My general advice is "don't sue" the FDA. The reason is pure economics. A lawsuit will delay your product from clearance/approval. Courts are backlogged, and delays can be substantial. Say you have a product whose potential revenues are $12 million a year—not an unrealistic estimate for many drugs worth pursuing. If you lost even six months (an unrealistically short time) in a court proceeding, you have lost $6 million. Even a day's delay would cost you more than $32,876. If you can work out something that the FDA will allow, some resubmission that you can do in six weeks, the six-week delay would have cost only $1.3 million compared with the $6 million loss for the court delay. And that $6 million assumes you win in court, and the FDA doesn't appeal. If the case drags on for three years, you have lost $36 million and, more than likely, three valuable years of patent exclusivity. So, unless you are manufacturing cigarettes, you don't have much to gain by suing.

18. Which Is More Important—a Law or a Regulation?

The problem for regulators is that both are equally important. Violation of laws can result in criminal penalties, but hopefully no one is reading this chapter with an eye to "cutting it close on the out-of-jail" end of things. Violation of regulations results in warning letters, which is why a lot of "old-timers" in the industry insist that "a regulation is a law you follow."

19. What Is the Difference Between the USC and the CFR?

The USC stands for the United States Code and contains *laws*. The CFR stands for the Code of Federal Regulations and contains *regulations*. The CFR does *not* have laws, and the USC does *not* have regulations. The USC is enacted by Congress and the CFR is the domain of the executive branch, in our case, HHS.

A CRF has nothing to do with either one of them. CRF stands for "Case Report Form."

20. How Do I Find a Current Regulation?

You can find current regulations by *always* checking the revision date of the Web page you are reading. You'll be surprised to know that the FDA doesn't always have the most current regulation available via its Web site.

In the year 2007, each time I checked the regulation on prescription drug advertising using the FDA Web page, CFR link,[15] the link connected me with an old version, which did not have any of the language concerning Internet advertisements. This regulation did have the FDA logo across the top. This does not mean that the FDA is only enforcing the old version of the regulation, and you would have freedom to post whatever you wanted. It means only that a careful regulator knows to check the date, which is in the upper left corner most of the time, to be sure the date is within 12 months of your access.

This graphic[16] shows where to find the version date.

```
Code of Federal Regulations]
[Title 21, Volume 4]
[Revised as of April 1, 2007]
[CITE: 21CFR202.1]
```

TITLE 21—FOOD AND DRUGS
CHAPTER I—FOOD AND DRUG ADMINISTRATION
DEPARTMENT OF HEALTH AND HUMAN SERVICES
SUBCHAPTER C—DRUGS: GENERAL

PART 202 – PRESCRIPTION DRUG ADVERTISING
Sec. 202.1 Prescription-drug advertisements.

In using this method, you must remember that the CFR title governing the FDA is updated only once a year, on April 1. This is important for historic reasons, to determine what regulation was in effect at the time a new drug application (NDA) was submitted, for example, or what part 50 required when

---

[15] Accessible from www.fda.gov.

[16] See www.accessdata.fda.gov/scripts/cdrh/cfdocs/cfcfr/CFRSearch.cfm?fr=202.1.

you were conducting the investigation. For information on which regulation is in effect today, the government has developed an electronic code of federal regulations site,[17] which is reflected in the following graphic:

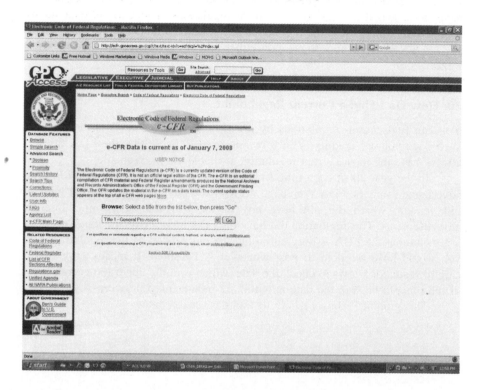

If you are not using the e-CFR (because you need the more robust text search engine at the CFR main page from GPOAccess), you will see that there are specific revision dates for each chapter. For 21 CFR, it is April 1. That date tells you that the version you are looking at contains regulations published and in effect up to March 31.

To determine whether or not there are any changes to a particular regulation, search the *Federal Register* for any published changes to the regulation, from April 1 through the date that is important to you. You can also use e-CFR.

It is good to know that all new regulations, guidances, proposals, and drafts must be printed in the *Federal Register*. However, the *Federal Register* link from the FDA home page does not access the actual register. The FDA link brings you to a calendar, with notations of docket numbers. The docket numbers are printed in the calendar days when the FDA has some activity on the *Federal Register*. This is a great reference if you are interested in meetings, but won't help you

---

[17] See http://ecfr.gpoaccess.gov/cgi/t/text/text-idx?c=ecfr&tpl=%2Findex.tpl.

find a new regulation or guidance. To do that, you need the GPOAccess page, found at www.gpoaccess.gov/fr/index.html. From there, you can insert your regulation citation ("21 CFR Part XX") or keyword, and see what has happened. A "No" or "0" result does *not* mean that the regulation no longer exists; it means that there were no changes to the regulation during the time period you have specified.

This *Federal Register* page is one of my favorite haunts. I use it to see if there are any regulation changes in the offing, find older versions of regulations (you will need these to establish what the rules were when you started a trial, process, etc.), and also keep abreast of what guidances FDA has contemplated or issued that may be relevant. This is one of the best government sites around. Take some time to learn the advanced search features; you won't be sorry.

You can usually buy hard copies of the code, whether on disk or in paper. Many professionals I admire continue to make these purchases, despite the fact that regulations are available electronically. The same reasons apply here as for purchasing the code—you must click through each section, cannot easily go forward or back, and can't write in the margins.

21. How Do I Find Older Regulations?

For example, say you want to know what regulation was in effect on June 30, 2003. The current edition of 21 CFR goes up to April 1, 2003. That leaves the period between April and June 30 out. You can go to the *Federal Register* and refine your search to the dates between April 1, 2003 and June 30, 2003 to determine if there were any changes. I like to overlap my date searches, so that I catch any changes that are in progress on the edition date. It is more than likely that the April 1 edition will contain regulations that become effective on April 1, but by starting my *Federal Register* search on March 31, I overlap a day and remove all doubt.

22. What Is "Guidance"?

The FDA issues guidance on a number of subjects. As the lead paragraph says, the guidance represents the agency's thinking, but is not binding. That means you should read it to determine what the agency's view on a subject is or was at a particular time. The disclaimer also means that following a guidance does not guarantee that your application will be filed. Some guidances are, by the agency's own admission, hopelessly out of date, but it just hasn't gotten around to revising them yet.

You should discuss what guidances to follow at the preliminary meetings you hold with your FDA reviewers. This removes all doubt about what you are expected to do, and hopefully makes the job easier. You should always read and understand a relevant guidance before your preliminary meeting, so you can ask intelligent questions about how the guidance impacts your application. There is a central listing of guidances available from the FDA's Web site. You can check your results by searching your center for applicable guidances.

23. Tips For Using Search Engines

A "search engine" is a computer program that looks for information on the Internet, also known as the worldwide Web. Most search engines use "text searches," which means that you type in a topic or a few words that you want to find (called a "search string"—a "string" of words) and the search engine then takes that text and looks in various Web sites for the same text. When the search engine finds your text on a Web site, you have a "hit."

Search engines are sometimes called "spiders" by their programmer inventors, playing off the worldwide Web image. (Spiders spin webs and then crawl over them, looking for prey.)

Most engines use "text," that is, words, to find things. You list a word, and then the engine generally goes to the title line of a Web page to see if your word is in the title, or somewhere on that page. If your search word is there, the spider will usually bring the page back to you and display it.

Lucky for us, the spider doesn't bring back *every* page that matches your word. First, there are simply too many pages on the Web, and more are added every day. It may take a search engine a month to check all of the Web pages that exist, so unless you are willing to wait 30 days or more, you won't get all of the most recent Web pages in your search. Next, not all Web pages are accessible to spiders.

I recommend the tutorial at the University of California Berkley Web site; the same page refers scholars to Wikipedia for information on the "Deep Web," where no search engines go. Know the limitations and use the tutorial to determine what information is worth getting.

While Google is one of the best-known search engines, competition is heating up. Be aware of ranking and how it works (ranking is how low a hit number a site has, the lower being the more frequently accessed). The low number can indicate a high number of hits, but also a hefty payment to improve visibility. Try doing the same search string with several engines, including the so-called "mega-search" engines, like Dogpile (www.dogpile.com), which combines Google, Yahoo!®, and Ask™ to name a few.

For a critique of Google, an analysis of its rankings, discussion of privacy issues, and essentially another perspective, check out Google-Watch, at www .google-watch.org. Addresses without the hyphen are commercial and will not get you the same results.

So, user beware. A big thing to remember about search engine results— just because you didn't find the information you were looking for doesn't mean the information doesn't exist. It only means you didn't find it.

There are a couple of reasons why you didn't find what you were looking for. One, the information simply may not be posted on a Web site that you can access for free. This is unfortunately true with many court decisions and regulations. As state funding is cut back, fewer and fewer states go to the expense of putting all their laws and court decisions online. Two, you may not have plugged in the right text for your search or chosen the right search engine.

A couple of things can go wrong with any search. You can get way too many hits, you can get the wrong hits, and you can get nothing. So, let's deal with the easy things first. Like getting too many hits. Say I want to know how much a parking fine is in the Town of Arlington, Massachusetts. I type in "fine" and "Arlington." I end up with "fine arts," "fine art framing," Arlington Heights, Virginia, Arlington, Texas, fine homes, fine dining, fine weather—you get the picture. A search engine can't distinguish between different meanings for words in a text search. So, the spider on my Google search is replete with success, having found about 347,000 hits for me to peruse. I, however, have not gotten the information I wanted. I can only have gotten the information I wanted if the Town of Arlington, Massachusetts had a Web site and that Web site has the information about parking fines, and if I limited my search to "parking fines" *and* "Arlington, Massachusetts." This time, the search was successful. Google produced 763 hits, and the first one was "Traffic Rules, Article 10, Arlington, Massachusetts." When I hit on the link, I was thwarted. The message was that the Web page was temporarily out of order, had moved, etc., etc. However, Google has a feature that bailed me out. I moved the cursor to the "cached" line, and lo and behold, a list of parking fines appeared (it is $10 for all night parking; same as for an expired meter). Google has this neat feature of putting into memory—its cache—copies of the Web pages. So, as long as I know the Arlington selectmen didn't vote to increase parking fines last night, looking at the old, Google-saved cache worked just fine.

A search engine will not substitute synonyms or concepts for your text. If you want to find out the gross sales of Tylenol® and its generic equivalents, you must know that "acetaminophen" is the active ingredient in Tylenol. More to the point, you must be aware of specific terms or names used to identify concepts, laws, and regulations. Many industry folks refer to the 21 CFRs part 50 as the "Informed Consent Regulation." In fact, the true title of part 50 is "Protection of Human Subjects." Your brain can make the connection between the two titles, but a search engine using text cannot. So, sometimes you have to peruse a table of contents to find what you are really looking for. Lastly, a text search engine will not correct spelling. So, even if you know the correct title for part 50, and type in "protection for humane subjects," the search won't succeed.

In conclusion, time spent learning these terms and citations should give you a great start in getting and keeping your products in regulatory compliance!

13

FDA Advisory Committees

Christina A. McCarthy and David S. Mantus
Cubist Pharmaceuticals, Inc., Lexington, Massachusetts, U.S.A.

INTRODUCTION

An integral part of the Food and Drug Administration's (FDA) mission is to protect the public health by assuring the safety, efficacy, and security of human drugs, biological products, and medical devices. Because of the great magnitude and implication of this mission, the FDA occasionally calls upon external experts for advice and counsel. One of the ways that the FDA can access external scientific expertise is through the use of the FDA advisory committee system. Advisory committees have been under considerable scrutiny over the past decade and the system has been a focus of congressional oversight. According to 21 Code of Federal Regulations (CFR) 14.5(a), "An advisory committee is utilized to conduct public hearings on matters of importance that come before FDA, to review the issues involved, and to provide advice and recommendations to the Commissioner." Utilizing advisory committees, the FDA can seek advice and input from scientific and medical experts, consumers, and patient advocacy groups on a number of issues ranging from approvals of new medical products to providing guidance on appropriate methods of clinical investigation. The advisory committee system is most frequently employed in reviewing products or topics that are controversial; however, the FDA is not bound to the recommendations of the advisory committee.

According to Dr. Linda A. Suydam, D.P.A., former senior associate commissioner of the FDA:

"The FDA advisory committee system was established to provide independent expertise and technical assistance related to the development and evaluation of products regulated by the FDA; to lend credibility to the product review process; to speed the review of products by providing a visible sharing of the responsibility for evaluation and judgment; to provide a forum for public discussion on matters of significant public interest; to allow sponsors and consumer to stay current with trends in the product development and review process and changes in regulations and guidelines related to FDA-regulated industries; and to provide external review of FDA intramural research programs."[1]

HISTORICAL AND REGULATORY FRAMEWORK

Informally, the FDA's practice of seeking external scientific and consumer advice began in 1964.[2] An early example of this practice includes a series of meetings held by the FDA, in which it consulted manufacturing and nutritional experts, as well as the general population, regarding what types of ingredients should be included in white bread.[3] Formal implementation of the system as we know it today, however, did not occur until the enactment of the Federal Advisory Committee Act of 1972 (FACA).

FACA was passed by Congress in 1972 to provide federal agencies with a formal mechanism for seeking external expertise and advice. The purpose of federal advisory committees is to "provide independent, expert, and objective advice on policy, the funding of research, and other issues."[4,5] This act was passed in part because of concern by some legislators that there were too many informal and secret advisory committees within sectors of the federal government.[5] FACA created a formal system that allowed government agencies to seek external advice, ensuring appropriate checks and balances. FACA also defines the operation of federal advisory committees and emphasizes the importance of public involvement in the advisory committee system.

In 1997, the Food and Drug Administration Modernization Act (FDAMA) amended the Food, Drug, and Cosmetic Act [21 United States Code (USC) 355],

[1] Department of Health and Human Services Web site. Assistant secretary for legislation (ASL). Testimony on vaccine advisory committees by Linda A. Suydam, D.P.A., senior associate commissioner, Food and Drug Administration, Department of Health and Human Services, before the Committee on Government Reform, U.S. House of Representatives. June 15, 2000. Available at: http://www.hhs.gov/asl/testify/t000615a.html. Accessed January 17, 2006.

[2] Farley D. Getting outside advice for close calls. FDA consumer special report. January 1995. Available at: http://www.fda.gov/fdac/special/newdrug/advice.html. Accessed January 10, 2006.

[3] Lewis C. Advisory committees: FDA's primary stakeholders have a say. FDA Consumer Magazine September-October 2000. Available at: http://www.fda.gov/fdac/features/2000/500_adv.html. Accessed January 10, 2006.

[4] Federal Advisory Committee Act. 5 USC App. 1 Publ L. 92-463. Available at: http://www.accessreports.com/statutes/FACA.htm. Accessed January 14, 2006.

[5] Steinbrook R. Science, politics, and federal advisory committees. N Engl J Med 2004; 350(14): 1454–1460. Available at: http://content.nejm.org/cgi/content/full/353/2/116. Accessed January 20, 2006.

directing the FDA to establish or use panels of experts to provide advice on the research and approval of drugs.[6] FDAMA focused on advisory board membership, including improving training and defining conflicts of interest, as well as stressing the need for timely considerations and notifications of committee deliberations.[7] Inclusion of provisions for use of advisory committees in FDAMA reinforced the importance of the advisory committee system within the FDA.

Most recently, the Food and Drug Administration Amendments Act of 2007 (FDAAA) included additional provisions for the advisory committee system. Most notably, FDAAA stipulates that before a new drug (specifically, "a drug no active ingredient (including any ester or salt of the active ingredient) of which has been approved in any other application") is approved, the Secretary must refer the new drug for review at an advisory committee. If the drug is not referred to an advisory committee for review prior to approval, the action letter must include the reasons stating why.[8] The effect of this stipulation on the advisory committee system, as well as on industry as a whole, may be significant. Delays may be experienced if advisory committees are regulatory held prior to each new drug approval. As the FDA begins to implement FDAAA's new requirements, we will be able to better assess the impact of this provision on the new drug approval process.

The advisory committee system is highly regulated. 21CFR14 describes almost every operational aspect of the advisory committee system. The detailed regulation provides a platform for uniform application of the advisory committee system throughout the government. Since the enactment of FACA, the FDA has also issued a number of guidance documents on the advisory committee system, ranging from guidance detailing the impact of FDAMA on the advisory committee system to multiple documents discussing disclosure of confidential information and management of conflicts of interest.

The FDA advisory committee Web site includes general information, such as guidance documents, frequently asked questions (FAQs), meeting schedules, and transcripts from previous meetings. Detailed information on each committee, including financial status and membership rosters, are available for public review on the federal advisory committee database Web site.[9]

STRUCTURE

As detailed in 21CFR14.100, the FDA has 35 standing advisory committees. In addition to the standing advisory committees, the FDA uses policy and technical advisory committees. While all of the centers at the FDA each have at least one

---

[6] FDA Modernization Act of 1997. Publ. L. 105–115. November 1997. S. 830.

[7] U.S. Food and Drug Administration Web site. FDA advisory committees. Available at: http://www .fda.gov/oc/advisory/default.htm. Accessed January 9, 2006.

[8] Food and Drug Administration Amendments Act of 2007. Available at: http://www.fda.gov/oc/ initiatives/advance/fdaaa.html. Accessed December 27, 2007.

[9] Federal Advisory Committee Database Web site. Available at: http://www.fido.gov/facadatabase/. Accessed January 6, 2006.

advisory committee, 90% of standing FDA advisory committees can be found within the FDA's three major centers handling human medicinal products. While there are only 35 standing advisory committees detailed in the regulations, review of the FDA advisory committee Web site indicates that there are additional active advisory committees.[7]

Those FDA advisory committees that are not mandated by law are created at will by the Department of Health and Human Services (DHHS). Committees are chartered for two years; at the end of the two-year term, the FDA, in conjunction with DHHS, must determine whether the committee should continue its service. If the committee is no longer useful to the FDA, it is dissolved.

Each FDA center is responsible for the general administration of its advisory committees. However, because there may be variability between the centers in regard to how advisory committees are managed, there is a central office, which is responsible for the general administration of the FDA advisory committee system. The Advisory Committee Oversight and Management Staff is an office within the FDA, whose primary function is to ensure that the advisory committee system runs smoothly. This office handles member training as well as administrative aspects such as organizing travel and reimbursement for committee members.

COMPOSITION

The FDA advisory committees are made up of various individuals who range from practicing clinicians to individual patients/consumers. The membership roster includes those individuals who are considered standing members, but the law also provides the opportunity to call upon other individuals on a temporary basis. At certain types of meetings, depending on the type of input that the FDA is seeking, a vote may be necessary; however, not all members are voting members. Regulations explicitly define which members can vote; voting status is dependent upon the type of committee (standing, policy, or technical) on which members serve (21CFR14.80).

FACA requires that all advisory committee members be appropriately trained. As such, the Advisory Committee Oversight and Management Staff provides training to all advisory committee members.

Membership Type

In general, the role of an FDA advisory committee member is to provide independent advice and expertise to questions asked by the FDA on a particular topic or product. FACA mandates diverse committee membership representing the general public. The FDA takes measures to ensure the diversity of its advisory committees with regard to demography as well as professional/scientific expertise. All outside members who are hired by the FDA for their input on advisory committees, except for industry representatives, are considered special government employees

(SGEs).[10] Members are paid per day of committee meeting service and are reimbursed for travel, food, and lodging expenses. The payment, however, is minimal. According to a consumer special report article published by the FDA in 1995, members only receive $150 a day during meeting service.[2]

For each advisory committee there is an executive secretary and a committee chairperson. The executive secretary is an FDA employee who is assigned to oversee the general administration of the advisory committee. The executive secretary does not participate as an advisory committee member, but rather as a liaison between the FDA and the committee. The executive secretary ensures that all regulations are followed in committee conduct. In contrast, the committee chairperson, mandated by 21CFR14.30, is a committee member and is most often one of the more experienced members, and has the authority to conduct hearings and meetings.

With the implementation of FDAMA, advisory committee membership is divided between core membership and ad hoc membership. Core members are those individuals who are appointed by the commissioner on the basis of scientific expertise, while ad hoc members are those that are asked to serve on committees when needed. The standard term of service is usually four years, and membership extensions are rarely given.[11]

Members of the FDA advisory committees include scientists/academicians/practitioners, consumers, patients, and industry representatives. Each of these types of members plays a different and important role on the advisory committee panel. According to a 2001 FDA survey, 80% of advisory committee members are scientists, followed by consumers, industry representatives, and then patient representatives.[12] The academicians/practitioners are frequently employed as chairperson because of their expertise in the field. The role of an industry representative is to provide advice and address concerns from an industry standpoint. While any one industry member will have individual ties to a particular company, their role is not to represent that specific company, but rather to represent the industry as a whole.[13] Industry representatives are permitted membership on advisory committees, but because of conflict of interest concerns, industry members are by law always nonvoting.[7]

---

[10] Sherman, L.A. Looking through a window of the Food and Drug Administration: FDA's advisory committee system. Preclinica: A BioTechniques Publications March/April 2004. 2(2). Available at: http://www.preclinica.com/default.asp?page=articles&issue=0304. Accessed January 6, 2006.

[11] U.S. Food and Drug Administration Web site. Advisory committee 101: member selection. Available at: http://www.fda.gov/oc/advisory/Presentations/NMT05/NMT05TalkShermanLinda. pps#395,39,Member Selection (Varies Somewhat by Member Type). Accessed January 10, 2006.

[12] U.S. Food and Drug Administration Web site. FDA advisory committee new member training. April 20, 2005. Available at: http://www.fda.gov/oc/advisory/Presentations/NMT05/NMT2005 Agenda.html. Accessed January 10, 2006.

[13] Rados, C. Advisory committees: critical to the FDA's product review process. FDA Consumer Magazine. January-February 2004. Available at: http://www.fda.gov/fdac/features/2004/104_adv.html. Accessed January 10, 2006.

One of the most important aspects of the FDA advisory committee system is public involvement in important and/or controversial issues, products, and policies that the FDA is considering. The public is formally involved in advisory committees through consumer representative membership. The FDA is careful to ensure that the consumer representative is well qualified to handle the scientific nature of the discussions, as well as be a true representative of the public, and not simply provide an individual opinion.[14]

Patient representatives are intended to bring a unique and humanistic viewpoint to advisory committees. Patient representation allows for the input of those individuals who are directly affected by the issue or product being discussed. Historically, it was the HIV/AIDS patient advocacy groups that lobbied the FDA for representation in the decisions being made regarding drug approvals. Committee members were initially resistant to the inclusion of patient representatives; however, patient members provided valuable input, and today their representation is highly respected.[3] Currently, patient representatives are predominantly used on advisory committees handling HIV/AIDS and oncology issues; however, the FDA requests patient representation on other advisory committees, discussing serious and/or life-threatening illnesses on an ad hoc basis.[15] Patient representatives usually have had direct experience, individually or through a family member, with the disease being discussed, and can articulate how the disease affects quality of life. Oftentimes, the patients are well informed and have formal affiliations with advocacy groups.[16] While patient representatives can be both voting and nonvoting, patient representatives who are members on advisory committees that review oncology products/therapies are voting members, and those representatives serving on most other nononcologic advisory committees are nonvoting. The FDA maintains a comprehensive Web site on patient representation for those individuals interested in participating in the program.[15]

Qualification Requirements

21CFR14.80 details membership qualifications; these are dependent on the type of committee represented, and the regulation mandates that members have diverse interests, education, training, and experience. However, technical expertise, unless as a member on a technical committee, is not a formal requirement.

---

[14] U.S. Food and Drug Administration Web site. Advisory committee consumer representatives. Available at: www.fda.gov/oc/advisory/consumer.html. Accessed January 10, 2006.

[15] U.S. Food and Drug Administration Web site. FDA patient representative program. Available at: http://www.fda.gov/oashi/patrep/patientrep.html#apply. Accessed January 10, 2006.

[16] Meadows, M. Bringing real life to the table: Patient reps help FDA review products. FDA Consumer Magazine. January-February 2002. Available at: http://www.fda.gov/fdac/features/2002/102_real.html. Accessed January 10, 2006.

Appointment Process

The nomination and selection process of committee advisory members is highly regulated. For voting members of standing advisory committees, the process begins with the commissioner publishing a notice in the Federal Register requesting nominations. Nominations are then screened by the appropriate product divisions within the Centers to ensure that the nominee possesses the required expertise and to screen for potential conflicts of interest.[11] Persons nominated and selected in this manner serve on the committee as an individual and not as an advocate for a larger organization (e.g., consumer representative).

For consumer and industry representatives, a request for nomination is published in the Federal Register. For consumer representatives, the regulations urge that nominations be filtered through consumer advocacy groups. For industry representatives, regulations state that the industry organizations with corresponding member nominees are to decide among themselves who is to be the representative. If no decision is made, then the commissioner selects the industry representative.

Anyone can nominate a candidate to serve as a patient representative.[15] Nominations are sent to the FDA patient representative program where the selection process is vetted.

Membership Training

The FDA is required by law to provide training to every advisory committee member prior to participation in a committee meeting. All members undergo a comprehensive training program run by the FDA staff. The FDA advisory committee new member training program is available for public review on the FDA Web site.[11] In addition to the formal member training, patient representatives are oriented by the Office of Special Health Issues. According to the FDA's patient representative Web site, newly selected patient members receive training on an individual basis, which includes observing an advisory committee meeting and discussions with previous patient representatives.

CONFLICTS OF INTEREST

While many aspects of the FDA's advisory committee system have been scrutinized, nothing has been more controversial and closely examined than member conflict of interest. Because many of the advisory committee members are also experts in their respective fields, they are often closely involved with cutting edge research. It is because of their direct knowledge of new research and/or products that the FDA seeks their advice. Sometimes, however, members' involvement in research is closely linked to the development of specific products, which can become an issue when it is on those products that the FDA is seeking advice. While there can be many types of conflicts of interest, the primary conflict with which the

FDA is concerned is financial. Prior to every advisory meeting, committee members are sent a confidential questionnaire (FDA form 3410, "Conflict of Interest Disclosure Report for SGEs"), which asks about financial interests in regard to the product or the product's sponsor to be discussed at the meeting. Along with the form, a list of all products and sponsors associated with the meeting is sent. Using this information, the member is asked to determine if they have financial interest in anything that is being reviewed. Financial interests can range from direct investments in a particular company to receiving research grants from a sponsor whose product is under review.[1]

Once the FDA receives the completed financial disclosure form, it is then determined whether, and to what extent, a member has a conflict of interest. If there is a conflict, the FDA staff determines if the conflict qualifies for a waiver, or, if it is too significant, the conflicted member should be excluded from the meeting. Most often this decision is made by the FDA official from the division or office, requesting the advisory committee's assistance.[1] The Director of Advisory Committed Oversight and Management is also closely involved in the determination of conflicts of interest.[17] Furthermore, if there is any question about any waivers that are granted, an independent review by the FDA Ethics office is conducted.

Advisory committee members are subject to two conflict of interest laws, under which criminal prosecution is possible. The Criminal Conflict of Interest statute regulates conflict of interest for all federal government employees, including SGEs; since voting advisory committee members are considered SGEs, these members are subject to the law (18 USC 208). FDAMA included provisions for conflict of interest management, and more recently, FDAAA expanded on those provisions in an attempt to make the process simpler and more transparent.[6,8]

Conflict of Interest Waivers

According to the Criminal Conflict of Interest statute, if an SGE has a financial conflict of interest then they are not allowed to participate in related advisory committee meetings unless a waiver of exclusion is granted.[18] The Criminal Conflict of Interest statute, FDAMA, and FDAAA, however, include provisions which allow for waivers of conflicts of interest.

18 USC 208 (b) allows for three types of waivers to be granted to advisory committee members with conflicts of interest. The first type of waiver is for federal employees serving on an advisory committee and experts who are performing tasks

---

[17] U.S. Food and Drug Administration Web site. Draft guidance for the public, FDA advisory committee members, and FDA staff on procedures for determining conflict of interest and eligibility for participation in FDA advisory committees. Available at: http://www.fda.gov/oc/advisory/waiver/COIguidedft.html. Accessed October 20 2007.

[18] U.S. Food and Drug Administration Web site. Guidance for FDA advisory committee members and other special government employees on conflict of interest 2000. Available at: http://www.fda.gov/oc/advisory/conflictofinterest/waiver.html. Accessed January 24, 2006.

other than serving on an advisory committee. This waiver is granted when the financial interest is determined not to be significant enough to affect outcomes. The second type of waiver is for committee members participating in meetings; this waiver is slightly more lax than the first waiver. This waiver is granted when it is determined that "the need for the individual's services outweighs the potential for a conflict of interest." The third type of waiver is for financial interests that are determined by regulation to be minimal by the Office of Government Ethics.

FDAMA included a provision for a waiver [which only applies to advisory committee members for Center for Drug Evaluation and Research (CDER) and Center for Biologics Evaluation and Research (CBER) panels], which allowed committee members to vote in a particular matter, from which they or an immediate family member may receive financial gain, if their expertise is essential (i.e., no one else has the needed expertise) to the committee.[5]

With the implementation of FDAAA, additional, more detailed requirements detailing how the FDA should address conflicts of interest for advisory committees have been enacted. Members, or their immediate family members, with financial interests with potential to affect the meeting, are prohibited from participating in the FDA advisory committee meetings. And while FDAAA maintains that the FDA has the authority to grant a waiver if the member's expertise is essential to the advisory committee, it does limit how many waivers the FDA can grant annually, and requires the publication of an annual report. Furthermore, FDAAA requires that the FDA review potential conflicts of interest when initially considering new members for advisory committees. In addition, FDAAA requires that all members of advisory committees disclose to the public any conflicts of interest in regard to the meeting's subject matter. In October 2007 draft guidance, the FDA states that prior to an advisory committee meeting each member must disclose the type, nature, and magnitude of any financial conflicts of interest, and stipulates that members cannot participate until this disclosure is made. The FDA will post the disclosure, along with any waiver granted by the agency, on the FDA Web site.[19]

In 1994, the FDA issued a guidance document titled "FDA Waiver Criteria," which outlined how, when, to whom, and under which conditions waivers may be granted for committee members with conflicts of interest. That document was updated in 2000 (titled "Waiver Criteria 2000"),[20] and more recently in 2007.[17] Because of the scrutiny of its financial conflict of interest policies, the FDA issued a draft guidance document in March 2007, which attempts to simplify the process by which the FDA assesses conflicts of interests and determines meeting participation, including the granting of waivers. In part, the guidance was intended to "enhance public trust" in the

---

[19] U.S. Food and Drug Administration Web site. Guidance for the public, FDA advisory committee members, and FDA staff: public availability of advisory committee members' financial interest information and waivers. Available at: http://www.fda.gov/oc/advisory/waiver/ACdisclosure1007 .html#_ftn1. Accessed December 13, 2007.

[20] U.S. Food and Drug Administration Web site. Conflict of interest. Available at: http://www.fda .gov/oc/advisory/conflictofinterest/intro.html. Accessed January 24, 2006.

advisory committee function by better describing the algorithm for determining when waivers for conflicts of interest are granted.[17] This algorithm is presented in Figure 1. The March 2007 draft guidance sets forth the following stipulations:

- Members should not participate in advisory committee meetings, regardless of need for expertise, if their disqualifying financial interest exceeds $50,000.
- When the disqualifying financial interest is less than $50,000, members can only participate when the need for the member's service outweighs the potential conflict, and can only participate as nonvoting members.
- The FDA can limit participation when there may be a perceived conflict of interest, even if none have been determined under law.

The FDA focuses primarily on individual financial conflicts of interest. While there are other types of conflicts, like previous involvement with a particular product/industry sponsor or an SGE's institutional potential financial gain, the FDA is often not required to grant a waiver in those broader situations; instead, only a public disclosure is made.[18]

FDA-Initiated Conflict of Interest Studies

Periodically, the FDA conducts surveys in which conflicts of interest in the advisory committee system are explored. In 2001, the FDA sent a survey out to 400 advisory committee members (SGEs). The survey asked general questions about members' attitudes toward conflicts of interest, particularly regarding public disclosure.[21] The FDA received answers from 73% of the members polled.[21] Member attitudes toward public disclosures is important because anytime a waiver is granted for a conflicted member, public disclosure is legally required. Of note, 65% of the respondents indicated that additional disclosure did not add credibility to the process, whereas 33% said it did.[22] Also notable were members' response to the question, "If FDA asked for more disclosure, I would. . . . " To this question, 58% answered that they would "act dependent on what was required" and 36% answered that they would "do what was asked."[22] Interestingly, 5% of the respondents answered that they would consider resignation, and one committee member responded that he or she would resign if the FDA asked for more disclosure.[22] Again, this is important information for the agency to know and consider when making policies on how far public disclosure should be taken. The FDA concluded

---

[21] U.S. Food and Drug Administration Web site. Brief report: SGE financial disclosure survey. Available at: http://www.fda.gov/oc/advisory/conflictofinterest/2001Survey/COISurveyRslts2001Q1 Intro.pdf. Accessed January 10, 2006.

[22] U.S. Food and Drug Administration Web site. Brief report: SGE financial disclosure survey. Q7. Available at: http://www.fda.gov/oc/advisory/conflictofinterest/2001Survey/COISurveyRslts2001Q7 ToQ11.pdf. Accessed January 10, 2006.

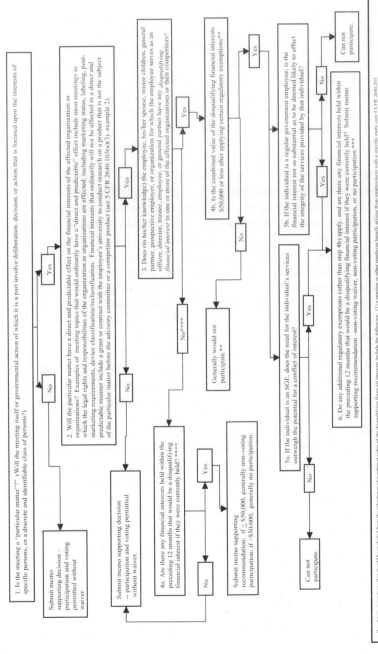

Figure 1 Algorithm for considering advisory committee member participation. *Source:* From http://www.fda.gov/oc/advisory/waiver/ACAlgorithm.pdf.

from the survey results that most members would be willing to publicly disclose more of their financial information; however, they also concluded that about half of the members indicated that continuation of membership was dependent on the severity of disclosure procedures.[23] While it is important to abide by the conflict of interest public disclosure laws, if the disclosures are so strict that committee members refuse to participate, then the system would be defunct.

In 2003, the FDA conducted a second survey titled "Conflicts of Interest and FDA Advisory Committee Meetings: A Study of Public Attitudes and Opinions."[24] The two-part study consisted of the FDA surveying attendees and advisory committee members from 11 advisory committee meetings throughout the spring of 2003. According to the study summary report, "The study's intent was to examine the perceived fairness and credibility of FDA advisory committee meetings related to FDA's management of real or potential conflicts of interest among advisory committee members."[24] The FDA was also interested in finding out how much audience members knew about the FDA's procedures to manage conflicts of interest, as well as how satisfied they were with the FDA's current conflict of interest procedures. Furthermore, the survey asked what aspect of the advisory committee meetings was most important to audience members and inquired about general satisfaction with the FDA.[24] The study summary stated that there was a 21% overall response rate by audience members polled and 66% response rate by the committee members who were polled.[24]

44.8% of the audience members indicated familiarity with the FDA's procedures for reviewing conflicts of interest of advisory committee members, but only 33.8% of the audience respondents considered themselves knowledgeable about how the FDA monitors conflicts of interest among its advisory committee members.[24] Furthermore, 75.1% of the audience indicated disagreement with the statement, "The FDA should not allow members with conflicts of interest to participate in any capacity at advisory committee meetings." Of note, 83.5% of audience respondents considered it "unreasonable to expect that advisory committee members won't have some conflicts of interest."[24] In regard to the most important aspects of advisory committee meetings, audience respondents stated that "Fairness of decision or outcomes" and "Committee members are top experts" were equally important aspects and of top importance. It is worth noting that 82% of the audience respondents were paid by an employer or organization to attend the meeting, and therefore it appears that the responses were industry heavy, and thus subject to bias.[24]

---

[23] U.S. Food and Drug Administration Web site. Comparing answers for all types of financial interest. Available at: http://www.fda.gov/oc/advisory/conflictofinterest/2001Survey/COISurveyRslts2001 AnlysCncl.pdf. Accessed January 10, 2006.

[24] U.S. Food and Drug Administration Web site. Conflicts of interest and FDA advisory committee meetings. Available at: http://www.fda.gov/oc/advisory/acstudy0904/JIFSANresearch.html. Accessed January 10, 2006.

In regard to the advisory committee member survey, while it was much shorter than the audience version, the overwhelming response was that the FDA's policies and procedures on conflicts of interest for the advisory committee system are impartial and are fair to both committee members and to the general public.

It is not evident what specific impact the two surveys have had on the FDA policies or decision making. Following the first survey, the FDA published a draft guidance titled "Draft Guidance on Disclosure of Conflicts of Interest for Special Government Employees Participating in FDA Product Specific Advisory Committees; Availability." It is important to note, however, that the FDA has not indicated that the guidance was a direct result of the SGE financial disclosure survey.

The FDA contracted Eastern Research Group, Inc. to assess the "relationship between expertise and financial conflicts of interest of FDA advisory committee members."[25] In October 2007, data on member expertise and conflict of interest were published. The study was based on a sample of advisory committee meetings held between December 2005 and October 2006. The study found that members with higher levels of expertise were more likely to have been granted waivers for conflicts of interest.[25] Of note, however, was that in the cases where expert members had financial conflicts of interest, alternative members with equal expertise, while easy to find, would also have similar conflicts of interest. For members granted waivers, it was reported that median total dollar value of financial interest was $14,500. The report concluded, "Overall we judge the ability to create alternative conflict-free advisory panels to be speculative. If possible, it would represent an uncertain and potentially substantial additional burden on the cost and the timeliness of advisory committee operations. Further, the FDA might not always be able to match the specialized expertise of some existing advisory committees."[25]

With the enactment of FDAAA, and the issuance of several draft guidance documents, it is evident that the FDA is taking matters of conflicts of interest in the advisory committee system seriously. The issue of conflicts of interest within the advisory committee system have been scrutinized and criticized by the public in the past several years, as evidenced by the many articles published on the topic. It can be speculated that with the new provisions and simpler algorithms provided by the FDA, the manner in which member conflict of interest is handled will become more transparent, and perhaps, therefore, less criticized by the public.

---

[25] U.S. Food and Drug Administration Web site. Measuring conflict of interest and expertise on FDA advisory committees ERG, Inc. Submitted to Nancy Gieser Office of Policy, Planning and Preparedness U.S. Food and Drug Administration; Submitted by Nyssa Ackerley, John Eyraud, Marisa Mazzotta, Eastern Research Group, Inc. October 27, 2007. Available at: http://www.fda.gov/oc/advisory/ERGCOIreport.pdf. Accessed December 17, 2007.

OPERATION

The primary function of the FDA advisory committee system is to provide the FDA with expertise on products and/or topics for which the agency is seeking external guidance. These recommendations are provided at formal meetings that are highly regulated. An integral part of the laws and regulations governing the advisory committee system is the inclusion of public involvement. As a result, advisory committee meetings are generally open to the public; however, regulations do permit full and/or partial closure of meetings under certain conditions.

Before the advisory committee can be held, it is important for members to be debriefed on the subject matter under deliberation. In cases where a specific product is to be reviewed, the FDA may request that the sponsor submit a written information summary (briefing document) detailing safety, efficacy, or other pertinent data. If written information is requested by the FDA, the sponsor (the company whose product is under review) is required to submit the summary at least three weeks before the meeting. The agency then distributes the sponsor's summary, in addition to its own summary of pertinent information, to the committee members. In addition to the briefing documents, the committee members are also given a list of questions that the FDA would like addressed. These questions are usually then posted in the Federal Register and on the FDA's Web site for public review (not public comment) in advance of the meeting (often no more than a couple of business days before the meeting).

The format in which the FDA advisory committee meetings are to be conducted is detailed in 21CFR14.25. Regulations stipulate that advisory committee meetings may have four portions: open public hearing, open committee discussion, closed presentation of data, and closed committee deliberations. Open meetings are those in which the public may attend and present information, whereas closed meetings are those in which the meeting is only open to the advisory committee members and associated support staff. It is important to note that not all committee meetings require all of the above four elements. In meetings at which topics of a general nature are discussed, there may be no need to close any portion of the meeting. As per regulation, all the FDA advisory committee meetings are published in the Federal Register at least 15 days before the meeting's date, thereby allowing anyone interested the opportunity to attend and speak at the meeting (21CFR14.20). Federal regulations also detail the required elements to be published in the Federal Register; items such as the meeting agenda, nature of topics to be discussed, as well as contact information for the FDA. People who wish to use the public forum are not required to contact the FDA in advance of the meeting, but they are urged to register beforehand. Preregistration of public speakers allows the FDA advisory committee oversight office to plan accordingly for speakers. According to 21CFR14.29, at least sixty minutes of each advisory committee meeting must be allotted for open public comment. However, if the public comment portion of the meeting does not take sixty minutes, then that time may be decreased. Alternatively, if the topic under discussion is of great public interest and sixty minutes is insufficient to hear all public comments, then the advisory committee chairperson is allowed to increase the time allotted.

In addition to presentations made by the public, during advisory committee meetings at which specific products are under review, the sponsor presents pertinent data. The sponsor's address to the committee is usually the most formal and well-rehearsed presentation. The preparation required for the sponsor presentation will be explored in further detail in the "Industry Perspective" section.

The purpose of advisory committees is for advisory members to provide the FDA with guidance on selected topics. As mentioned earlier, prior to the meeting the agency sends committee members a list of questions, which are to be addressed at the meeting. Therefore, an integral part of advisory committee meetings is the committee discussion of these questions. Frequently, committee deliberation of the FDA's questions occurs during the open portion of the meeting. From review of transcripts from previous advisory committee meetings, it is typical for the chairperson to go through each question and elicit a response from the members; however, depending on whether the agency is seeking product-specific or general policy guidance, the methodology for how the questions are answered varies. If a vote is required, the chairperson asks for the members' vote and then often summarizes the votes after all members have answered the question.

The FDA can ask advisory committee members to deliberate on a variety of topics, ranging from issues of general subject matter to advice regarding specific marketing applications. Depending on the type of advice that the FDA is seeking, the advisory committee can issue a number of different types of recommendations.

General topics reviewed typically include request for guidance on policy making, advice regarding clinical study design for certain disease indications or conditions, or input on safety of certain classes of products. When the FDA calls upon an advisory committee to review a particular marketing application, several recommendations are possible and are dependent on the type of advice the FDA is seeking. When the FDA is asking whether the committee concurs that the data presented are sufficient for marketing approval, the committee may concur and recommend approval, or they may issue recommendations for additional information prior to final approval. These recommendations may include additional studies, more safety or efficacy data, population/age restrictions, and changes to the proposed indication/labeling.

The FDA is not bound to the recommendations made by the advisory committee members; however, recommendations are taken under serious consideration. It is difficult to predict whether the FDA will concur with an advisory committee recommendation; however, data tend to suggest that there is a positive correlation between the determinations; or at minimum, the FDA takes the recommendations into consideration in their own deliberations. While one must consider that there are a multitude of other factors affecting the FDA determination of final action, the impact of an advisory committee determination cannot be discounted. Furthermore, in light of the referral provisions included in the FDA Amendments Act of 2007 referred to earlier in this chapter, the impact of advisory committee determinations may significantly impact the new drug approval process.

INDUSTRY PERSPECTIVE

The very public and important nature of advisory committee meetings and their content makes them one of the most resource-intensive interactions between sponsor companies and the FDA. The future of a product's development, a company, and even an industry may be impacted by the recommendations of a particular advisory committee. A sponsor company can attempt to manage and optimize the advisory committee process in three key areas: (*i*) influencing when advisory committees are used, (*ii*) preparing for advisory committee meetings, and (*iii*) once a committee has met and provided guidance to the FDA, a sponsor company must then manage the impact of the meeting.

Affecting FDA'S Decision to Call a Meeting

Since the FDA calls on its advisory committee system for guidance when the internal expertise of the agency is insufficient to either decide on an issue or provide more general guidance for product development, the back-and-forth between the FDA and a sponsor company can increase the likelihood of an advisory committee consultation. For example, if the FDA and a sponsor company cannot reach agreement on a particular issue, including the factors that influence market approval of a product, the sponsor may ask the FDA to bring the issue to an advisory committee. Even without such a request, the FDA may bring an issue to committee because discussions with a sponsor are no longer progressing and the opinion of an external and expert panel may aid in reaching mutual understanding. Even if there are no contentious issues between the FDA and a sponsor company, a particular product development path, or an entire class of products, may be so novel as to require the assistance of an advisory committee to provide guidance on paths forward to both the FDA and industry.

When a sponsor company has not asked for an advisory committee meeting, it is common for the FDA to provide advance notice to a company before publicly announcing an advisory committee meeting. While this notice provides a company with the theoretical opportunity to influence the FDA's decision, in general the FDA's initial decision to convene a committee meeting is final.

Preparing for Advisory Committee Meetings

A sponsor company may have as long as one year or as little as two months to prepare for an FDA advisory committee meeting. The amount of time depends on whether or not the guidance needed from the committee is part of a long-term development program (or group of programs) that is years away from approval, or a group of approved products or product classes, or whether committee input is needed urgently on a time-sensitive subject, such as safety, or as part of a user-fee driven review timeline. The least amount of preparation time for advisory committee meetings are usually the result of meetings called as part of priority product reviews, in which the FDA targets total review times of six months or less. During product reviews, the FDA usually makes the decision to call an advisory committee after two to three months of review has been completed, thus leading to meetings that often (*i*) have very short lead times for preparations and (*ii*) occur only weeks before action dates (approval, approvable, or not approved decisions).

Successful preparation for advisory committee meetings is not achieved via a single approach, and each meeting is unique. In general, the following principles are critical to success, and the approaches described have proven successful in some instances.

Success Criteria: Dedicated Team

A sponsor should form a team of employees and consultants who will be dedicated to planning and carrying out advisory committee meeting functions. It is important that the team working on the advisory committee meeting be experienced and extremely knowledgeable of the product under review. In general, this means the team is the same team that has led product development to date, or a subteam, but additional team members and leadership may be required. Proactive team leadership is vital to success, as preparations are required on a variety of fronts, from reanalyses of data to logistics.

Each speaker on behalf of the sponsor company should have a dedicated support team to aid in presentation development and in response to questions from the committee. These support teams should have as intimate a knowledge of the data as the speaker. Each speaker should also have an assigned backup, in case of last minute emergencies that prevent their participation in the meeting.

Success Criteria: External Expertise

All advisory committee meetings include challenges of content and logistics. It is unlikely that any company has all the content experts required for successful presentation of data, and perspective on that data, to the committee. Experts with a level of technical accomplishment and global recognition at the same level as committee members (or beyond) are usually present at these meetings. This is not to say that such experts present all of the data. Normally, they are used to present either key findings or help place findings in the perspective of medical standard of care and medical need. Using such experts brings the communication of data to the peer-to-peer level with the committee.

In addition to outside content experts, most companies facing the challenge of an advisory committee meeting employ experts in an array of logistical and style challenges of presenting vast quantities of data in a short time period (often 90 minutes or less), to a relatively unfamiliar audience, and respond to questions from the committee. There are a number of firms that specialize in the preparation, cataloging, and presentation of slides for advisory committee meetings. These companies provide staff expert at presenting data, managing thousands of slides, and retrieving slides in a manner of seconds for display in answering questions. It is important for the sponsor company to develop a strong working relationship with the presentation vendor as early as possible and to demand a dedicated staff presence on the committee meeting team. Additional outside experts can be called upon to help hone the presentation skills of speakers, the overall flow and messaging of the data presentations, as well as the logistics of practices (see below) and last-minute preparations.

Success Criteria: Rehearsal

Rehearsing for advisory committee meetings can be highly analogous to practices in American football. Early rehearsals are loosely organized with the intent of working out timing, general flow, and allowing the speakers to refine their presentations. Each presentation should be scripted, so that eventually, every word is documented to allow for last-minute replacements in case of emergency. Every rehearsal should have an audience. Early on, these can be other team members, but eventually they should be external experts who play the role of committee members. As practices continue, a log should be maintained of all questions, and brainstorming sessions to consider all possible questions should be held. Special rehearsal of individual presentations, or just focused on one set of technical issues, may also occur. Eventually, mock committee meetings should be held. Some companies go to the extreme of simulating the room in which the meeting is scheduled, so as to acclimate the speakers and support staff to the logistical realities of the day of the meeting. Some rehearsals are staged with all the aspects of a real meeting, including assigned roles for the audience, an agenda that matches the day, presentations by the mock FDA staff, and rules that no one breaks until the practice is concluded. As in football, all of these practices are intended to make the team comfortable with all the possible twists of the day. Effective practices lead to high-quality presentations of data, and quick and accurate responses to committee questions.

Briefing document and slides. As mentioned earlier, sponsors are usually required to submit summary data of pertinent information, typically referred to as a briefing document. The summary is a comprehensive compilation of all information and data that are relevant for the committee member review. Typically, the briefing document should be about 20 to 30 pages long. It is important to remember that this document is used by the committee as a reference in considering their guidance to the FDA and that often the committee only has a few weeks to prepare for the meeting. This heightens the need for clear, concise, and accurate summaries of data, and a flow to the document that anticipates, to the degree possible, potential questions committee members might have and potential points of contention with the FDA. It is also important to remember that this document is posted publicly, and will be in the public domain forever. The sponsor is also given the opportunity to review the briefing information created by the agency and to request changes, if errors are noted.

The slides accompanying the oral presentations given by the sponsor company are also critical documentation, and will be presented publicly, and be archived as a public record of the meeting. Slides are carefully prepared to present data that are integral to the committee members' deliberations, specifically in regard to those questions that the FDA has asked the committee to answer. A key component to the sponsor presentation is the ability to anticipate what questions committee members or agency representatives may ask. Backup slides, as many as several thousand, are created as backup for potential questions. The speakers must learn every backup slide and be able to recall appropriate data on the spot to address questions at the meeting.

After the Advisory Committee Meetings

The outcome of an advisory committee meeting is usually some form of guidance to the FDA, often in the form of a vote on key questions. As has been stated, these recommendations are nonbinding, but as a matter of public record, they can have significant impact on a company, or even an industry. In terms of regulatory follow-up, it is important for a sponsor company to quickly digest the questions raised at the meeting, committee's recommendations, and the potential impact on the FDA's ongoing review(s) of product applications. In some instances, the positive recommendations of the committee can be leveraged to improve the chance of a successful review. However, this leverage is unlikely to come from simply quoting a positive tally of the committee votes. Arguments should be based on the justifications presented by the committee for the vote, new insight from the committee on the data, and the broader perspective the committee often brings to the discussion. In the case of a negative vote, a sponsor company should continue to work with the FDA to resolve issues and present, or re-present, their data to support their arguments. Whether the cumulative response from the committee is positive or negative, their feedback on the data, and their revelation of potential previously unaddressed issues, should be considered. The goal should be seamless inclusion of the advisory committee meeting into the review process.

CONCLUSION

The FDA advisory committee system is a significant part of the FDA's decision-making process and can be a highly charged component of the process. As a public forum, advisory committees have the potential to impact the political and commercial environment of entire industries. Even when considering a single product application, a committee can have the power to halt development and change the course of a company's future. These factors make it imperative that sponsor companies fully understand the advisory committee process and are well prepared to be part of that process. This chapter has attempted to outline the process and provide guidance on how to maneuver successfully within the process. A typical regulatory professional may only have a few opportunities in a career to have projects reviewed at an advisory committee, and therefore any and all references, including this chapter and the counsel of experienced consultants, should be used in preparations. A well-prepared company, with a well-rehearsed and scientifically strong presentation of the issues, should not only receive a fair and balanced review by an advisory committee but also present an image of the company to the public as a diligent, compassionate, and rigorously datacentric player in the public health industry.

14

Biologics

Timothy A. Keutzer

Cubist Pharmaceuticals, Inc., Lexington, Massachusetts, U.S.A.

BIOLOGICS

Though employed in traditional medicine over the millennia, biologics, as we know them today, may trace their evolution to the scientific and social developments of the late-19th and early 20th centuries. It was at this time that novel discoveries in the fields of immunology—such as those of Koch and Pasteur— and epidemiology combined with increased interest in public health to support campaigns focused on the elimination of certain infectious diseases. As has often been the case in the history of drug development, it was a tragedy that highlighted an incomplete understanding of the science and technology employed, and the subsequent need for regulatory oversight, in this case over biologics. In this chapter, we will review the FDA's (Food and Drug Administration) oversight of biologics, identify similarities and differences to small molecule drugs as these relate to their development and licensure, and provide an overview of the regulatory processes that govern their entry to the market.

At the dawn of the 20th century, Americans saw great improvements in medicine, and significant reductions in childhood mortality, through the intro-duction of vaccines and blood-based antitoxin treatments. It was in this context that in 1901, in St. Louis, 13 children died as a result of receiving a horse-derived diphtheria antitoxin that was contaminated with tetanus toxin. Reviews of records in these cases tracked the antitoxin back to a single horse, Jim, that was destroyed when it was found to be infected with tetanus. Serum harvested from the horse was not properly tested, and subsequently distributed for use to tragic results.[1]

What followed was a change in the U.S. government's approach to biologics oversight. The Biologics Control Act of 1902 established a board composed of the surgeon generals of the Marines, the Army, and the Navy and mandated that the board create regulations directed at licensing facilities involved in the "preparation of viruses, serums, toxins, and anti-toxins" for sale.[2] In 1944, the Public Health Service Act added licensure of the biologic products themselves in addition to the facilities engaged in their manufacture. This fundamental approach—that both the facility making the biologic and the biologic itself be licensed—held until 1999,[3] when the FDA issued a final rule to implement a single biologics license that combined the two schema, with particular emphasis on analytical characterization.

CURRENT FDA OVERSIGHT

As is noted elsewhere in this book, the FDA is organized into centers with specific areas of responsibility (e.g., Center for Food Safety and Applied Nutrition versus the Center for Veterinary Medicine). For the purposes of biologics, we will consider the Center for Biologics Research and Evaluation and the Center for Drug Evaluation and Research. In the interest of clarity and space, we will leave aside the combination products (in the context of this chapter, either a biologic/device or a biologic/drug combination), except to note that the choice of centers for regulation is product dependent, and relies on the identification of primary mode of action (Figs. 1,2).

Before consideration is given to which center is responsible for specific biologics, the current definition for a biological product must be understood:

> "Biological products, like other drugs, are used for the treatment, prevention or cure of disease in humans. In contrast to chemically synthesized small molecular weight drugs, which have a well-defined structure and can be thoroughly characterized, biological products are generally derived from living material–human, animal, or microorganism–are complex in structure, and thus are usually not fully characterized.

Section 351 of the *Public Health Service (PHS) Act* defines a biological product as a "virus, therapeutic serum, toxin, antitoxin, vaccine, blood, blood component or derivative, allergenic product, or analogous product, ... applicable to the prevention, treatment, or cure of a disease or condition of human beings."

[1] Suzanne White Junod, Biologics Centennial: 100 Years of Biologics Regulation, from the "Making History" column of the November-December 2002 issue of Update, the bimonthly publication of the Food and Drug Law Institute.

[2] Ibid.

[3] Federal Register October 20, 1999 (Volume 64, Number 202).

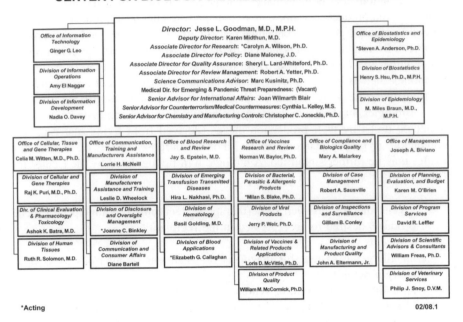

Figure 1 Organization chart for the Center for Biologics Research and Evaluation.

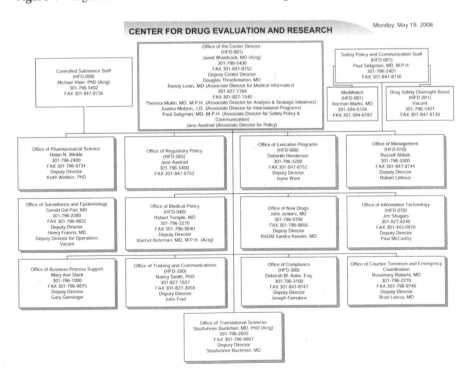

Figure 2 Organization chart for the Center for Drug Evaluation and Research.

FDA regulations and policies have established that biological products include blood-derived products, vaccines, in vivo diagnostic allergenic products, immuno-globulin products, products containing cells or microorganisms, and most protein products. Biological products subject to the *PHS Act* also meet the definition of *drugs* under the *Federal Food, Drug and Cosmetic Act (FDC Act)*. Note that hormones such as insulin, glucagon, and human growth hormone are regulated as drugs under the *FDC Act*, not biological products under the *PHS Act*."[4]

Biologics, in short, are drugs by definition. They are contrasted with small molecule drugs by their production means (derived from living material) and complexity (typically macromolecules). For the purposes of this discussion, the matter may be further simplified. A biologic will be regulated by the Center for Biologics if it is:

- a gene therapy product. Gene therapies are vectors coding-specific gene products desired to be expressed in the recipient
- a vaccine
- an allergenic extract for diagnosis or treatment of allergies as well as allergin patch tests
- an antitoxin, antivenin, or venom
- blood or blood products (e.g., IVIG, albumin), the recombinant analogues thereof (e.g., clotting factors), and the devices used in the collection, testing, and processing of blood
- a human cell, tissue, or cellular and tissue-based product.
- a xenotransplant (i.e., cells, tissues, or organs from a nonhuman source, or human cells, tissues, or organs that have had ex vivo contact with non-human live animal cells)

With the advent in 1996 of the concept of a "well-characterized biologic," it became possible for CDER to regulate certain biologics, among them:

- Monoclonal antibodies for in vivo use
- Immunomodulators (except vaccines or allergenic compounds, as noted above)
- Most proteins for therapeutic use (except those specifically noted as being regulated within CBER, above), including cytokines, enzymes, hema-topoietic factor, and growth factors, be they plant- or animal-derived or recombinant in nature.

From the point of view of an organization engaged in biologics develop-ment, the center at which the product is regulated is largely secondary to the rules and guidance documents laid down by FDA governing biologics. While there exist differences in the legal governing authority under which CBER and

---

[4] See www.fda.gov/cder/biologics/qs.htm.

CDER are organized (in the case of CBER, it is the Public Health Service Act that governs, and for CDER it is the Food, Drug, and Cosmetic Act), one engaged in the development of a biologic will have a similar experience with either center. Therefore, for purposes of the rest of this chapter, we will focus on biologics generally, be they regulated by CBER or CDER, as the issues related to them are common across both centers.

BIOLOGICS DEVELOPMENT

The development process for a biologic is essentially the same as that for a traditional, small molecule drug. That is, it is a systematic process whereby the structure and function of a molecule is studied relative to the effect that is sought. In the case of a small molecule, this may be in the form of high-throughput screening in an enzyme interference assay. For a biologic, it may be cloning a specific antibody and demonstrating that it binds its ligand *in vitro*. If sufficient evidence of activity is obtained, additional studies are planned and executed, and formal toxicity testing is performed. These data, along with manufacturing data and a proposed clinical plan, are assembled into an investigational new drug (IND) and filed to the FDA. As with all things, and especially with pharmaceutical development, the devil is in the details.

A primary complicating factor—and one that creates differences from small molecules—is that biologics by their nature are complex molecules not given to precise structural elucidation (Table 1).

As a function of this complexity, the specific of development of biologics differs from that of traditional drugs in significant ways. Again, the formal steps to both IND and market application are the same—the sponsor will produce and test the material, enroll it into formal safety studies, and finally test it in humans—but the approaches to these steps necessitated by the complexity of a

Table 1 Characteristics of Drugs and Biologics[5]

Characteristic	Drug	Biologic
Composition	Dozens of atoms	Potentially millions of atoms
Molecular weight	Measured in the hundreds of Daltons	Measured in kilodaltons or hundreds of kilodaltons
Structure	Described by a fixed chemical formula	Often incompletely understood or cannot be fully described
Production	Chemical synthesis	Synthesized by cells in culture
Starting materials	Defined chemicals	DNA inserted to cells grown in complex media

---

[5] From the testimony of Dr. William Hancock, Bradstreet Chair of Bioanalytical Chemistry, Northeastern University, June 23, 2004, United States Senate Committee on the Judiciary.

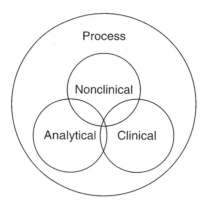

Figure 3 Venn diagram of relationship of process, analytical methods, nonclinical, and clinical studies.

biologic differ. Below, we will consider process development, analytical development and testing, and nonclinical testing as they relate to biologics, and how these are treated in regulatory filings (Fig. 3).

The above is a simplified diagram of the connections among the various disciplines related to biologics development. Process is inclusive of the development and manufacture of drug substance and drug product. Subtle changes to process may have profound impact on the entire program. Analytical refers to the myriad assays and techniques brought to bear both on characterization of the active molecule and in vivo quantification of drug levels and/or biological effects. For example, a change to the fermentation parameters for the growth of production cells can lead to the introduction of a new species of the protein of interest (e.g., a new glycoform). Absent detailed analytical characterization of the new process-derived material, the change could go unnoticed by routine release testing, and result in the introduction of a novel immunogen to the final product.

Process Development and Manufacturing

Requirements for chemistry, manufacturing, and controls (CMC) are discussed elsewhere in this book, and so we will here focus on those elements related to CMC that differ significantly from a drug, and how these are managed for a biologic. For purposes of example, we will focus on a protein therapeutic coded by a human gene and expressed in a nonhuman, mammalian cell line. The manufacturer will need to submit to the FDA:

- identification of species from which the gene was cloned (in this case, human)
- description of the methods used to identify and clone the gene of interest. Is this a humanized antibody using sequences from nonhuman species? Was the gene synthesized *in silico* from a known sequence?

- a detailed description of the vector into which the gene is inserted. This will include a map of the plasmid used, identifying other genes carried; other active sequences (e.g., promoters and enhancers); and selection markers employed such as a gene conferring antibiotic resistance
- a description of the techniques used to transfect the plasmid into the host (production) cell. Methods for amplification of the copy number of the plasmid, as well as how the clones are selected, must also be provided

Upon transfection and selection of a clone with which to proceed, the manufacturer will establish a master cell bank (MCB), from which working cell banks (WCB) will ultimately be produced. The banks are typically kept frozen in ampoules under defined conditions (e.g., in the vapor phase of liquid nitrogen). Each ampoule contains a standard cell density from the single clone. The history of the cells laid down for the MCB should be described, including the passage number or generation number of the cells when frozen, as well as any selection markers used. While there are a number of cell lines suitable for production, the manufacturer should carefully consider the needs of the protein product and the regulatory history of the host line when selecting a cell line candidate. For example, Chinese Hamster Ovary (CHO) cells have a long history of recombinant product production that a primary, recently immortalized cell line will lack. In the latter case, much additional cell line characterization will need to be performed and submitted to the agency.

The MCB will need to be tested for incorporation and maintenance of the expression system. In broad terms, the expression system may be either incorporated to the host cell genome or maintained extrachromosomally. In either case, the stability of the transfectant will need to be demonstrated, as well as the fidelity of the copy to the original construct. It is possible that the newly incorporated gene can mutate in the same manner as any other gene. The manufacturer will therefore need to either re-clone or isolate the gene from the MCB, sequence it, and compare the results with those from the original construct used in transfection. The nucleic acid sequences should be identical. Finally, the limits of *in vitro* age must be established to define an acceptable generation number for production use. This is verified by comparison of end-of-production cells to the original MCB, as noted above.

Having established the production cell line, the manufacturer will need to describe the conditions under which the cells are grown for production. As with a small molecule, the detail to which this is described will increase with the product's proceeding through the development process. The media used to grow the cells will need to be described fully, and it is advisable for the manufacturer to use fully defined media where possible. As our example cell line is of mammalian origin, it is theoretically possible for it to harbor viruses that may be harmful to humans. For purposes of safety, it is advisable to limit this theoretical exposure to the cell line itself. Any human- or animal-derived proteins or components used in the growth media—indeed, any such components used in any stage of the production process—should be fully described and their sources verified. In practice, the use of such components should be minimized to provide the highest theoretical assurance of safety from adventitious viruses or other potentially infective agents.

The purification of small molecules is often performed under conditions unsuitable for a biologic. Crystallization, extraction with organic solvents, or the use of physiologically harsh conditions are frequently employed with small molecules, and these would typically be associated with the destruction or inactivation of a protein. Until the mid-1980s, when improved screening and testing was developed, plasma fractionation for the production of coagulation factors effectively partitioned infective viruses along with the final product. As a result, many patients receiving these products were infected with HIV, hepatitis B, and hepatitis C. It is against this backdrop, and in vigilance against the introduction of new diseases such as the transmissible spongiform encephalopathies, that guidance for the demonstration of virus removal has been developed for biologics. In short, the manufacturer will need to show that the purification techniques used would effectively remove viruses that may be present in the cell line used, the raw materials employed, or introduced to the production from an external source (e.g., production personnel). Validation of viral removal will need to be performed prior to licensure, but should be considered early in the program in selecting or developing purification processes.

Less dramatic but still important to the purification process is the removal of nonproduct proteins and other biomolecules. Proteins of host cell origin may be co-purified with the protein of interest, and acceptable limits for these must be established. The composition of host cell proteins will be specific to a given production cell line and the conditions under which it is grown. Therefore, specific methods will be developed over time to characterize and quantify host cell protein in a given product. Moreover, residual DNA from the production cell line may be present in the final product; specific purification steps are therefore employed to minimize the presence of this contaminant.

We have so far been concerned with what is not in the final product—viruses, host cell contaminants—but we cannot lose sight of what must be in the final product, i.e., a fully active biologic of sufficient purity and potency. Biologics tend to be large, complex molecules with significant secondary, tertiary, and often quaternary structures. The process must yield a final material having the correct conformational state and any modifications necessary to its biological activity. Protein denatured or otherwise inactivated in processing may be co-purified with fully active material, and the presence of such impurities must be understood. Additional purification methods may be included to exclude such material or current methods may be refined to limit them. In all cases, the process will need to be characterized at each stage of production to understand the status of the active component. The presence and quantities of inactive forms or active isoforms will be qualified in non-clinical testing.

Select Guidance Documents:

International Conference on Harmonization (ICH) Q5B: Quality of Biotechnological Products: Analysis of the Expression Construct in Cells Used for Production of rDNA Derived Protein Products. November 30, 1995.

ICH Q5D: Derivation and Characterisation of Cell Substrates Used for Production of Biotechnological Products. July 16, 1997.

FDA: Content and Format of Chemistry, Manufacturing, and Controls Information and Establishment Description Information for a Vaccine or Related Product. January 1999.

FDA: Compliance Program Guidance Manual Chapter 45 – Biological Drug Product Development. December 1, 2004.

FDA: For the Submission of Chemistry, Manufacturing, and Controls and Establishment Description Information for Human Plasma-Derived Biological Products, Animal Plasma or Serum-Derived Products. February 1999.

FDA: Monoclonal Antibodies Used as Reagents in Drug Manufacturing. May 1999.

Analytical Development

As noted earlier, the complexity of biologics adds significantly to the complexity of their analysis. Where a relatively small set of techniques might be used to assess the purity and potency of a small molecule, a more extensive set of techniques will be employed for a biologic. Moreover, multiple methods may need to be employed to characterize a given attribute of the product. Purity may be defined by several methods, each of which contributing information on a different molecular characteristic of the product. Size-exclusion HPLC may provide data on the molecular weight of the protein, and will demonstrate the presence of higher molecular weight species (such as aggregates) or lower weight species (such as fragments). Similarly, reverse-phase HPLC and ion-exchange HPLC will expose variations in hydrophobicity and charge, respectively, and may demonstrate the presence of isoforms or degradants in the product. No single method will capture the full heterogeneity of the compound, and therefore several may be employed to fully characterize a given attribute of the protein. The data will be assessed as a whole, and will provide a composite picture of the compound in development. The rationale for method selection—what information is provided and the relevance thereof—will be submitted to the FDA.

Further complicating the analytical picture for a biologic is the inherent variability of the methods used. As potency is often a function of biologic response in a living system, cell-based assays may be employed. Acceptable specifications may therefore be in the range of 50% to 150% of a standard response, a function of

Table 2 Example of Methods Employed in Monoclonal Antibody
Production and Release

Test	Method
Appearance	Visual
Concentration (mg/mL)	UV A280
Purity(%)	SDS-PAGE
Isoelectric focusing	IEF Gel
Molecular weight	SEC-HPLC
Specific activity (IU/mL)	Protein specific—this may need to be developed by the manufacturer
Heavy and light chains	SDS-PAGE and Western blot
Protein A (used in purification of a monoclonal antibody)	SDS-PAGE and Western blot
Isotype/subclass	ELISA
pH	Standard
Endotoxin (EU/mL)	USP
Bioburden (CFU/mL)	USP
Particulates	USP
Sterility	USP

the inherent variability of living systems. This argues further for the use of orthogonal methodology to describe specific attributes under consideration. Table 2 outlines a number of methods used in the characterization of a monoclonal antibody therapeutic drug product.

Depending on the purpose for the analyses of the hypothetical monoclonal antibody, additional attributes may be examined, such as V/J subgroups, assessment of affinity constant, tissue cross-reactivity, and glycoforms. In some cases, whole animal systems will be needed to test a particular attribute.

Methods used in nonclinical and clinical studies are often based on the same platform, but must be assessed against the matrices in which the drug sample is presented. New reagents for these studies may be required, and crossover studies should be performed to demonstrate the applicability of data from one species to another. Of particular concern will be the methods selected to demonstrate the immunogenic potential of the compound in development, and specific assays for the detection of the presence of total antibody directed against the compound versus the presence of antibodies that neutralize biologic activity are needed. As this is a key safety issue, these methods must be carefully chosen and extensively developed. Neutralizing antibodies cannot only alter of limit the biologic activity of the test compound at a given dose, but may also cross-react with endogenous protein with negative results. Coagulation factors in the treatment of hemophilia elicit a neutralizing antibody response in some patients, which severely limits the treatment options for the condition.[6] Exogenous erythropoietin may elicit an antibody response that cross-reacts with endogenously produced protein, resulting in pure red cell aplasia or severe anemia.[7] Assessing the potential for a biologic to elicit such a response is critical to demonstrating its safety profile.

Select Guidance Documents:
FDA: Analytical Procedures and Methods Validation. Chemistry, Manufacturing, and Controls Documentation. August 2000.
ICH Q6B: Specifications : Test Procedures and Acceptance Criteria for Biotechnological/Biological Products.
ICH Q5C: Quality of Biotechnological Products: Stability Testing of Biotechnological/Biological Products. September 1995.

Comparability

We have briefly reviewed above some of the needs and complications for biologics process and analytical development. During the development of any pharmaceutical product, and in fact well into the market phase, there will often be the need to make process changes. These may be for reasons of scale-up in mid-development (e.g., between phase 1 and phase 2, when increased quantities are required), as a response to new regulatory guidance, or in the quest for improved manufacturing efficiency. For small molecules, many roads can lead to the same end—a variety of processes can yield the same final product. In the case of biologics, the changes may be subtle and difficult to observe. Extended comparability studies may therefore be enlisted. The intent is to compare the product at the appropriate stage of manufacture where changes may be best captured from both the new and the old process. Such comparisons are prospective in nature, and may include additional nonclinical and/or clinical testing to ensure that there is no change to the pharmacokinetic or safety profile of the compound. In all cases, the intent is to demonstrate that the product has maintained its overall safety and efficacy. The potential for serious impact of seemingly minor changes to process was demonstrated recently by Johnson & Johnson's epoietin product, Eprix[R]. In keeping with guidance, the company replaced the stabilizer human serum albumin (a plasma-derived product) with Polysorbate 80. Subsequently, increased rates of reports for pure red cell anemia were received by the company. Investigations have shown that the surfactant may have leached an organic compound from uncoated stoppers used in prefilled syringes. The resulting material was associated with increased antigenicity. Routine testing for release did not identify the new impurity.[8]

---

[6] Package Insert for ADVATE (antihemophilic factor, recombinant), Baxter Healthcare Corporation.
[7] Package Insert for Procrit[R] (epoietin alfa), Amgen, Inc.
[8] Biotechnology Industry Organization White Paper. The Difference with Biologics: The Scientific, Legal, and Regulatory Challenges of any Follow-on Biologics Scheme. April 25, 2007.

Select Guidance Documents:

FDA: Comparability Protocols - Protein Drug Products and Biological Products -
    Chemistry, Manufacturing, and Controls Information. September 2003.

ICH Q5E: Comparability of Biotechnological/Biological Products Subject to
    Changes in Their Manufacturing Process. February 2002.

FDA: Guidance Concerning Demonstration of Comparability of Human Bio-
    logical Products, Including Therapeutic Biotechnology-derived Products,
    Center for Biologics Evaluation and Research (CBER), Center for Drug
    Evaluation and Research (CDER). April 1996.

Nonclinical Evaluation

The requirements for nonclinical evaluation of pharmaceuticals naturally extend
to biologics. Before human testing may be performed, adequate safety in the
predicted dosing range and duration must be demonstrated in model species.
However, there exist unique challenges in the design and execution of nonclinical studies for a biologic. These challenges result from both the variety of
molecules that are considered biologics (a gene therapy nonclinical program will
by its nature differ from that for a peptide) and the variety of biological effects
possible in multiple species. No single toxicology program can be applied to all
pharmaceuticals, and this is magnified in the case of biologics.

International Conference on Harmonization (ICH) guideline S6[9] offers the
following as elements to consider in the design of nonclinical studies:

*   selection of the relevant animal species;
*   age;
*   physiological state;
*   the maner of delivery, including dose, route of administration, and treat-
    ment regimen; and
*   stability of the test material under the conditions of use.

Primary consideration must be given to the nature of the biological effect
and the validity or availability of relevant model systems. For many viral diseases and certain malignancies, the only relevant species for a human therapeutic
is humans. Animal models of disease may be incomplete or may not offer direct
comparison to the human. Certain cytokines, e.g., may have profound effects
on murine models of cancer, which have not yet been shown to be fully predictive of human response.[10] Basic proof of concept data may therefore be

---

[9] Preclinical Safety Evaluation of Biotechnology-Derived Pharmaceuticals; July 16, 1997.

[10] Robertson MJ, Ritz J. Interleukin 12: basic biology and potential applications in cancer treatment.
Oncologist 1996; 1(1–2):88–97.

provided by *in vitro* systems alone, with little or no whole animal experience that may be predictive of a human response. Some molecules, such as cytokines, trigger a complex series of physiologic events, and these events may differ in their specifics among species. Cell culture data are extremely useful in elucidating the molecular events at the level of a single cell type, but may not be predictive of a whole animal response. It is possible to clone and produce the animal analogue of the protein of interest and use this in pharmacology or mechanistic studies; however, consideration must be given to both the homology of the protein and the similarity of biological effect in the human and animal species. Alternatively, cell lines from the target nonclinical species may be screened for biological activity of the protein to support or discount the validity of the species chosen. The affects of age on the physiological state of the animal species being tested will also be considered as they might impact the usefulness of the species chosen. Differences may be seen in the pharmacokinetics of a particular molecule as a function of the developmental status of the animal to which the biologic is given. The approach taken for these studies and the rationale behind the approach should be described in IND submissions.

Safety assessments are similarly clouded. As always, consideration must be given to the product being used and its impurity profile at the given stage of development; however, impurities are often product related and may be active. Of great concern is the potential for a given product to elicit an immune response in humans, a response that cannot be predicted confidently through nonhuman studies. By definition, a human protein administered to a nonhuman is a foreign protein, and would be expected to elicit an immune response (here, the assumption is <100% homology among the species). Moreover, a human protein produced in nonhuman mammalian cells may carry posttranslational modifications that differ from the endogenously produced protein because of inherent differences in cellular processing machinery. Depending on the extent to which the molecule is understood in terms of its activity, and depending on the nature and extent of anticipated human dosing, it may not be possible to maintain test animals without an immune response that renders null the data from long studies. Often complicating matters is the long lead time associated with assay development for quantifying antibody responses in animals. Another factor impacting the relative immunogenicity of a compound will be the route of administration. In general, intravenous delivery is associated with less immunogenic potential than subcutaneous or intramuscular delivery. As we have seen, the effects of formulation excipients or the presence of contaminants may also play a role in the development or absence of an immune response as well.

Specific nonclinical safety studies may be required as a function of the mechanism of action of the product studied. Monoclonal antibodies, by their nature, bind a specific epitope on a target. However, antibodies may bind to other epitopes that offer a similar conformational or structural presentation. It will therefore be necessary to perform tissue cross-reactivity studies *in vitro* to demonstrate that the antibody does not bind to tissues unrelated to the pharmacological effect of the antibody.

Carcinogenicity studies are not typically required for biologics, but this must be justified on the basis of knowledge of the specific function of the molecule under development. If the product is associated with hyperplasia, it may be necessary to perform such studies. In general, long-term studies are difficult because of the likelihood of an immune response. Any product likely to be given to women of childbearing potential will require some degree of reproductive toxicology studies; however, this will vary on the basis of both the likely extent of dosing and the specific disease being treated.

Finally, the stability of the test article for use in nonclinical studies must be described. Early in development, test article will often be supplied as a nonformulated product in solution. Studies should be performed to demonstrate that the product is stable and active in the period of use, and dosing materials should be analyzed to confirm that the animals receive the appropriate exposure. As the program matures, and as the formulation of the biologic is refined, these data will provide a foundation upon which to assess the nonclinical effect of the material over time.

Select Guidance Documents:
ICH S6: Preclinical Safety Evaluation of Biotechnology-Derived Pharmaceuticals.

Clinical Development

As is the case for small molecules, the clinical indication for which a biologic is developed will drive the design and execution of the clinical trials aimed at demonstrating safety and efficacy. Similar to certain oncology products that are toxic, the administration of some biologics to persons other than those suffering from the target disease may be unethical or impractical. Traditional phase 1 trials in healthy volunteers aimed at assessing pharmacokinetics and safety may offer data of limited value. In any event, the sponsor will need to demonstrate the safety and efficacy of the biologic, and will need to submit the proposed clinical plan, with statistical considerations where appropriate, to FDA. The biological activity of the product, the limits on measurement and assessing efficacy (as through the use of surrogate markers), and the availability of patients suitable for clinical trials must all be weighed in designing these trials.

It cannot be emphasized enough that the potential for immunogenicity for a biologic is of great concern. Baseline, pre-exposure samples must be drawn from patients exposed to the biologic, and the possibility of interference by the biologic in subsequent samples must be considered in determining the optimal frequency of sampling upon dosing commencement. The potential for anaphylaxis or anaphylactoid reactions must be considered, and appropriate steps to ameliorate these reactions must be taken.

Of particular concern is the unpredictability of a human response to a biologic despite nonclinical studies that may predict no adverse effect level doses in man. Recently, the development of an anti-CD28 humanized monoclonal antibody was halted after severe adverse reactions were noted in a phase 1 trial of healthy volunteers, at a starting dose of approximately 1/500th of the predicted efficacious dose.[11] The potential for unforeseen side effects by biologics must be given careful consideration, and changes to routine approaches to initial dosing, dose escalation, and patient versus volunteer selection may be indicated. The rationale for such selection will be submitted as part of an initial IND and subsequent updates.

BIOLOGICS APPROVAL PROCESS

For products of biological origin defined for regulatory purposes as a biologic (e.g., gene therapy and vaccines), the sponsor will submit a biologics license application (BLA) (Fig. 4). This form is the same as will be used to submit a new drug application (NDA); the applicant simply notes which type of product is being submitted in a check box under "Applicant Information." The format and submission details are in a state of change currently, with the FDA now moving to a common technical document (CTD) format, and mandating that new submissions be filed electronically (the eCTD).

Regardless of the format used, the information conveyed in the final application will remain the same. Review timelines by the FDA are dictated by Prescription Drug User Fee Act (PDUFA) guidelines that are described elsewhere in this book. The extent to which these timelines are met is almost wholly dependent on the adequacy and completeness of the data and reasoning that the sponsor submits to the FDA. We have here highlighted elements of biologics development that require special consideration in developing a registration strategy, such consideration that may help or hinder the biologic's navigation through the approval pathway. In every case, an early and open dialog with the FDA, coupled with excellence in execution of agreed upon development, will only serve to aid in ensuring that the biologic is brought to market in a timely manner accompanied by demonstrated safety and efficacy.

---

[11] MHRA. "Press release: Latest findings on clinical trial suspension," Press Release, April 5, 2006.

DEPARTMENT OF HEALTH AND HUMAN SERVICES	Form Approved: OMB No. 0910-0338

DEPARTMENT OF HEALTH AND HUMAN SERVICES
FOOD AND DRUG ADMINISTRATION

APPLICATION TO MARKET A NEW DRUG, BIOLOGIC, OR AN ANTIBIOTIC DRUG FOR HUMAN USE
(Title 21, Code of Federal Regulations, Parts 314 & 601)

Form Approved: OMB No. 0910-0338
Expiration Date: September 30, 2008
See OMB Statement on page 2.

FOR FDA USE ONLY

APPLICATION NUMBER

APPLICANT INFORMATION

NAME OF APPLICANT

DATE OF SUBMISSION

TELEPHONE NO. *(Include Area Code)*

FACSIMILE *(FAX) Number (Include Area Code)*

APPLICANT ADDRESS *(Number, Street, City, State, Country, ZIP Code or Mail Code, and U.S. License number if previously issued)*

AUTHORIZED U.S. AGENT NAME & ADDRESS *(Number, Street, City, State, ZIP Code, telephone & FAX number)* IF APPLICABLE

PRODUCT DESCRIPTION

NEW DRUG OR ANTIBIOTIC APPLICATION NUMBER, OR BIOLOGICS LICENSE APPLICATION NUMBER *(If previously issued)*

ESTABLISHED NAME *(e.g., Proper name, USP/USAN name)*

PROPRIETARY NAME *(trade name)* IF ANY

CHEMICAL/BIOCHEMICAL/BLOOD PRODUCT NAME *(If any)*

CODE NAME *(If any)*

DOSAGE FORM:

STRENGTHS:

ROUTE OF ADMINISTRATION:

(PROPOSED) INDICATION(S) FOR USE:

APPLICATION DESCRIPTION

APPLICATION TYPE *(check one)*
☐ NEW DRUG APPLICATION (CDA, 21 CFR 314.50)   ☐ ABBREVIATED NEW DRUG APPLICATION (ANDA, 21 CFR 314.94)
☐ BIOLOGICS LICENSE APPLICATION (BLA, 21 CFR Part 601)

IF AN NDA, IDENTIFY THE APPROPRIATE TYPE   ☐ 505 (b)(1)   ☐ 505 (b)(2)

IF AN ANDA, OR 505(b)(2), IDENTIFY THE REFERENCE LISTED DRUG PRODUCT THAT IS THE BASIS FOR THE SUBMISSION
Name of Drug   Holder of Approved Application

TYPE OF SUBMISSION *(check one)* ☐ ORIGINAL APPLICATION   ☐ AMENDMENT TO A PENDING APPLICATION   ☐ RESUBMISSION
☐ PRESUBMISSION   ☐ ANNUAL REPORT   ☐ ESTABLISHMENT DESCRIPTION SUPPLEMENT   ☐ EFFICACY SUPPLEMENT
☐ LABELING SUPPLEMENT   ☐ CHEMISTRY MANUFACTURING AND CONTROLS SUPPLEMENT   ☐ OTHER

IF A SUBMISSION OF PARTIAL APPLICATION, PROVIDE LETTER DATE OF AGREEMENT TO PARTIAL SUBMISSION:

IF A SUPPLEMENT, IDENTIFY THE APPROPRIATE CATEGORY   ☐ CBE   ☐ CBE-30   ☐ Prior Approval (PA)

REASON FOR SUBMISSION

PROPOSED MARKETING STATUS *(check one)*   ☐ PRESCRIPTION PRODUCT (Rx)   ☐ OVER THE COUNTER PRODUCT (OTC)

NUMBER OF VOLUMES SUBMITTED   THIS APPLICATION IS ☐ PAPER   ☐ PAPER AND ELECTRONIC   ☐ ELECTRONIC

ESTABLISHMENT INFORMATION (Full establishment information should be provided in the body of the Application.)
Provide locations of all manufacturing, packaging and control sites for drug substance and drug product (continuation sheets may be used if necessary). Include name, address, contact, telephone number, registration number (CFN), DMF number, and manufacturing steps and/or type of testing (e.g. Final dosage form, Stability testing) conducted at the site. Please indicate whether the site is ready for inspection or, if not, when it will be ready.

Cross References (list related License Applications, INDs, NDAs, PMAs, 510(k)s, IDEs, BMFs, and DMFs referenced in the current application)

FORM FDA 356h (10/05)   PAGE 1 OF 4

Figure 4a FDA Form 356h. Application to market a new drug, biologic, or an antibiotic drug for human use.

This application contains the following items: *(Check all that apply)*	

☐ 1. Index

☐ 2. Labeling *(check one)* ☐ Draft Labeling ☐ Final Printed Labeling

☐ 3. Summary (21 CFR 314.50 (c))

☐ 4. Chemistry section

☐   A. Chemistry, manufacturing, and controls information (e.g., 21 CFR 314.50(d)(1); 21 CFR 601.2)

☐   B. Samples (21 CFR 314.50 (e)(1); 21 CFR 601.2 (a)) (Submit only upon FDA's request)

☐   C. Methods validation package (e.g., 21 CFR 314.50(e)(2)(i); 21 CFR 601.2)

☐ 5. Nonclinical pharmacology and toxicology section (e.g., 21 CFR 314.50(d)(2); 21 CFR 601.2)

☐ 6. Human pharmacokinetics and bioavailability section (e.g., 21 CFR 314.50(d)(3); 21 CFR 601.2)

☐ 7. Clinical Microbiology (e.g., 21 CFR 314.50(d)(4))

☐ 8. Clinical data section (e.g., 21 CFR 314.50(d)(5); 21 CFR 601.2)

☐ 9. Safety update report (e.g., 21 CFR 314.50(d)(5)(vi)(b); 21 CFR 601.2)

☐ 10. Statistical section (e.g., 21 CFR 314.50(d)(6); 21 CFR 601.2)

☐ 11. Case report tabulations (e.g., 21 CFR 314.50(f)(1); 21 CFR 601.2)

☐ 12. Case report forms (e.g., 21 CFR 314.50 (f)(2); 21 CFR 601.2)

☐ 13. Patent information on any patent which claims the drug (21 U.S.C. 355(b) or (c))

☐ 14. A patent certification with respect to any patent which claims the drug (21 U.S.C. 355 (b)(2) or (j)(2)(A))

☐ 15. Establishment description (21 CFR Part 600, if applicable)

☐ 16. Debarment certification (FD&C Act 306 (k)(1))

☐ 17. Field copy certification (21 CFR 314.50 (l)(3))

☐ 18. User Fee Cover Sheet (Form FDA 3397)

☐ 19. Financial Information (21 CFR Part 54)

☐ 20. OTHER *(Specify)*

CERTIFICATION

I agree to update this application with new safety information about the product that may reasonably affect the statement of contraindications, warnings, precautions, or adverse reactions in the draft labeling. I agree to submit safety update reports as provided for by regulation or as requested by FDA. If this application is approved, I agree to comply with all applicable laws and regulations that apply to approved applications, including, but not limited to the following:

1. Good manufacturing practice regulations in 21 CFR Parts 210, 211 or applicable regulations, Parts 606, and/or 820.
2. Biological establishment standards in 21 CFR Part 600.
3. Labeling regulations in 21 CFR Parts 201, 606, 610, 660, and/or 809.
4. In the case of a prescription drug or biological product, prescription drug advertising regulations in 21 CFR Part 202.
5. Regulations on making changes in application in FD&C Act section 506A, 21 CFR 314.71, 314.72, 314.97, 314.99, and 601.12.
6. Regulations on Reports in 21 CFR 314.80, 314.81, 600.80, and 600.81.
7. Local, state and Federal environmental impact laws.

If this application applies to a drug product that FDA has proposed for scheduling under the Controlled Substances Act, I agree not to market the product until the Drug Enforcement Administration makes a final scheduling decision.

The data and information in this submission have been reviewed and, to the best of my knowledge are certified to be true and accurate.

Warning: A willfully false statement is a criminal offense, U.S. Code, title 18, section 1001.

SIGNATURE OF RESPONSIBLE OFFICIAL OR AGENT	TYPED NAME AND TITLE	DATE:

ADDRESS *(Street, City, State, and ZIP Code)*	Telephone Number

Public reporting burden for this collection of information is estimated to average 24 hours per response, including the time for reviewing instructions, searching existing data sources, gathering and maintaining the data needed, and completing and reviewing the collection of information. Send comments regarding this burden estimate or any other aspect of this collection of information, including suggestions for reducing this burden to:

Department of Health and Human Services
Food and Drug Administration
Center for Drug Evaluation and Research
Central Document Room
5901-B Ammendale Road
Beltsville, MD 20705-1266

Department of Health and Human Services
Food and Drug Administration
Center for Biologics Evaluation and Research (HFM-99)
1401 Rockville Pike
Rockville, MD 20852-1448

An agency may not conduct or sponsor, and a person is not required to respond to, a collection of information unless it displays a currently valid OMB control number.

Figure 4b *(Continued).*

SUMMARY

Following the St. Louis tragedy of 1901, in which tetanus toxin contaminated diphtheria antitoxin harvested from a horse, the U.S. government began to regulate biologics production facilities, and, later, the products themselves. Over the course of the century since, we have seen advances in the elucidation of biological activity and identity for biologics, and concomitant improvements in the analytical characterization of these macromolecules. Though the basic framework of drug development as applied to small molecules applies to biologics, there exist key differences between the two therapeutic types that must be considered and managed to achieve success. These differences are related to:

- the relative molecular complexity of a biologic relative to that of a small molecule. Analytical methods and production processes must take into account the heterogeneity of molecular species produced in living systems, and strategies for the management or reduction of these species must be in place;
- the complex and often poorly understood nature of biological activity. While the introduction of any therapeutic may have unforeseen effects, this is especially true for biologics. A protein may be associated with an enzymatic cascade that is not fully elucidated, or there may be feedback-regulatory mechanisms for the production of endogenous proteins, or there may even be nonspecific effects on tissues or organs distant from the target. Couple this with the frequent lack of relevant animal models, and it becomes evident that clinical studies are the only means by which to fully demonstrate a product's activity. This is in contrast to many small molecules, where the biologic effect will be fully described prior to entry to humans; and
- the intersection of the two points above, namely, the potential for process-related isoforms to dramatically affect clinical outcomes. The methods developed for a biologic may not fully differentiate seemingly minor differences in structure of a given molecule or may not identify at all a novel contaminant. The analytical net must be cast wide for any given biologic to protect against these risks, for the alternative is to enable, e.g., a novel antigen to enter clinical trial or market patients.

Each year brings significant and important advances to our understanding of basic biology and the role of biologics in public health. Since the approval of the first recombinant product in 1982, methods for the production and analysis of biologics have greatly improved, understanding of basic biology and physiology has skyrocketed, and whole new fields of study—genomics and proteomics to name two—have emerged. Drug regulation has adapted to these realities, keeping pace with the rapid changes and novel requirements for new classes of therapeutics.

Index